Acute Pancreatitis

AF137762

John Albert Windsor
Savio George Barreto
Anthony Ronald John Phillips

Editors

Acute Pancreatitis

A Practical Guide for Clinicians

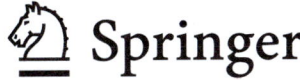 Springer

Editors
John Albert Windsor
Department of Surgery
Faculty of Medical and Health Sciences
Surgical and Translational Research
Centre
Auckland, New Zealand

Savio George Barreto
College of Medicine and Public Health
Flinders University
Bedford Park, SA, Australia

Anthony Ronald John Phillips
Surgical and Translational Research
Centre, Faculty of Medical and Health
Sciences, School of Biological Sciences
Faculty of Science
University of Auckland
Auckland, Auckland, New Zealand

ISBN 978-981-97-3134-3   ISBN 978-981-97-3132-9   (eBook)
https://doi.org/10.1007/978-981-97-3132-9

© The Editor(s) (if applicable) and The Author(s), under exclusive license to Springer Nature Singapore Pte Ltd. 2024, corrected publication 2024
This work is subject to copyright. All rights are solely and exclusively licensed by the Publisher, whether the whole or part of the material is concerned, specifically the rights of translation, reprinting, reuse of illustrations, recitation, broadcasting, reproduction on microfilms or in any other physical way, and transmission or information storage and retrieval, electronic adaptation, computer software, or by similar or dissimilar methodology now known or hereafter developed.
The use of general descriptive names, registered names, trademarks, service marks, etc. in this publication does not imply, even in the absence of a specific statement, that such names are exempt from the relevant protective laws and regulations and therefore free for general use.
The publisher, the authors and the editors are safe to assume that the advice and information in this book are believed to be true and accurate at the date of publication. Neither the publisher nor the authors or the editors give a warranty, expressed or implied, with respect to the material contained herein or for any errors or omissions that may have been made. The publisher remains neutral with regard to jurisdictional claims in published maps and institutional affiliations.

This Springer imprint is published by the registered company Springer Nature Singapore Pte Ltd. The registered company address is: 152 Beach Road, #21-01/04 Gateway East, Singapore 189721, Singapore

If disposing of this product, please recycle the paper.

Preface

This book is written for all those involved in the care of patients with acute pancreatitis. Each of you know how challenging this disease can be. Characterized by a wide spectrum of severity; from a self-limiting disease that does not always result in hospital admission through to being rapidly fatal from fulminant multiple organ failure in the intensive care unit. You also know that a specific and effective drug treatment is not available. Despite that we have made progress. The overall mortality of acute pancreatitis has been dropping through many incremental evidence-based advances. Together these have had a positive impact on the clinical outcome of patients with acute pancreatitis. However, major challenges remain and disruptive thinking based on new paradigms are necessary if we are to subdue this common and serious disease.

Experimental and clinical research to understand the key pathophysiological events in acute pancreatitis continues around the world. Knowledge gaps are being filled, risk factors and disease mechanisms are being defined and dissected, biomarkers and potential treatment targets are being highlighted. While the history of drug trials in acute pancreatitis has been a litany of failure, there are many reasons for hope. There are so many potential treatment opportunities that derive from our rapidly expanding knowledge of what drives severe acute pancreatitis. But the clinical translation and implementation of this new knowledge requires a concerted and collaborative commitment, with robust and well-powered clinical trials. These trials need to ensure that interventions are timely. The success observed with treating acute coronary syndrome and stroke highlights the importance of intervention timing. The same urgency and hope should be applied to finding the appropriate treatment for acute pancreatitis, which when severe has a mortality risk like that of these diseases.

This book has been structured in two sections with the express purpose of making the contents more readily accessible to the diversity of readership. The first section is more theoretical, providing chapters that cover key mechanisms driving acute pancreatitis and its panoply of complications, as currently understood. The significant gaps in our knowledge offer avenues for future research. The second section provides the best practical advice on key aspects of management of acute pancreatitis in your patients. These include determining the etiology of acute pancreatitis, predicting the severity, identifying those who require early transfer, optimizing fluid therapy, selecting analgesia, providing safe and effective nutritional support, deciding when to intervene with ERCP, deciding when and how to intervene for infected pancreatic necrosis, and how best to support patients with organ dysfunction and failure.

One could argue that the separation between knowledge and practice is artificial and that these two sections should be combined. We think that for those who want practical advice about the steps in the management of patients with acute pancreatitis, this concise approach is helpful. We also think that those with questions and disappointments arising from the management of their patients and who see that progress requires new thinking and further research will find this approach helpful. This structure also highlights how much of our research acquired understanding of acute pancreatitis has still to make a difference in how we treat patients. Examples of this abound. The elegantly described mechanisms within the acinar cell at the onset of acute pancreatitis still await clinical application. The complexities of the cytokine storm have been mapped, but a treatment to tame that storm has yet to be implemented. The mechanisms driving organ failure are beginning to be understood, but still await definitive proof of clinical impact.

The lead authors of the chapters in this book are all internationally acclaimed experts who were carefully selected based on their recent and notable contributions to the field. These contributions reflect cutting-edge science and substantial clinical experience. They have delivered a book that is both stimulating and useful. It has been a pleasure working with them and with our publisher.

John Albert Windsor
Savio George Barreto
Anthony Ronald John Phillips

Contents

Part I

Clinically Relevant Science

Epidemiology of Acute Pancreatitis

Jeffrey J. Easler and Dhiraj Yadav

Key Points

- AP is among the most common gastrointestinal disorders responsible for hospital admission. The incidence of AP is increasing worldwide.
- The common etiologies of AP include gallstones, heavy alcohol consumption, hypertriglyceridemia, medications, and ERCP. The distribution of etiologies varies based on age, sex, ethnicity, and underlying risk factors. The severity and mortality of AP increase with age due to a higher prevalence of risk factors and comorbidities.
- Minimum work-up to determine the etiology of the first attack of AP includes the following—a thorough history, laboratory testing for liver function tests, calcium and triglycerides, and trans-abdominal ultrasound. In about one in five patients, no etiology is detected.
- About one in five patients with AP develops recurrent acute pancreatitis and 10% progresses to chronic pancreatitis. Alcohol etiology, tobacco use, and severe acute pancreatitis

are risk factors for recurrence. The best strategy to reduce the risk of disease progression is identification of etiology and addressing it, if possible.
- Diabetes and exocrine pancreatic insufficiency each develop in about one-third of AP patients during follow-up.
- Necrotizing and severe AP negatively impact quality of life and may lead to disability, which in some patients last for many months or even longer.

J. J. Easler
Division of Gastroenterology and Hepatology,
Indiana University School of Medicine,
Indianapolis, IN, USA
e-mail: jjeasler@iu.edu

D. Yadav (✉)
Division of Gastroenterology and Hepatology,
University of Pittsburgh Medical Center,
Pittsburgh, PA, USA
e-mail: yadavd@upmc.edu

1 Introduction

Acute pancreatitis (AP) is an important public health problem. It ranks among the most common causes of hospitalizations for gastrointestinal illnesses. In 2014, in the USA, there were 351,526 emergency room visits, 279,145 inpatient hospitalizations, and 1840 in-hospital deaths from AP with a total expenditure for inpatient care of $2.64 billion [1]. A number of population-based and large single or multicenter studies have clarified various aspects of the epidemiology of AP. The use of standardized definition and classification of severity proposed by the Revised Atlanta Classification in 2012 has brought uniformity to reporting and made it easier to compare results between studies [2]. Well-conducted systematic reviews and meta-analyses help in synthesizing information from published literature while highlighting their strengths and weak-

© The Author(s), under exclusive license to Springer Nature Singapore Pte Ltd. 2024
J. A. Windsor et al. (eds.), *Acute Pancreatitis*, https://doi.org/10.1007/978-981-97-3132-9_1

nesses. In this chapter, we have attempted to use information from population-based studies, systematic reviews, and meta-analyses as much as possible. The chapter is organized into a discussion of population trends, the impact of demographic and socioeconomic factors, relevant discussion of individual etiologies or risk factors, and the sequelae of AP. Finally, we review the concept of holistic prevention of pancreatitis and its application in disease prevention [3].

2 Global Incidence and Temporal Trends

A recent systematic review and meta-analysis of 44 population-based studies published between 1961 and 2016 evaluated global temporal trends in AP incidence [4]. Although the mean incidence varied widely (2.71–134.90 per 100,000 persons), in more than half of the studies, the mean incidence was more than 30 per 100,000. Over 70% of studies reported a significant average annual percentage change in AP incidence, which in pooled analysis showed an increase of 3.07% per year. The majority of studies (80%) originated from Europe and North America. Few data were available from Asia, South America, and Oceania, and none from the Middle East and Africa, suggesting the critical need for studies from these populations to better understand the global population burden of AP. An increasing temporal trend was observed for both sexes, in adult as well as pediatric age groups, and in all geographic regions except Asia. Etiologically, an increase from the two most common etiologies, i.e., gallstone—and alcohol-related AP, were considered to be the major contributors to the increasing incidence, which in turn are related to rising obesity, metabolic syndrome, and alcohol consumption in different populations [4]. Increasing use and exposure to medications is also a potential contributor, although establishing a cause and effect is challenging [5, 6]. Increasing awareness of the disease, wide availability of serum testing for pancreatic enzymes, and imaging studies are also likely contributors, but their relative contribution is difficult to assess [7–9].

Plateauing of incidence observed in some of the recent studies likely points to a saturation of the effects of many of the aforementioned factors [4].

3 Demographic and Socioeconomic Factors

The incidence of AP increases in a progressive fashion after the age of 50 years. In one cohort study, the incidence rate per 100,000 in the age groups <50, 50–69, and ≥70 years increased from 16.8 to 64.2 and 122.3, respectively, among men, and 18.3 to 46.4 and 96.5, respectively, among women [10]. Increasing incidence with age is related to the prevalence of risk factors, e.g., in middle age from a higher prevalence of gallstones and alcohol use and in the elderly from a higher prevalence of gallstones and exposure to medications. The incidence of AP is roughly similar in men and women [11]. However, the proportional distribution of etiologies differs by sex—women have a higher prevalence of gallstone-related AP, while men are more likely to have AP related to alcohol, hypertriglyceridemia, and diabetes [12–14]. The incidence of AP also varies by race. In a meta-analysis of three studies, the incidence of AP per 100,000 was the highest among indigenous peoples (Maori: 93.6, Native American: 43, Pacific Islander: 35.6) and the lowest among Asian population (11.8). The incidence of AP was lower in Caucasians (19.7) when compared with African American (28.6) and Hispanic (23.1) populations [15].

A systematic review and meta-analysis of 33 studies also noted a similar relationship between increasing age and risk of severity (3.7% for ages <40 years to 16.1% for those aged 60+ years) and mortality from AP (~1% in those <40 years to 13.9% in those aged 60+ years) [16]. The increase in mortality is related to a higher burden of comorbidities with age [17].

Obesity is associated with an increased risk of AP. In a meta-analysis, estimates from 9 population-based studies demonstrated the relative risk of AP to increase by 18% for every 5 kg/m² increase in body mass index (BMI) and 36% for every 10 cm increase in waist circumference. The association remained significant after stratification for sex and controlling for confounding factors. The risk was nonlinear with BMI and linear with waist circumference, suggesting a stronger association between central adiposity and AP [18]. Obesity is also associated with increased severity of and mortality from AP. In a meta-analysis of 19 studies, patients with severe AP were more likely to have a higher BMI (mean difference 1.79, 95% CI 0.89–2.70). When compared with individuals with a normal BMI, those with a BMI of >25 were almost 3 times more likely to have severe AP (OR 2.87, 95% CI 1.90–4.35). Obese patients (BMI >30) had significantly higher mortality when compared to those with BMI <30 (OR 2.89, 95% 1.10–7.36) [19].

There are limited data on the role of social determinants of health on the burden of AP. In a population-based study from Wales, UK, the presence of social deprivation was associated with an increased risk of AP. This association was stronger for alcohol-related AP vs. gallstone or other etiologies of AP (3.9-fold vs. 1.5—and 1.6-fold, respectively) [20].

4 Relevant Discussion by Etiology (Table 1)

4.1 Gallstone-Related AP

Gallstone disease is the most frequent cause of AP worldwide accounting for 42% of cases [11]. The rate of gallstone-related AP increases with age. Gallstone disease is also more common in women, and there is an increased comparative prevalence of gallstones for women (vs. men) within each age group [21]. The rate of gallstone-related AP is higher in certain ethnic groups and in the presence of risk factors for gallstone disease, such as obesity or pregnancy [22, 23]. The diagnosis of gallstones as the cause of AP is often circumstantial; the likelihood of coexisting gallstones to have caused an episode of AP is greater with concurrent elevation in liver function tests. According to a meta-analysis, the positive predictive value for an elevation in serum alanine transaminase of more than 3 times normal for biliary AP was 95% (and somewhat lower for elevations in aspartate transaminase and bilirubin) [24]. Except for a small fraction of patients

Table 1 Clinical features of the select etiologies of acute pancreatitis

Etiology	Demographic factors	Clinical, lab, and imaging finding(s)	Other clinical pearls
Gallstones	• Increases with age • More common in females than males	• Elevation in serum liver function tests (positive predictive value of elevated ALT of >3 times normal is ~95%) • Gallstones and/or bile duct dilation on imaging	• Abdominal ultrasound has higher sensitivity than a CT scan to detect gallstones • History of antecedent biliary colic or other biliary complications (e.g., cholecystitis)
Alcohol	• More common in middle-age • More common in males than females	• Elevation in serum liver function tests; AST to ALT ratio • Elevated MCV • Positive blood/urine metabolites (e.g., PeTH)	• Risk increases with the amount of alcohol consumption, binge drinking • Coexistent fatty liver or features of cirrhosis
Hypertriglyceridemia	• More common in young and middle-aged • More common in males than females	• Elevation in serum triglyceride levels (usually >500–1000mg/dL)	• Common clinical scenarios (diabetes, alcoholism, metabolic syndrome, medications, pregnancy) • Risk of HTG-related AP increased even with milder elevations in serum triglycerides

(continued)

Table 1 (continued)

Etiology	Demographic factors	Clinical, lab, and imaging finding(s)	Other clinical pearls
Medications	• Likely more common with increasing age (due to exposure to medications)	• Appropriate latency period with the initiation of medication • Recurrent pancreatitis with rechallenge	• Antineoplastic, antibiotics, and anticonvulsants account for a large proportion of reports
Post-ERCP pancreatitis	• More common in young and middle-aged • More common in females than males	• Symptom onset soon after undergoing ERCP • Serum amylase or lipase 3 or more times normal 24 h after ERCP • Hospital stay lasting or increased by more than 48 h New imaging findings consistent with AP after ERCP	• Patient factors that increase risk: sphincter of Oddi dysfunction, female gender, younger age, history of AP, and post-ERCP pancreatitis • Procedure factors that increase risk: pancreatic duct injection(s) and manipulations, pancreatic sphincterotomy, cannulation difficulty • Risk decreased by: appropriate patient selection, operator expertise, rectal NSAIDS, periprocedural fluid administration, prophylactic pancreatic duct stent
Pancreas divisum	• Female dominance in clinically diagnosed cases	• Pancreas divisum morphology on imaging (s-MRCP)	• Often co-prevalent with other risk factors (tobacco, alcohol, genetic polymorphisms) • Prevalence enriched with idiopathic and recurrent AP
Pancreatic cancer	• More common in elderly	• Jaundice, weight loss, new-onset diabetes • Elevation in serum liver function tests • Pancreatic mass, biliary, and/or pancreatic duct dilation on imaging	• Other neoplasms (IPMN, neuroendocrine tumors, etc.) can also present as AP
Genetic polymorphism(s)	• More frequently discovered in idiopathic AP and recurrent acute pancreatitis	• Pathogenic polymorphisms in pancreatitis susceptibility genes (PRSS1, SPINK1, CFTR, CTRC)	• Family history of pancreatitis, pancreatic cancer, or cystic fibrosis • Short stature, infertility, recurrent sinopulmonary infections, and male infertility may suggest the presence of CFTR polymorphism(s)
Autoimmune pancreatitis	• More common after age 50 years • More common in males	• Jaundice • Elevated serum IgG4, imaging—diffuse enlargement, focal mass, pancreatic duct stricture(s)	• Resolution of symptoms and imaging findings with corticosteroids often verifies the diagnosis • Features of other organ involvement • Inflammatory bowel disease

with retained stones or the formation of new stones in the common bile duct, the performance of cholecystectomy virtually eliminates the risk of future episodes of gallstone-related AP. Substantial level 1 evidence based on randomized clinical trials and meta-analyses recommend cholecystectomy to reduce the risk of recurrent attacks, and cholecystectomy should preferably performed during the index hospitalization or soon thereafter [25, 26].

4.2 Alcohol-Related AP

Alcohol is the second most common cause of AP accounting for 21% of cases [11]. The risk of alcohol-related AP is higher in middle-aged individuals and in men (vs. women) due to higher alcohol consumption in these groups [27]. The primary determinant for pancreatitis is the amount and duration of alcohol consumption— roughly one in 20 individuals who drink heavily develop pancreatitis [28, 29]. Two meta-analyses have evaluated the risk of pancreatitis based on alcohol consumption [30, 31]. Overall, the risk appears to be linear, especially at levels above ~4 drinks/day. Lower levels of consumption may be associated with a lower risk of pancreatitis, especially in women [31, 32]. Available data are mixed regarding the effect of alcohol consumption patterns and the type of alcohol on the risk of pancreatitis [33–35].

A diagnosis of alcohol-related AP relies on obtaining a good history and if/as needed corroboration from family members and/or friends. Certain laboratory tests, such as the pattern of serum aspartate transaminase (AST) and alanine transaminase (ALT), elevations in gamma-glutamyl transferase (GGT), high mean corpuscular volume (MCV) of red cells, and imaging findings of fatty liver and/or cirrhosis, can provide a clue toward alcohol etiology [36]. When suspicion of alcohol as an etiology is high with unclear clinical history, the blood level of phosphatidyl ethanol (PeTH) can help uncover occult alcohol consumption. PeTH are abnormal phospholipid metabolites of alcohol that accumulate in cell membranes and can be detected for up to 2–3 weeks after moderate-heavy alcohol consumption [37].

Aggressive and repeat counseling can help to reduce alcohol consumption, the risk of recurrences, and progression to chronic pancreatitis. In a randomized control trial, when compared with a single inpatient session, repeated counseling for alcohol cessation led to a lower rate of recurrent AP (RAP) (21% vs. 8%, $p = 0.042$) and fewer AP episodes in those with recurrent acute pancreatitis over 2 years of follow-up [38]. Outpatient pharmacotherapy for alcohol cessa-tion is beneficial with a number needed to treat ranging from 12 to 20 [39]. Currently, there is no such data for alcohol-related AP.

4.3 Hypertriglyceridemia (HTG)-Related AP

HTG accounts for 2–5% of AP cases in most published studies, except for those originating from China, where multiple studies over the years have consistently reported a much higher prevalence (up to 20%) [11, 40] [41]. HTG is an underrecognized cause of AP: the most common reasons being a lack of recognition of the association between serum triglycerides and AP and a delay in the measurement of serum triglyceride levels after admission. Typically, HTG-related AP is defined by a serum triglyceride level of 1000 mg/dL during hospital admission [42]. It is being recognized that the risk may be elevated even at much lower levels of serum triglycerides. Two population-based studies have observed a dose-dependent increase in the risk of AP with serum triglyceride levels [43, 44]. In the study from Scotland, when compared with individuals with a serum triglyceride of <150 mg/dL, the risk of incident AP was significantly higher in those with triglyceride between 150 and 499 mg/dL (hazard ratio, HR 1.50, 95% CI, 1.14–1.97) and ≥ 500 mg/dL (HR 3.20, 95% CI, 1.99–5.16). The incidence of AP increased by 4% for every 100 mg/dL increase in triglyceride levels after adjusting for such covariates as biliary disease and alcohol-related morbidities. Importantly, the population-attributable risk of AP was greater for moderate than severe hypertriglyceridemia (18.37% vs. 7.74%) [43]. In the other study from Denmark, when compared with individuals with a serum triglyceride level of <89 mg/dL, a progressive increase in incident AP was found for each 88 mg/dL increase in triglyceride levels. The adjusted risk for AP was over eightfold (HR 8.7 95% CI, 3.7–20.0) for those with levels >443 mg/dL [44].

Clinicians need to be aware of the scenarios associated with HTG-related AP. In decreasing frequency, these include poorly controlled diabetes, alcoholism, concurrent use of medications that increase serum triglyceride levels, and the third trimester of pregnancy. Extremely uncommon are scenarios where there is a single polymorphism (e.g., lipoprotein lipase, LPL deficiency) as the cause of HTG [42]. These are all secondary causes of HTG in individuals with an underlying, often polygenic disorder [45]. Frequently, patients have more than one risk factor, e.g., a patient with diabetes also has obesity, metabolic syndrome, poor dietary habits, and/or alcohol consumption, which all contribute to the increase in serum triglyceride levels [13].

Empiric data from carefully performed studies have documented poorly controlled triglyceride levels to be associated with an increased risk of recurrence. In one such study from Kaiser Permanente, the risk of recurrent AP was 8.45-fold (95% CI 2.55–27.96) among patients with the highest triglyceride levels (>500 mg/dL) [46]. Control of serum triglyceride levels may reduce the risk of recurrences [47].

4.4   Medication-Induced AP

Adverse effects of medications account for less than 5% of cases of AP [11]. Medication-induced AP is an idiosyncratic event. The mechanisms for injury by which AP occurs from medications are multiple [48]. A good history is helpful to demonstrate a temporal relationship between the initiations of a medication, usually in the weeks or months prior to AP. Before making a diagnosis, work-up for other etiologies should be undertaken to ensure that another potentially treatable cause (e.g., gallstones) is not missed. Diagnostic uncertainty may also exist in situations where other known risk factors are present in a patient presumed to have medication-induced AP. Badalov et al. proposed a classification system, which offers guidance for assessing the likelihood that a medication associated with AP. Within this framework, medication is highly implicated for AP if supported by a combination of multiple reports, rechallenge evidence, and a temporal relationship between drug exposure and AP, including a reasonable latency period in at

least four reports, and by publications describing a process of exclusion of other AP etiologies [49]. Drug reaction probability scales have also been repurposed and refined to determine the likelihood of a given medication having caused AP [50].

A recent systematic review of over 1000 cases revealed antineoplastic agents (17%), antibiotics (12%), and anticonvulsant (10%) accounted for the greatest proportion of medication-induced pancreatitis, while valproic acid (7.64%) and L-asparaginase (6.42%) were the most frequent individual agents [51]. AP severity (18.4 vs. 5.63%) and mortality (7.3 vs. 2.2%) in medication-induced AP were noted to be higher than other etiologies [51]. While this in part may be related to reporting bias, another possibility is that individuals who develop medication-induced AP also have comorbidities, which place them at greater risk for severity.

One class of medications increasingly recognized for medication-induced AP is immune checkpoint inhibitors (ICI) (see Autoimmune Pancreatitis, AIP section).

4.5   Post-ERCP Pancreatitis (PEP)

PEP is the most frequent complication of endoscopic retrograde cholangiopancreatography (ERCP) and accounts for ~2% of all AP cases [11, 52]. The risk of PEP can increase to greater than 15% based on modifiable and non-modifiable risk factors [53]. Pre-procedure factors that increase risk include an indication (e.g., sphincter of Oddi dysfunction, minor papilla endotherapy in the setting of pancreas divisum, intraductal papillary mucinous neoplasm), female sex, younger age, prior history of PEP, and AP of any cause. Intra-procedure factors include pancreatic duct injection, pancreatic duct manipulations and therapy, precut sphincterotomy, papillary balloon dilation, placement of metallic biliary stent, and cannulation difficulty. Other factors associated with increased risk include the experience of the endoscopist [54–57]. Consequently, careful patient selection, utilizing high-quality pancreaticobiliary imaging (e.g., magnetic resonance cholangiopancreatography [MRCP] and endoscopic ultrasound [EUS]) to verify pathology, performing ERCP only for therapeutic purposes, and concentrating complex procedures in the hands of experts are strategies that mitigate pre-procedure risk [58]. Evidenced-based prophylactic interventions that reduce the risk of post-ERCP pancreatitis include placement of a temporary pancreatic duct stent, administration of rectal nonsteroidal anti-inflammatory agents, and aggressive peri-procedure hydration [59–61]. A recent randomized clinical trial found rectal indomethacin alone to be inferior to the combination rectal indomethacin and prophylactic pancreatic duct stent placement in preventing PEP in high-risk patients [62].

5 Other Causes and Risk Factors for AP

5.1 Pancreas Divisum

The most common congenital anatomic variant of the pancreatic duct noted in up to 10% of the population is "complete" pancreas divisum [63, 64]. It is characterized by the failure of fusion during the development of the main pancreatic duct segments of the dorsal (Santorini) and ventral anlage (Wirsung). In pancreas divisum, since more than 70% of the functional pancreas relies on the minor papilla orifice for exocrine pancreas secretion, it is believed to increase the risk of AP by causing functional obstruction to the pancreatic duct outflow [65]. Secretin-MRCP offers the ideal balance of accuracy, reproducibility, and safety for the diagnosis of pancreas divisum [66]. Evaluation for pancreas divisum is typically considered in patients with recurrent acute pancreatitis. Pancreas divisum is noted to be overrepresented in patients with recurrent acute and chronic pancreatitis, especially in individuals with certain genetic polymorphisms [67]. Although minor papillotomy or serial pancreatic duct stent placements are reported to benefit up to 76% of patients with recurrent pancreatitis and pancreas divisum, due to methodological issues, the true benefit of intervention on the natural

course of disease in this condition remains unclear [68, 69]. The effectiveness of minor papillotomy is currently undergoing a rigorous evaluation in the form of a multicenter randomized sham-controlled trial [70] The role of endotherapy in pancreas divisum in the setting of a single episode of AP is limited to the management of AP-related complications.

5.2 Neoplasia

Neoplasms are an infrequent cause of AP accounting for <5% of cases [11]. The mechanism of AP in these patients is obstruction of the pancreatic duct. Among patients with pancreatic ductal adenocarcinoma, ~10% present with AP as the initial manifestation [71]. In a patient with AP, the presence of certain clinical and imaging features, especially in the absence of another obvious cause, should raise the possibility of underlying malignancy and prompt further workup with contrast-enhanced CT scan and endoscopic ultrasound. These high-risk features include older age (>50 years), history of smoking, weight loss, jaundice, new-onset diabetes, presence of a mass on an imaging study, and pancreatic duct dilatation associated with atrophy [72–74].

Among patients with AP, the risk of detection of pancreatic cancer is the greatest within the first year after diagnosis (14.5 per 1000 person-years), which increases with age (7.69 among those <40 years vs. 28.67 per 1000 person-years among those 70 years and older) [71]. A Swedish national health registry study evaluated the risk of pancreatic cancer following an episode of AP. When compared with controls, during a median of 5.3 years of follow-up, incident pancreatic cancer was much higher in the AP cohort (1.1% vs. 0.1%), with the risk being greatest in the first 2 months after the AP event (HR 172.84, 95% CI 54.85–544.66). The majority of cancer cases (>89%) were also diagnosed within the first 5 years following the index AP attack and declined to the baseline after 10 years [75].

Intraductal papillary mucinous neoplasm, especially those affecting the main pancreatic duct, can present with AP due to ductal obstruction from thick mucinous secretion [76]. Other neoplasms, such as mucinous cystic neoplasm, neuroendocrine tumors, or other uncommon tumors, can also cause AP by causing obstruction of the pancreatic duct [77–79]. Diagnosis is established by a combination of distinctive findings on cross-sectional imaging (e.g., neuroendocrine tumors appear hypervascular during the arterial phase of a triphasic computed tomography [CT] scan) and EUS-guided sampling.

5.3 Celiac Disease and Other Autoimmune Diseases

Celiac disease increases the risk of pancreatitis. In a population-based study from Sweden, 28,908 individuals with celiac disease were matched with 143,746 controls. During a mean follow-up of 11+/−6.5 years, individuals with celiac disease had an increased risk of pancreatitis of about threefold (HR 2.85, 95% CI 2.53–3.21) with an excess risk of 81/100,000 per year. The risk of gallstone-related AP and non-gallstone AP in individuals with celiac disease was increased by 1.59-fold (95% CI 1.06–2.40, excess risk 3/100,000 person-years) and 1.86-fold (95% CI 1.52–2.26, excess risk of 19/100,000 per years), respectively [80]. One proposed mechanism of pancreatitis in these patients is peri-ampullary inflammation, leading to papillary stenosis [81]. In clinical practice, a celiac panel should be considered in patients with AP without an identifiable cause. The presence of other autoimmune disorders such as hypo—or hyperthyroidism and diabetes (especially early onset) could provide a clue to the diagnosis.

AP is also reported in case reports and series in individuals with other autoimmune disorders, such as inflammatory vasculitis and systemic lupus erythematosus [82, 83].

5.4 Autoimmune Pancreatitis (AIP)

A detailed discussion of AIP is beyond the scope of this review. AP can be an uncommon manifestation of AIP. In a series of 63 AIP patients from a tertiary care center, 24% met the Revised Atlanta Classification criteria for AP. AIP patients with AP (vs. without AP) tended to be younger (50.3 vs. 62.8 years), more likely to be male (100 vs. 73%), have abdominal pain (100 vs. 37%), and more likely to have Type 2 AIP (33 vs. 4%). The was no difference in the prevalence of disease-specific manifestations, such as obstructive jaundice, elevated transaminases, elevation in serum IgG4 levels, and response to steroids. On cross-sectional imaging, none had a focal mass, 47% had diffuse, 27% had focal pancreatic enlargement, and none had pancreatic necrosis [84].

In the past few years, a new form of AIP called Type 3 AIP has come to attention as a side effect of immune checkpoint inhibitors (ICIs) used for the treatment of a variety of malignancies. ICIs are antibodies designed to inhibit programmed death receptor 1 (PD-1) and its ligand 1 (PD-L1) or cytotoxic T lymphocyte-associated protein 4 (CTLA-4). The most frequent clinical presentation of ICI-related pancreatic injury (ICI-PI) is asymptomatic elevation in pancreatic enzymes, while the remainder have epigastric pain, nausea, vomiting with or without imaging changes of AP, and/or local complications [85] In a systematic review of 50 randomized control trials encompassing 35,223 patients, the incidence of ICI-PI was 2.22% (95% CI 1.94–2.53), and severe ICI-PI (grade ≥ 3) was 2.08% (95% CI 1.70–2.46). The incidence was higher when a combination of two ICIs was used (overall, 3.76 vs. 2.25%; severe 2.32 vs. 1.95%). ICI-PI varied by the type of ICI (in decreasing %—PD-L1, CTLA-4, PD-1), and the agent with the highest risk was pembrolizumab (7.23%, 95% CI = 1.69–30.89%) [86]. The role of steroids in the management of ICI-PI is unclear. A recent review organized the clinical presentation according to the Revised Atlanta Classification and proposed management of ICI-PI [85].

5.5 Genetic Factors

Polymorphisms in a variety of genes have been associated with increased susceptibility to pancreatitis, and a detailed discussion is beyond the scope of this chapter. Testing for many of these (PRSS1, SPINK1, CFTR, CTRC) is commercially available. Assessment for genetic factors as the cause is typically reserved for patients who have RAP [87, 88].

5.6   Infectious Causes

Infectious agents are a rare cause of AP in adults. Infectious pancreatitis is suspected in a patient with AP who also meets the clinical criteria for a given infection; the infection is verified by biochemical, serologic, and/or culture results; and, most importantly, common causes of AP (e.g., biliary, alcohol) have been excluded. A systematic review including 320 patients found viral infections to account for most cases of infectious AP (65%), followed by parasitic infections (19%). In this cohort, the mean age of patients was 40.5 years, the majority were male (2:1 ratio), and a significant proportion were immunocompromised (18.5%). Of note, patients with viral AP (vs. those with nonviral infections) were significantly younger (39.3 vs. 43.8 years), more likely to be immunocompromised (24.9 vs. 3.5%), and had higher mortality (21.8 vs. 7%) [89]. With the advent of severe acute respiratory syndrome coronavirus 2 (SARS-CoV2 virus) in 2019 as the cause of COVID-19, there has been an interest in pancreatic injury in these patients. In a systematic review, among >150,000 reported cases of COVID-19, the incidence rate of AP confirmed by clinical and imaging criteria was 0.16% [90].

5.7   Hypercalcemia

Hypercalcemia accounts for less than 1% of cases of AP [11, 91]. While the exact threshold of serum calcium elevation at which risk AP elevates is unclear, hypercalcemia is believed to accelerate the conversion of intrapancreatic trypsinogen to trypsin, leading to pancreatitis. Conditions such as hyperparathyroidism, paraneoplastic, and sarcoidosis have been reported as causes of hypercalcemia-induced AP [92, 93].

5.8   Tobacco Use

Although the literature mainly evaluates cigarette smoking, it is likely that tobacco use in all forms increases the risk of AP. Unlike the causal association with alcohol, smoking is considered a risk factor. In a meta-analysis of eight prospective studies, the risk of AP was increased in current smokers (relative risk, RR 1.49, 95% CI 1.20–1.72), former smokers (RR 1.24, 95% CI 1.15–1.34), and ever smokers (RR 1.39, 95% CI 1.25–1.54) when compared with nonsmokers [94]. The relative risk per 10 cigarettes/day increased by 30% (RR 1.30, 95% CI 1.18–1.42) and per 10 pack years by 13% (RR 1.13, 95% CI 1.08–1.17) in current smokers. As discussed in a subsequent section in this chapter, smoking is an important cofactor for disease progression. Clinicians should be aware of the relationship between tobacco use and AP, and all patients who use tobacco should be counseled toward the risk of progression and encouraged to quit.

5.9   Diabetes

There is growing recognition of the bidirectional relationship between diabetes and AP. A meta-analysis of six observational studies noted the relative risk of AP in individuals with diabetes to be 1.84 (95% CI 1.45–2.33) [95]. While a subset of patients with diabetes may develop AP due to co-existent risk factors, such as metabolic syndrome, and HTG, the exact pathophysiology of how diabetes increases the risk of AP is unclear. A population-based analysis noted that the risk of AP was reduced among diabetic patients with better control of blood sugar levels [96].

5.10 End-Stage Renal Disease (ESRD) and Renal Replacement Therapy

Several studies suggest an increased risk for AP in patients with ESRD undergoing peritoneal and hemodialysis [97, 98]. A study that followed 2603 hemodialysis patients found a 3.4-fold (95% CI 2.5–4.7) increased risk of AP (vs. 773,140 controls) over a 3-year period [99]. Retrospective and case-control studies also suggest the risk for AP to be ~three-fold higher in ESRD patients managed with peritoneal compared to hemodialysis [100]. Multiple factors including metabolic abnormalities (e.g., hyperparathyroidism) and comorbidities of ESRD, hemodynamic shifts with dialysis, and toxicity from dialysate are mechanisms for AP in these populations [100].

5.10.1 Idiopathic AP

Idiopathic AP is the third most common etiologic category after gallstones and alcohol. Idiopathic AP is diagnosed when no obvious etiology is identified. The proportion of AP patients that are idiopathic depends in part on the extent of etiologic work-up performed. In a systematic review and meta-analysis of 46 studies from 36 countries published between 2006 and 2017, 18% (95% CI 15–22) patients were noted to be assigned to idiopathic category [11]. The International Association of Pancreatology guidelines on the management of AP published in 2013 recommends the minimum etiologic work-up after the first attack of AP to include a thorough history, laboratory tests (serum liver function tests, triglycerides, calcium), and an abdominal ultrasound (Table 2) [101]. Additional testing should be considered in specific situations. As an example, a contrast-enhanced CT scan is not indicated in all patients with AP. However, in individuals aged 50 years or older who have no other identifiable etiology, a contrast-enhanced CT scan can help to detect a pancreatic mass (pancreatic cancer or other neoplasms) presenting as AP. In our practice, when the outlined work-up is negative, we order a celiac panel, and in select cases, serum IgG4

Table 2 Minimum recommended work-up for acute pancreatitis

Index attack	Subsequent attack(s)
• Detailed history with attention to prior history of pancreatic disease and/or pancreaticobiliary procedures (e.g., ERCP, surgery), history of gallstone disease or symptoms of biliary colic, family history (pancreatic disease, cystic fibrosis, celiac disease), risk factors (alcohol consumption, tobacco use, metabolic syndrome), medication history • Laboratory tests: serum liver function tests, calcium, triglycerides • Right upper quadrant ultrasound *Optional (select cases)* • Contrast-enhanced CT scan • Serum IgG4 levels • PeTH testing • Celiac panel	• Repeat trans-abdominal ultrasound • Contrast-enhanced CT scan • Endoscopic ultrasound (EUS) • MRI with contrast/MRCP with secretin if available • Genetic testing for polymorphisms in pancreatitis susceptibility genes (PRSS1, SPINK1, CFTR, CTRC)

(when imaging findings are suggestive of AIP), PeTH testing (when there is a concern for alcohol etiology in the absence of a corroborative history), and a EUS to evaluate for microlithiasis or an occult cancer in older individuals or when contrast-enhanced CT shows suggestive or concerning findings.

Further etiologic work-up is usually completed after the second or subsequent episodes of AP. Appropriate studies include EUS, MRI, and MRCP (with secretin, if possible) and testing for genetic polymorphisms that increase susceptibility to pancreatitis [101]. EUS can help detect microlithiasis, an occult pancreatic mass, and parenchymal and ductal changes of chronic pancreatitis. MRCP can help to assess for pancreatic ductal abnormalities, such as pancreas divisum, intraductal papillary mucinous neoplasm, pancreatic duct stricture, and pancreas secretory function after secretin administration [102].

A post hoc analysis of 1632 patients treated at 19 Dutch Hospitals from 2008 to 2015 evaluated the yield of further work-up for presumed idiopathic AP (first attack) in a community setting.

The authors identified 12% (191/1632) of patients with idiopathic AP after initial work-up. Of these, 176 (92%) underwent further work-up during a median follow-up of 4 years. An etiology was uncovered in 36% (64/176) patients with biliary (36/64, 56%) and neoplasm (12/64, 19%), being the two most common etiologies identified [103]. In a single tertiary care center study, among 201 patients with presumed idiopathic AP ($n = 80$) or RAP ($n = 121$), further work-up identified microlithiasis/cholelithiasis in 21 (10%), pancreas divisum in 43 (21%), CP in 21 (10%), sphincter of Oddi dysfunction in 61 (25%), and miscellaneous cases in 3% [104]. Differences in etiologic distribution between the two studies reflect the study setting (community vs. tertiary care center) and referral population.

5.10.2 Geographic Differences in AP Phenotype

The previously mentioned systematic review and meta-analysis evaluated geographic differences in AP etiology from 36 countries [11]. Two distinct differences were noted—although gallstones (pooled estimate 41.7%) and alcohol (pooled estimate 20.5%) were the two most common etiologies of AP worldwide, the proportion of gallstone-related AP (pooled estimate 68.5%) was much higher, and alcohol-related AP was lower (pooled estimate 5%) in studies published from Latin America. In the sole study from South Africa, the dominant etiology was alcohol (70%).

A multicenter, prospective, international registry from 22 centers in four continents reported on the clinical phenotype of AP in 1612 patients treated between 8/2015 and 1/2018. Although not population-based and with the limitations of bias from a selection of participating centers and referral patterns, the study provides insights into geographic differences that are relevant. In addition to etiology, distinct differences were noted based on age, BMI, prevalent comorbidities, and severity, which are summarized in Table 3 [105].

5.10.3 Recurrent Acute Pancreatitis

Recurrent pancreatitis is defined as another AP attack after complete resolution of symptoms and an intervening asymptomatic period (1–3 months). The risk of recurrence is determined by the duration of observation, etiology, and severity of the AP attack. Consequently, identification and elimination of the inciting cause of AP, if possible, provides the best opportunity to prevent or reduce the risk of recurrences.

The incidence and prevalence of recurrent acute pancreatitis is unknown and was estimated to be 8–10 per 100,000 people per year and 110–140 per 100,000 population, respectively, in an expert review [106]. A number of studies have assessed the risk of recurrences after an initial episode. In a meta-analysis of 11 studies with over 8000 patients, the risk was estimated to be 21% (95% CI 17–26%) after the first attack. The

Table 3 Geographic differences in select clinical features of AP

Variable	European centers	Indian centers	Latin American centers	North American centers
Age, years, median (IQR)	58 (45, 74)	39 (30, 50)	43 (29, 50)	52 (37, 65)
Gender, male %	49.6	74.9	33.5	50.6
Etiology, %				
Biliary	50.4	27.9	78.1	45.3
Alcohol	19.1	44.5	1.9	20.9
Idiopathic	18.1	21.0	6.9	16.5
Hypertriglyceridemia	4.6	1.9	6.0	4.7
Post-ERCP	3.2	2.2	4.7	8.3
Other	4.6	2.5	2.5	4.2
Severe AP, %	11.9	22.5	7.4	7.5
Mortality, %	5.7	3.3	2.3	0.6

Data reported from Ref 105: Matta B, Gougol A, Gao X, et al. Worldwide Variations in Demographics, Management, and Outcomes of Acute Pancreatitis. Clin Gastroenterol Hepatol. 2020 Jun;18(7):1567-1575.e2. doi: 10.1016/j.cgh.2019.11.017. Epub 2019 Nov 9. PMID: 31712075; PMCID: PMC9198955

risk was higher in patients with alcohol than in biliary etiology (38 vs. 17%) [107]. A more recent meta-analysis evaluated the relationship between the four most common etiologies with recurrent acute pancreatitis. The risk was similar for alcohol and HTG-related AP; it was higher for HTG-related AP (vs. biliary AP, OR 2.69, 95% CI 1.55–4.65) and alcohol-related AP (vs. biliary AP, OR 2.98, 95% CI 2.22–4.01). The recurrence rate was similar for biliary and post-ERCP pancreatitis [108].

The risk of recurrence is also associated with tobacco use and the severity of AP attacks. In a cross-sectional survey of a multicenter cohort, the risk of recurrent acute pancreatitis was greatest among those with active alcohol and tobacco use (50% after 5 years). On multivariable analysis, tobacco use (OR 2.77, 95% CI 1.69–4.53), pancreatic necrosis (OR 2.53, 95% CI 1.48–4.33), and APACHE II score (OR 0.91, 0.86–0.96) were independently associate with risk of RAP [109]. In a population-based study, during a median follow-up of 4.6 years in 1457 patients after first attack of AP, the risk of recurrences was significantly higher in smokers (HR 1.42, 95% CI 1.03–1.95), alcohol-related AP (HR 1.58, 95% CI 1.25–2.23), organ failure (HR 1.46, 95% 1.05–2.03), and systemic (HR 1.88, 95% CI 1.27–2.79) or local complications (HR 1.66, 95% CI 1.22–2.27) [110]. Similar observations were observed in another recent population-based study from Iceland [111].

5.10.4 Chronic Pancreatitis

According to the mechanistic definition, acute and recurrent pancreatitis represent earlier stages of chronic pancreatitis, and a subset of them transition to chronic pancreatitis during follow-up [112]. Similar to RAP, the risk of progression from AP and RAP to CP is dependent on the duration of follow-up, etiology, severity of AP episodes, and other risk factors, such as tobacco use.

In the meta-analysis focusing on progression from acute to chronic pancreatitis previously discussed, the risk of progression from a single episode of AP to chronic pancreatitis was 10% (95% CI 6–15%), while the risk of progression from

recurrent acute pancreatitis to chronic pancreatitis was 35% (95% CI 20–53%) [107]. In other large studies published after the systematic review and discussed in the previous section, recurrent acute pancreatitis was noted to be the most important determinant for progression with risk estimates as high as sevenfold (HR 6.74, 95% CI 4.02–11.3) with chronic pancreatitis occurring in up to 32% of patients [109–111] The other important risk factors were alcohol etiology (risk estimates, 2.29–4.8-fold), smoking (risk estimates 1.62–2.9-fold), and disease severity including pancreatic necrosis (1.37–8.78-fold).

Another way to evaluate the relationship between acute and chronic pancreatitis is the prevalence of AP among patients with chronic pancreatitis. In a study from the Mayo Clinic, among 499 patients, 50.1% of patients were diagnosed with AP prior to chronic pancreatitis diagnosis. Among those with AP prior to chronic pancreatitis, 45% had a single episode, while 55% had recurrent acute pancreatitis [113]. In another multicenter study from the USA, among patients with chronic pancreatitis, the prevalence of prior AP was higher (71%). Most of the patients in this study with AP had recurrent acute pancreatitis (86.5%) [114]. These data suggest that a subset of patients with chronic pancreatitis have clinically diagnosed episodes of AP and transition between stages as outlined in the mechanistic definition.

6 Long-Term Sequalae of AP

6.1 Diabetes

About one in five patients with AP have preexisting diabetes [14, 115]. Among those with no known diabetes, a subset is diagnosed with diabetes either during hospitalization or follow-up. In population-based studies, after adjusting for age and sex, the risk of incident diabetes is noted to be 2–2.5-fold greater when compared with controls [116, 117]. Importantly, the risk is not limited to patients with severe AP [14, 115]. In a meta-analysis that included 31 studies, the pooled prevalence of new-onset diabetes after AP was 30% (95% 27–33%) [118]. The pooled estimates for diabetes were higher in severe (39 vs. 14% in non-severe AP) and necrotizing AP (37 vs. 11%), suggesting that physical destruction of the pancreatic parenchyma leads to increased risk. Diabetes risk was higher based on etiology (alcohol-related AP 28%, biliary AP 12%, other etiologies 24%) and with the duration of follow-up (20% with follow-up <5 years, 37% with follow-up of >5 years).

In a prospective study of 152 patients with AP who underwent assessment for diabetes every 6 months for 2 years, the risk of new-onset diabetes and prediabetes at 1 year was 7.2% and 33.9%, respectively, and at 2 years was 11% and 45%, respectively [119]. Only a small fraction of patients in this study had necrotizing AP (5%). Incident diabetes was not associated with demographic and other disease-related factors, which in part may be related to a small sample size of the cohort. In a subsequent analysis, the authors stratified patients into three risk groups and identified those with high glucose variability during hospital admission to be at the greatest risk of new-onset diabetes during follow-up [120].

The mechanisms of diabetes developing after AP, especially in patients with mild or non-necrotizing AP are unknown. A large multicenter study in the USA is currently enrolling patients with AP for longitudinal assessment of the risk and determinants of diabetes and the mechanisms of diabetes in these patients [121–123].

6.2 Exocrine Pancreatic Insufficiency (EPI)

A systematic review and meta-analysis comprehensively evaluated the rates of EPI rates in patients with AP during index hospitalization ($n = 370$, 10 studies) and with long-term follow-up ($n = 1795$, 39 studies), some of which had follow-up of more than 60 months [124]. EPI was assessed by studies using a variety of direct and indirect measures. Overall, the pooled estimates for EPI during hospitalization was 62% (95% CI 39–82%), and during follow-up was 35% (CI 27–43%). When the analysis was restricted to studies that reported both rates, the prevalence of

EPI was 71% during hospitalization and 33% during follow-up. These data suggest that pancreatic function is suppressed during the acute and early recovery phase of the disease, which returns to normal in a sizeable fraction of patients. The risk of EPI after AP was also affected by disease severity, presence of necrosis, and etiology. Pooled estimates during follow-up were higher in patients with moderate-severe AP (27–30% vs. 16% in mild AP), necrotizing AP (47% vs. 24% in interstitial AP), and alcohol-related AP (44% vs. 22% in biliary AP, 19% in other etiologies). In 26 or 39 studies, new-onset diabetes and/or prediabetes were also assessed. A subset analysis of these studies showed similar pooled prevalence of EPI and new-onset diabetes and/or prediabetes (32% and 38%, respectively). Currently, there are no guidelines for which patients with AP should be tested for EPI or receive pancreatic enzyme replacement therapy. The authors of this meta-analysis concluded by recommending the performance of EPI testing during admission and at 3 and 6–12 months to determine the need and continuation of pancreatic enzyme replacement therapy [124].

6.3 Quality of Life (QOL) and Disability

Mild AP is self-limited, and most patients recover within a few days after disease onset. The impact of AP on QOL is primarily determined by disease severity, and most published literature has evaluated QOL in such patients, either individually or comparing different modalities of treatment (surgery vs. endoscopic therapy) [125–127]. In general, a reduction in QOL, more so for physical component score, is observed earlier in the disease course, which improves over time. A systematic review evaluating the impact of endoscopic vs. surgical management on QOL noted wide variability in the results to draw firm conclusions but acknowledged that endoscopic necrosectomy may have an advantage at least in the short term due to early recovery [127]. A similar observation was made in the long-term follow-up of patients in the randomized trial published by the Dutch Pancreatitis Study Group [128]. Similar to QOL, long-term disability in patients with AP is linked with disease severity and can be as high as 53% in patients with necrotizing pancreatitis [129].

7 Holistic Prevention of Pancreatitis

The Holistic Prevention of Pancreatitis model builds upon the mechanistic definition of CP and proposes opportunities for primary, secondary, and tertiary prevention as they apply to different stages of pancreatitis [3, 112]. In the context of AP, primary prevention applies to prevention of the first attack of AP at a population level, secondary prevention by reducing disease severity and risk of recurrences, while tertiary prevention addresses the reduction of sequelae such as diabetes, EPI, and poor bone health. The current framework for the management of AP focuses on secondary prevention. Although a common gastrointestinal condition, AP is still a low-incidence disease overall, so challenges in developing policies for primary prevention may be difficult, which is understandable. However, within this limitation, measures applicable to other common diseases (e.g., heart disease), such as counseling for reducing high-risk behaviors, and adopting healthy lifestyle with better diet and exercise can also have beneficial effects on the risk of AP [130, 131]. Future research should also focus on identifying patients with AP who are at risk for developing diabetes, EPI, and poor bone health and taking measures to reduce the risk of such events. As an example, since the incidence of AP is far greater than that of CP, or pancreatic cancer, the population burden of diabetes related to exocrine pancreatic disease is far greater than that of AP than another exocrine disease, and measures to mitigate such risk would have important public health benefits.

References

1. Peery AF, Crockett SD, Murphy CC, et al. Burden and cost of gastrointestinal, liver, and pancreatic diseases in the United States: update 2018. Gastroenterology. 2019;156(1):254–272 e11. https://doi.org/10.1053/j.gastro.2018.08.063.
2. Banks PA, Bollen TL, Dervenis C, et al. Classification of acute pancreatitis—2012: revision of the Atlanta classification and definitions by international consensus. Gut. 2013;62(1):102–11. https://doi.org/10.1136/gutjnl-2012-302779.
3. Petrov MS, Yadav D. Global epidemiology and holistic prevention of pancreatitis. Nat Rev Gastroenterol Hepatol. 2019;16(3):175–84. https://doi.org/10.1038/s41575-018-0087-5.
4. Iannuzzi JP, King JA, Leong JH, et al. Global incidence of acute pancreatitis is increasing over time: a systematic review and meta-analysis. Gastroenterology. 2022;162(1):122–34. https://doi.org/10.1053/j.gastro.2021.09.043.
5. Oscanoa TJ, Lizaraso F, Carvajal A. Hospital admissions due to adverse drug reactions in the elderly. A meta-analysis. Eur J Clin Pharmacol. 2017;73(6):759–70. https://doi.org/10.1007/s00228-017-2225-3.
6. Delara M, Murray L, Jafari B, et al. Prevalence and factors associated with polypharmacy: a systematic review and meta-analysis. BMC Geriatr. 2022;22(1):601. https://doi.org/10.1186/s12877-022-03279-x.
7. Morinville VD, Barmada MM, Lowe ME. Increasing incidence of acute pancreatitis at an American pediatric tertiary care center: is greater awareness among physicians responsible? Pancreas. 2010;39(1):5–8. https://doi.org/10.1097/MPA.0b013e3181baac47.
8. Yadav D, Ng B, Saul M, Kennard ED. Relationship of serum pancreatic enzyme testing trends with the diagnosis of acute pancreatitis. Pancreas. 2011;40(3):383–9. https://doi.org/10.1097/MPA.0b013e3182062970.
9. Shinagare AB, Ip IK, Raja AS, Sahni VA, Banks P, Khorasani R. Use of CT and MRI in emergency department patients with acute pancreatitis. Abdom Imaging. 2015;40(2):272–7. https://doi.org/10.1007/s00261-014-0210-1.
10. Oskarsson V, Hosseini S, Discacciati A, et al. Rising incidence of acute pancreatitis in Sweden: national estimates and trends between 1990 and 2013. United European Gastroenterol J. 2020;8(4):472–80. https://doi.org/10.1177/2050640620913737.
11. Zilio MB, Eyff TF, Azeredo-Da-Silva ALF, Bersch VP, Osvaldt AB. A systematic review and meta-analysis of the aetiology of acute pancreatitis. HPB (Oxford). 2019;21(3):259–67. https://doi.org/10.1016/j.hpb.2018.08.003.
12. Yadav D, Lowenfels AB. Trends in the epidemiology of the first attack of acute pancreatitis: a systematic review. Pancreas. 2006;33(4):323–30. https://doi.org/10.1097/01.mpa.0000236733.31617.52.
13. Vipperla K, Somerville C, Furlan A, et al. Clinical profile and natural course in a large cohort of patients with hypertriglyceridemia and pancreatitis. J Clin Gastroenterol. 2017;51(1):77–85. https://doi.org/10.1097/MCG.0000000000000579.

14. Paragomi P, Papachristou GI, Jeong K, et al. The relationship between pre-existing diabetes mellitus and the severity of acute pancreatitis: report from a large international registry. Pancreatology. 2022;22(1):85–91. https://doi.org/10.1016/j.pan.2021.10.001.

15. Cervantes A, Waymouth EK, Petrov MS. African-Americans and indigenous peoples have increased burden of diseases of the exocrine pancreas: a systematic review and meta-analysis. Dig Dis Sci. 2019;64(1):249–61. https://doi.org/10.1007/s10620-018-5291-1.

16. Marta K, Lazarescu AM, Farkas N, et al. Aging and comorbidities in acute pancreatitis I: a meta-analysis and systematic review based on 194,702 patients. Front Physiol. 2019;10:328. https://doi.org/10.3389/fphys.2019.00328.

17. Frey CF, Zhou H, Harvey DJ, White RH. The incidence and case-fatality rates of acute biliary, alcoholic, and idiopathic pancreatitis in California, 1994-2001. Pancreas. 2006;33(4):336–44. https://doi.org/10.1097/01.mpa.0000236727.16370.99.

18. Aune D, Mahamat-Saleh Y, Norat T, Riboli E. High body mass index and central adiposity is associated with increased risk of acute pancreatitis: a meta-analysis. Dig Dis Sci. 2021;66(4):1249–67. https://doi.org/10.1007/s10620-020-06275-6.

19. Dobszai D, Matrai P, Gyongyi Z, et al. Body-mass index correlates with severity and mortality in acute pancreatitis: a meta-analysis. World J Gastroenterol. 2019;25(6):729–43. https://doi.org/10.3748/wjg.v25.i6.729.

20. Roberts SE, Akbari A, Thorne K, Atkinson M, Evans PA. The incidence of acute pancreatitis: impact of social deprivation, alcohol consumption, seasonal and demographic factors. Aliment Pharmacol Ther. 2013;38(5):539–48. https://doi.org/10.1111/apt.12408.

21. Everhart JE, Khare M, Hill M, Maurer KR. Prevalence and ethnic differences in gallbladder disease in the United States. Gastroenterology. 1999;117(3):632–9. https://doi.org/10.1016/s0016-5085(99)70456-7.

22. Kumar MP, Singh AK, Samanta J, et al. Acute pancreatitis in pregnancy and its impact on the maternal and foetal outcomes: a systematic review. Pancreatology. 2022;22(2):210–8. https://doi.org/10.1016/j.pan.2021.12.007.

23. Torgerson JS, Lindroos AK, Naslund I, Peltonen M. Gallstones, gallbladder disease, and pancreatitis: cross-sectional and 2-year data from the Swedish obese subjects (SOS) and SOS reference studies. Am J Gastroenterol. 2003;98(5):1032–41. https://doi.org/10.1111/j.1572-0241.2003.07429.x.

24. Tenner S, Dubner H, Steinberg W. Predicting gallstone pancreatitis with laboratory parameters: a meta-analysis. Am J Gastroenterol. 1994;89(10):1863–6. https://www.ncbi.nlm.nih.gov/pubmed/7942684.

25. Prasanth J, Prasad M, Mahapatra SJ, et al. Early versus delayed cholecystectomy for acute biliary pancreatitis: a systematic review and meta-analysis. World J Surg. 2022;46(6):1359–75. https://doi.org/10.1007/s00268-022-06501-4.

26. da Costa DW, Bouwense SA, Schepers NJ, et al. Same-admission versus interval cholecystectomy for mild gallstone pancreatitis (PONCHO): a multicentre randomised controlled trial. Lancet. 2015;386(10000):1261–8. https://doi.org/10.1016/S0140-6736(15)00274-3.

27. Collaborators GBDA. Population-level risks of alcohol consumption by amount, geography, age, sex, and year: a systematic analysis for the global burden of disease study 2020. Lancet. 2022;400(10347):185–235. https://doi.org/10.1016/S0140-6736(22)00847-9.

28. Lankisch PG, Lowenfels AB, Maisonneuve P. What is the risk of alcoholic pancreatitis in heavy drinkers? Pancreas. 2002;25(4):411–2. https://doi.org/10.1097/00006676-200211000-00015.

29. Yadav D, Eigenbrodt ML, Briggs MJ, Williams DK, Wiseman EJ. Pancreatitis: prevalence and risk factors among male veterans in a detoxification program. Pancreas. 2007;34(4):390–8. https://doi.org/10.1097/mpa.0b013e318040b332.

30. Irving HM, Samokhvalov AV, Rehm J. Alcohol as a risk factor for pancreatitis. A systematic review and meta-analysis. JOP. 2009;10(4):387–92. https://www.ncbi.nlm.nih.gov/pubmed/19581740.

31. Samokhvalov AV, Rehm J, Roerecke M. Alcohol consumption as a risk factor for acute and chronic pancreatitis: a systematic review and a series of meta-analyses. EBioMedicine. 2015;2(12):1996–2002. https://doi.org/10.1016/j.ebiom.2015.11.023.

32. Setiawan VW, Pandol SJ, Porcel J, et al. Prospective study of alcohol drinking, smoking, and pancreatitis: the multiethnic cohort. Pancreas. 2016;45(6):819–25. https://doi.org/10.1097/MPA.0000000000000657.

33. Phillip V, Huber W, Hagemes F, et al. Incidence of acute pancreatitis does not increase during Oktoberfest, but is higher than previously described in Germany. Clin Gastroenterol Hepatol. 2011;9(11):995–1000se3. https://doi.org/10.1016/j.cgh.2011.06.016.

34. Kristiansen L, Gronbaek M, Becker U, Tolstrup JS. Risk of pancreatitis according to alcohol drinking habits: a population-based cohort study. Am J Epidemiol. 2008;168(8):932–7. https://doi.org/10.1093/aje/kwn222.

35. Juliusson SJ, Nielsen JK, Runarsdottir V, Hansdottir I, Sigurdardottir R, Bjornsson ES. Lifetime alcohol intake and pattern of alcohol consumption in patients with alcohol-induced pancreatitis in comparison with patients with alcohol use disorder. Scand J Gastroenterol. 2018;53(6):748–54. https://doi.org/10.1080/00365521.2018.1455893.

36. Mundle G, Ackermann K, Munkes J, Steinle D, Mann K. Influence of age, alcohol consumption and abstinence on the sensitivity of carbohydrate-deficient transferrin, gamma-glutamyltransferase and mean corpuscular volume. Alcohol Alcohol.

1999;34(5):760–6. https://doi.org/10.1093/alcalc/34.5.760.

37. Viel G, Boscolo-Berto R, Cecchetto G, Fais P, Nalesso A, Ferrara SD. Phosphatidylethanol in blood as a marker of chronic alcohol use: a systematic review and meta-analysis. Int J Mol Sci. 2012;13(11):14788–812. https://doi.org/10.3390/ijms131114788.

38. Nordback I, Pelli H, Lappalainen-Lehto R, Jarvinen S, Raty S, Sand J. The recurrence of acute alcohol-associated pancreatitis can be reduced: a randomized controlled trial. Gastroenterology. 2009;136(3):848–55. https://doi.org/10.1053/j.gastro.2008.11.044.

39. Jonas DE, Amick HR, Feltner C, et al. Pharmacotherapy for adults with alcohol use disorders in outpatient settings: a systematic review and meta-analysis. JAMA. 2014;311(18):1889–900. https://doi.org/10.1001/jama.2014.3628.

40. Pu W, Luo G, Chen T, et al. A 5-year retrospective cohort study: epidemiology, etiology, severity, and outcomes of acute pancreatitis. Pancreas. 2020;49(9):1161–7. https://doi.org/10.1097/MPA.0000000000001637.

41. Lin XY, Zeng Y, Zhang ZC, Lin ZH, Chen LC, Ye ZS. Incidence and clinical characteristics of hypertriglyceridemic acute pancreatitis: a retrospective single-center study. World J Gastroenterol. 2022;28(29):3946–59. https://doi.org/10.3748/wjg.v28.i29.3946.

42. Scherer J, Singh VP, Pitchumoni CS, Yadav D. Issues in hypertriglyceridemic pancreatitis: an update. J Clin Gastroenterol. 2014;48(3):195–203. https://doi.org/10.1097/01.mcg.0000436438.60145.5a.

43. Murphy MJ, Sheng X, MacDonald TM, Wei L. Hypertriglyceridemia and acute pancreatitis. JAMA Intern Med. 2013;173(2):162–4. https://doi.org/10.1001/2013.jamainternmed.477.

44. Pedersen SB, Langsted A, Nordestgaard BG. Nonfasting mild-to-moderate hypertriglyceridemia and risk of acute pancreatitis. JAMA Intern Med. 2016;176(12):1834–42. https://doi.org/10.1001/jamainternmed.2016.6875.

45. Dron JS, Hegele RA. Genetics of Hypertriglyceridemia. Front Endocrinol (Lausanne). 2020;11:455. https://doi.org/10.3389/fendo.2020.00455.

46. Wu BU, Batech M, Dong EY, Duan L, Yadav D, Chen W. Influence of ambulatory triglyceride levels on risk of recurrence in patients with Hypertriglyceridemic pancreatitis. Dig Dis Sci. 2019;64(3):890–7. https://doi.org/10.1007/s10620-018-5226-x.

47. Christian JB, Arondekar B, Buysman EK, Johnson SL, Seeger JD, Jacobson TA. Clinical and economic benefits observed when follow-up triglyceride levels are less than 500 mg/dL in patients with severe hypertriglyceridemia. J Clin Lipidol. 2012;6(5):450–61. https://doi.org/10.1016/j.jacl.2012.08.007.

48. Barakat MT, Abu-El-Haija M, Husain SZ. Clinical insights into drug-associated pancreatic injury. Curr

Opin Gastroenterol. 2022;38(5):482–6. https://doi.org/10.1097/MOG.0000000000000865.

49. Badalov N, Baradarian R, Iswara K, Li J, Steinberg W, Tenner S. Drug-induced acute pancreatitis: an evidence-based review. Clin Gastroenterol Hepatol. 2007;5(6):648–61; quiz 644. https://doi.org/10.1016/j.cgh.2006.11.023.

50. Weissman S, Aziz M, Perumpail RB, Mehta TI, Patel R, Tabibian JH. Ever-increasing diversity of drug-induced pancreatitis. World J Gastroenterol. 2020;26(22):2902–15. https://doi.org/10.3748/wjg.v26.i22.2902.

51. Meczker A, Hanak L, Parniczky A, et al. Analysis of 1060 cases of drug-induced acute pancreatitis. Gastroenterology. 2020;159(5):1958–1961 e8. https://doi.org/10.1053/j.gastro.2020.07.016.

52. Andriulli A, Loperfido S, Napolitano G, et al. Incidence rates of post-ERCP complications: a systematic survey of prospective studies. Am J Gastroenterol. 2007;102(8):1781–8. https://doi.org/10.1111/j.1572-0241.2007.01279.x.

53. Kochar B, Akshintala VS, Afghani E, et al. Incidence, severity, and mortality of post-ERCP pancreatitis: a systematic review by using randomized, controlled trials. Gastrointest Endosc. 2015;81(1):143–149 e9. https://doi.org/10.1016/j.gie.2014.06.045.

54. Keswani RN, Qumseya BJ, O'Dwyer LC, Wani S. Association between Endoscopist and center endoscopic retrograde Cholangiopancreatography volume with procedure success and adverse outcomes: a systematic review and meta-analysis. Clin Gastroenterol Hepatol. 2017;15(12):1866–1875 e3. https://doi.org/10.1016/j.cgh.2017.06.002.

55. Cotton PB, Garrow DA, Gallagher J, Romagnuolo J. Risk factors for complications after ERCP: a multivariate analysis of 11,497 procedures over 12 years. Gastrointest Endosc. 2009;70(1):80–8. https://doi.org/10.1016/j.gie.2008.10.039.

56. Cheng CL, Sherman S, Watkins JL, et al. Risk factors for post-ERCP pancreatitis: a prospective multicenter study. Am J Gastroenterol. 2006;101(1):139–47. https://doi.org/10.1111/j.1572-0241.2006.00380.x.

57. Ding X, Zhang F, Wang Y. Risk factors for post-ERCP pancreatitis: a systematic review and meta-analysis. Surgeon. 2015;13(4):218–29. https://doi.org/10.1016/j.surge.2014.11.005.

58. Obeidat AE, Mahfouz R, Monti G, et al. Post-endoscopic retrograde Cholangiopancreatography pancreatitis: what we already know. Cureus. 2022;14(1):e21773. https://doi.org/10.7759/cureus.21773.

59. Mazaki T, Mado K, Masuda H, Shiono M. Prophylactic pancreatic stent placement and post-ERCP pancreatitis: an updated meta-analysis. J Gastroenterol. 2014;49(2):343–55. https://doi.org/10.1007/s00535-013-0806-1.

60. Radadiya D, Devani K, Arora S, et al. Periprocedural aggressive hydration for post endoscopic retrograde Cholangiopancreatography (ERCP) pancreatitis Prophylaxsis: meta-analysis of randomized

controlled trials. Pancreatology. 2019;19(6):819–27. https://doi.org/10.1016/j.pan.2019.07.046.

61. Akshintala VS, Sperna Weiland CJ, Bhullar FA, et al. Non-steroidal anti-inflammatory drugs, intravenous fluids, pancreatic stents, or their combinations for the prevention of post-endoscopic retrograde cholangio-pancreatography pancreatitis: a systematic review and network meta-analysis. Lancet Gastroenterol Hepatol. 2021;6(9):733–42. https://doi.org/10.1016/S2468-1253(21)00170-9.

62. Elmunzer BJ, Foster LD, Serrano J, Coté GA, Edmundowicz SA, Wani S, Shah R, Bang JY, Varadarajulu S, Singh VK, Khashab M, Kwon RS, Scheiman JM, Willingham FF, Keilin SA, Papachristou GI, Chak A, Slivka A, Mullady D, Kushnir V, Buxbaum J, Keswani R, Gardner TB, Forbes N, Rastogi A, Ross A, Law J, Yachimski P, Chen YI, Barkun A, Smith ZL, Petersen B, Wang AY, Saltzman JR, Spitzer RL, Ordiah C, Spino C, Durkalski-Mauldin V; SVI Study Group. Indomethacin with or without prophylactic pancreatic stent placement to prevent pancreatitis after ERCP: a randomised non-inferiority trial. Lancet. 2024;403(10425):450–458. https://doi.org/10.1016/S0140-6736(23)02356-5. Epub 2024 Jan 11. PMID: 38219767; PMCID: PMC10872215.

63. Stimec B, Bulajic M, Korneti V, Milosavljevic T, Krstic R, Ugljesic M. Ductal morphometry of ventral pancreas in pancreas divisum. Comparison between clinical and anatomical results. Ital J Gastroenterol. 1996;28(2):76–80. https://www.ncbi.nlm.nih.gov/pubmed/8781998.

64. Bulow R, Simon P, Thiel R, et al. Anatomic variants of the pancreatic duct and their clinical relevance: an MR-guided study in the general population. Eur Radiol. 2014;24(12):3142–9. https://doi.org/10.1007/s00330-014-3359-7.

65. Fogel EL, Toth TG, Lehman GA, DiMagno MJ, DiMagno EP. Does endoscopic therapy favorably affect the outcome of patients who have recurrent acute pancreatitis and pancreas divisum? Pancreas. 2007;34(1):21–45. https://doi.org/10.1097/mpa.0b013e31802ce068.

66. Mosler P, Akisik F, Sandrasegaran K, et al. Accuracy of magnetic resonance cholangiopancreatography in the diagnosis of pancreas divisum. Dig Dis Sci. 2012;57(1):170–4. https://doi.org/10.1007/s10620-011-1823-7.

67. Bertin C, Pelletier AL, Vullierme MP, et al. Pancreas divisum is not a cause of pancreatitis by itself but acts as a partner of genetic mutations. Am J Gastroenterol. 2012;107(2):311–7. https://doi.org/10.1038/ajg.2011.424.

68. Liao Z, Gao R, Wang W, et al. A systematic review on endoscopic detection rate, endotherapy, and surgery for pancreas divisum. Endoscopy. 2009;41(5):439–44. https://doi.org/10.1055/s-0029-1214505.

69. Kanth R, Samji NS, Inaganti A, et al. Endotherapy in symptomatic pancreas divisum: a systematic review. Pancreatology. 2014;14(4):244–50. https://doi.org/10.1016/j.pan.2014.05.796.

70. Cote GA, Durkalski-Mauldin VL, Serrano J, et al. SpHincterotomy for acute recurrent pancreatitis randomized trial: rationale, methodology, and potential implications. Pancreas. 2019;48(8):1061–7. https://doi.org/10.1097/MPA.0000000000001370.

71. Munigala S, Kanwal F, Xian H, Scherrer JF, Agarwal B. Increased risk of pancreatic adenocarcinoma after acute pancreatitis. Clin Gastroenterol Hepatol. 2014;12(7):1143–1150 e1. https://doi.org/10.1016/j.cgh.2013.12.033.

72. Tummala P, Tariq SH, Chibnall JT, Agarwal B. Clinical predictors of pancreatic carcinoma causing acute pancreatitis. Pancreas. 2013;42(1):108–13. https://doi.org/10.1097/MPA.0b013e318254f473.

73. Bartell N, Bittner K, Vetter MS, Kothari T, Kaul V, Kothari S. Role of endoscopic ultrasound in detecting pancreatic cancer missed on cross-sectional imaging in patients presenting with pancreatitis: a retrospective review. Dig Dis Sci. 2019;64(12):3623–9. https://doi.org/10.1007/s10620-019-05807-z.

74. Jeon CY, Chen Q, Yu W, et al. Identification of individuals at increased risk for pancreatic cancer in a community-based cohort of patients with suspected chronic pancreatitis. Clin Transl Gastroenterol. 2020;11(4):e00147. https://doi.org/10.14309/ctg.0000000000000147.

75. Sadr-Azodi O, Oskarsson V, Discacciati A, Videhult P, Askling J, Ekbom A. Pancreatic cancer following acute pancreatitis: a population-based matched cohort study. Am J Gastroenterol. 2018;113(11):1711–9. https://doi.org/10.1038/s41395-018-0255-9.

76. Morales-Oyarvide V, Mino-Kenudson M, Ferrone CR, et al. Acute pancreatitis in intraductal papillary mucinous neoplasms: a common predictor of malignant intestinal subtype. Surgery. 2015;158(5):1219–25. https://doi.org/10.1016/j.surg.2015.04.029.

77. Chikuie E, Fukuda S, Tazawa H, Nishida T, Sakimoto H. A solid pseudopapillary neoplasm of the pancreas in a man presenting with acute pancreatitis: a case report. Int J Surg Case Rep. 2017;31:114–8. https://doi.org/10.1016/j.ijscr.2017.01.026.

78. Tejedor Bravo M, Justo LM, Lasala JP, Moreira Vicente VF, Ruiz AC, Scapa ML. Acute pancreatitis secondary to neuroendocrine pancreatic tumors: report of 3 cases and literature review. Pancreas. 2012;41(3):485–9. https://doi.org/10.1097/MPA.0b013e318227adef.

79. Ladd AD, Cho JJ, Hughes SJ. Relapsing acute pancreatitis caused by a mucinous cystic neoplasm. J Gastrointest Surg. 2020;24(5):1215–6. https://doi.org/10.1007/s11605-019-04429-0.

80. Sadr-Azodi O, Sanders DS, Murray JA, Ludvigsson JF. Patients with celiac disease have an increased risk for pancreatitis. Clin Gastroenterol Hepatol. 2012;10(10):1136–1142 e3. https://doi.org/10.1016/j.cgh.2012.06.023.

81. Patel RS, Johlin FC Jr, Murray JA. Celiac disease and recurrent pancreatitis. Gastrointest Endosc. 1999;50(6):823–7. https://doi.org/10.1016/s0016-5107(99)70166-5.

82. Yang Y, Ye Y, Liang L, et al. Systemic-lupus-erythematosus-related acute pancreatitis: a cohort from South China. Clin Dev Immunol. 2012;2012:568564. https://doi.org/10.1155/2012/568564.

83. Du L, Liu C, Wang X, Mu J, Yang Y. Acute pancreatitis associated with immunoglobulin a vasculitis: report of fifteen cases. Clin Rheumatol. 2022;42(3):839–47. https://doi.org/10.1007/s10067-022-06398-3.

84. Sah RP, Pannala R, Chari ST, et al. Prevalence, diagnosis, and profile of autoimmune pancreatitis presenting with features of acute or chronic pancreatitis. Clin Gastroenterol Hepatol. 2010;8(1):91–6. https://doi.org/10.1016/j.cgh.2009.09.024.

85. Sayed Ahmed A, Abreo M, Thomas A, Chari ST. Type 3 autoimmune pancreatitis (immune checkpoint inhibitor-induced pancreatitis). Curr Opin Gastroenterol. 2022;38(5):516–20. https://doi.org/10.1097/MOG.0000000000000873.

86. Zhang T, Wang Y, Shi C, et al. Pancreatic injury following immune checkpoint inhibitors: a systematic review and meta-analysis. Front Pharmacol. 2022;13:955701. https://doi.org/10.3389/fphar.2022.955701.

87. Gurakar M, Jalaly NY, Faghih M, et al. Impact of genetic testing and smoking on the distribution of risk factors in patients with recurrent acute and chronic pancreatitis. Scand J Gastroenterol. 2022;57(1):91–8. https://doi.org/10.1080/00365521.2021.1984573.

88. Jalaly NY, Moran RA, Fargahi F, et al. An evaluation of factors associated with pathogenic PRSS1, SPINK1, CTFR, and/or CTRC genetic variants in patients with idiopathic pancreatitis. Am J Gastroenterol. 2017;112(8):1320–9. https://doi.org/10.1038/ajg.2017.106.

89. Imam Z, Simons-Linares CR, Chahal P. Infectious causes of acute pancreatitis: a systematic review. Pancreatology. 2020;20(7):1312–22. https://doi.org/10.1016/j.pan.2020.08.018.

90. Babajide OI, Ogbon EO, Adelodun A, Agbalajobi O, Ogunsesan Y. COVID-19 and acute pancreatitis: a systematic review. JGH Open. 2022;6(4):231–5. https://doi.org/10.1002/jgh3.12729.

91. Prinz RA, Aranha GV. The association of primary hyperparathyroidism and pancreatitis. Am Surg. 1985;51(6):325–9. https://www.ncbi.nlm.nih.gov/pubmed/3994175.

92. Gebreselassie A, Mehari A, Dagne R, Berhane F, Kibreab A. Hypercalcemic pancreatitis a rare presentation of sarcoidosis: a case report. Medicine (Baltimore). 2018;97(2):e9580. https://doi.org/10.1097/MD.0000000000009580.

93. Rashmi KG, Kamalanathan S, Sahoo J, et al. Primary hyperparathyroidism presenting as acute pancreatitis: an institutional experience with review of the literature. World J Gastrointest Pharmacol Ther. 2022;13(4):47–56. https://doi.org/10.4292/wjgpt.v13.i4.47.

94. Aune D, Mahamat-Saleh Y, Norat T, Riboli E. Tobacco smoking and the risk of pancreatitis: a systematic review and meta-analysis of prospective studies. Pancreatology. 2019;19(8):1009–22. https://doi.org/10.1016/j.pan.2019.09.004.

95. Yang L, He Z, Tang X, Liu J. Type 2 diabetes mellitus and the risk of acute pancreatitis: a meta-analysis. Eur J Gastroenterol Hepatol. 2013;25(2):225–31. https://doi.org/10.1097/MEG.0b013e32835af154.

96. Lai SW, Muo CH, Liao KF, Sung FC, Chen PC. Risk of acute pancreatitis in type 2 diabetes and risk reduction on anti-diabetic drugs: a population-based cohort study in Taiwan. Am J Gastroenterol. 2011;106(9):1697–704. https://doi.org/10.1038/ajg.2011.155.

97. Chen HJ, Wang JJ, Tsay WI, Her SH, Lin CH, Chien CC. Epidemiology and outcome of acute pancreatitis in end-stage renal disease dialysis patients: a 10-year national cohort study. Nephrol Dial Transplant. 2017;32(10):1731–6. https://doi.org/10.1093/ndt/gfw400.

98. Lankisch PG, Weber-Dany B, Maisonneuve P, Lowenfels AB. Frequency and severity of acute pancreatitis in chronic dialysis patients. Nephrol Dial Transplant. 2008;23(4):1401–5. https://doi.org/10.1093/ndt/gfm769.

99. Hou SW, Lee YK, Hsu CY, Lee CC, Su YC. Increased risk of acute pancreatitis in patients with chronic hemodialysis: a 4-year follow-up study. PLoS One. 2013;8(8):e71801. https://doi.org/10.1371/journal.pone.0071801.

100. Barbara M, Tsen A, Rosenkranz L. Acute pancreatitis in chronic dialysis patients. Pancreas. 2018;47(8):946–51. https://doi.org/10.1097/MPA.0000000000001119.

101. Working Group IAPAPAAPG. IAP/APA evidence-based guidelines for the management of acute pancreatitis. Pancreatology. 2013;13(4 Suppl 2):e1–15. https://doi.org/10.1016/j.pan.2013.07.063.

102. Wan J, Ouyang Y, Yu C, Yang X, Xia L, Lu N. Comparison of EUS with MRCP in idiopathic acute pancreatitis: a systematic review and meta-analysis. Gastrointest Endosc. 2018;87(5):1180–1188 e9. https://doi.org/10.1016/j.gie.2017.11.028.

103. Hallensleben ND, Umans DS, Bouwense SA, et al. The diagnostic work-up and outcomes of 'presumed' idiopathic acute pancreatitis: a post-hoc analysis of a multicentre observational cohort. United European Gastroenterol J. 2020;8(3):340–50. https://doi.org/10.1177/2050640619890462.

104. Wilcox CM, Seay T, Kim H, Varadarajulu S. Prospective endoscopic ultrasound-based approach to the evaluation of idiopathic pancreatitis: causes, response to therapy, and long-term outcome.

Am J Gastroenterol. 2016;111(9):1339–48. https://doi.org/10.1038/ajg.2016.240.

105. Matta B, Gougol A, Gao X, et al. Worldwide variations in demographics, management, and outcomes of acute pancreatitis. Clin Gastroenterol Hepatol. 2020;18(7):1567–1575 e2. https://doi.org/10.1016/j.cgh.2019.11.017.

106. Machicado JD, Yadav D. Epidemiology of recurrent acute and chronic pancreatitis: similarities and differences. Dig Dis Sci. 2017;62(7):1683–91. https://doi.org/10.1007/s10620-017-4510-5.

107. Sankaran SJ, Xiao AY, Wu LM, Windsor JA, Forsmark CE, Petrov MS. Frequency of progression from acute to chronic pancreatitis and risk factors: a meta-analysis. Gastroenterology. 2015;149(6):1490–1500 e1. https://doi.org/10.1053/j.gastro.2015.07.066.

108. Balint ER, Fur G, Kiss L, et al. Assessment of the course of acute pancreatitis in the light of aetiology: a systematic review and meta-analysis. Sci Rep. 2020;10(1):17936. https://doi.org/10.1038/s41598-020-74943-8.

109. Ahmed Ali U, Issa Y, Hagenaars JC, et al. Risk of recurrent pancreatitis and progression to chronic pancreatitis after a first episode of acute pancreatitis. Clin Gastroenterol Hepatol. 2016;14(5):738–46. https://doi.org/10.1016/j.cgh.2015.12.040.

110. Bertilsson S, Sward P, Kalaitzakis E. Factors that affect disease progression after first attack of acute pancreatitis. Clin Gastroenterol Hepatol. 2015;13(9):1662–9 e3. https://doi.org/10.1016/j.cgh.2015.04.012.

111. Magnusdottir BA, Baldursdottir MB, Kalaitzakis E, Bjornsson ES. Risk factors for chronic and recurrent pancreatitis after first attack of acute pancreatitis. Scand J Gastroenterol. 2019;54(1):87–94. https://doi.org/10.1080/00365521.2018.1550670.

112. Whitcomb DC, Frulloni L, Garg P, et al. Chronic pancreatitis: an international draft consensus proposal for a new mechanistic definition. Pancreatology. 2016;16(2):218–24. https://doi.org/10.1016/j.pan.2016.02.001.

113. Hori Y, Vege SS, Chari ST, et al. Classic chronic pancreatitis is associated with prior acute pancreatitis in only 50% of patients in a large single-institution study. Pancreatology. 2019;19(2):224–9. https://doi.org/10.1016/j.pan.2019.02.004.

114. Singh VK, Whitcomb DC, Banks PA, et al. Acute pancreatitis precedes chronic pancreatitis in the majority of patients: results from the NAPS2 consortium. Pancreatology. 2022;22(8):1091–8. https://doi.org/10.1016/j.pan.2022.10.004.

115. Miko A, Farkas N, Garami A, et al. Preexisting diabetes elevates risk of local and systemic complications in acute pancreatitis: systematic review and meta-analysis. Pancreas. 2018;47(8):917–23. https://doi.org/10.1097/MPA.0000000000001122.

116. Lee YK, Huang MY, Hsu CY, Su YC. Bidirectional relationship between diabetes and acute pancreatitis: a population-based cohort study in Taiwan.

Medicine (Baltimore). 2016;95(2):e2448. https://doi.org/10.1097/MD.0000000000002448.

117. Shen HN, Yang CC, Chang YH, Lu CL, Li CY. Risk of diabetes mellitus after first-attack acute pancreatitis: a National Population-Based Study. Am J Gastroenterol. 2015;110(12):1698–706. https://doi.org/10.1038/ajg.2015.356.

118. Zhu X, Liu D, Wei Q, et al. New-onset diabetes mellitus after chronic pancreatitis diagnosis: a systematic review and meta-analysis. Pancreas. 2019;48(7):868–75. https://doi.org/10.1097/MPA.0000000000001359.

119. Bharmal SH, Cho J, Alarcon Ramos GC, et al. Trajectories of glycaemia following acute pancreatitis: a prospective longitudinal cohort study with 24 months follow-up. J Gastroenterol. 2020;55(8):775–88. https://doi.org/10.1007/s00535-020-01682-y.

120. Bharmal SH, Cho J, Ko J, Petrov MS. Glucose variability during the early course of acute pancreatitis predicts two-year probability of new-onset diabetes: a prospective longitudinal cohort study. United European Gastroenterol J. 2022;10(2):179–89. https://doi.org/10.1002/ueg2.12190.

121. Tirkes T, Chinchilli VM, Bagci U, et al. Design and rationale for the use of magnetic resonance imaging biomarkers to predict diabetes after acute pancreatitis in the diabetes RElated to acute pancreatitis and its mechanisms study: from the type 1 diabetes in acute pancreatitis consortium. Pancreas. 2022;51(6):586–92. https://doi.org/10.1097/MPA.0000000000002080.

122. Dungan KM, Hart PA, Andersen DK, et al. Assessing the pathophysiology of hyperglycemia in the diabetes RElated to acute pancreatitis and its mechanisms study: from the type 1 diabetes in acute pancreatitis consortium. Pancreas. 2022;51(6):575–9. https://doi.org/10.1097/MPA.0000000000002074.

123. Casu A, Grippo PJ, Wasserfall C, et al. Evaluating the Immunopathogenesis of diabetes after acute pancreatitis in the diabetes RElated to acute pancreatitis and its mechanisms study: from the type 1 diabetes in acute pancreatitis consortium. Pancreas. 2022;51(6):580–5. https://doi.org/10.1097/MPA.0000000000002076.

124. Huang W, de la Iglesia-Garcia D, Baston-Rey I, et al. Exocrine pancreatic insufficiency following acute pancreatitis: systematic review and meta-analysis. Dig Dis Sci. 2019;64(7):1985–2005. https://doi.org/10.1007/s10620-019-05568-9.

125. Hochman D, Louie B, Bailey R. Determination of patient quality of life following severe acute pancreatitis. Can J Surg. 2006;49(2):101–6. https://www.ncbi.nlm.nih.gov/pubmed/16630420.

126. Smith ZL, Gregory MH, Elsner J, et al. Health-related quality of life and long-term outcomes after endoscopic therapy for walled-off pancreatic necrosis. Dig Endosc. 2019;31(1):77–85. https://doi.org/10.1111/den.13264.

127. Psaltis E, Varghese C, Pandanaboyana S, Nayar M. Quality of life after surgical and endoscopic

management of severe acute pancreatitis: a systematic review. World J Gastrointest Endosc. 2022;14(7):443–54. https://doi.org/10.4253/wjge.v14.i7.443.

128. Onnekink AM, Boxhoorn L, Timmerhuis HC, et al. Endoscopic versus surgical step-up approach for infected necrotizing pancreatitis (ExTENSION): long-term follow-up of a randomized trial. Gastroenterology. 2022;163(3):712–722 e14. https://doi.org/10.1053/j.gastro.2022.05.015.

129. Umapathy C, Raina A, Saligram S, et al. Natural history after acute necrotizing pancreatitis: a large US tertiary care experience. J Gastrointest Surg. 2016;20(11):1844–53. https://doi.org/10.1007/s11605-016-3264-2.

130. Alsamarrai A, Das SL, Windsor JA, Petrov MS. Factors that affect risk for pancreatic disease in the general population: a systematic review and meta-analysis of prospective cohort studies. Clin Gastroenterol Hepatol. 2014;12(10):1635–44. e5. ;quiz e103. https://doi.org/10.1016/j.cgh.2014.01.038.

131. Oskarsson V, Sadr-Azodi O, Orsini N, Andren-Sandberg A, Wolk A. Vegetables, fruit and risk of non-gallstone-related acute pancreatitis: a population-based prospective cohort study. Gut. 2013;62(8):1187–92. https://doi.org/10.1136/gutjnl-2012-302521.

Genetic Factors in Acute Pancreatitis

David C. Whitcomb

Abbreviations

AP	Acute pancreatitis
CCY	Cholecystectomy
CP	Chronic pancreatitis
ERCP	Endoscopic retrograde cholangiopancreatography
EtOH	Alcohol
HTG	Hypertriglyceridemia
RAP	Recurrent acute pancreatitis

Key Points

- The inability to accurately predict the likelihood of acute pancreatitis and its clinical course or to predict the rate of progression to chronic pancreatitis or its complications indicates multiple "hidden variables" reside within each person.
- Susceptibility to acute pancreatitis is linked to factors that activate trypsinogen to trypsin, along with factors that protect the pancreas from the effects of active trypsin and the resulting immune response.
- The severity of the immune response is partially determined by host biological factors (e.g., obesity) and dysregulated cytokine release (cytokine storm) that is linked to genetic variants in immune-regulating cells.
- After the "sentinel acute pancreatitis event" (SAPE), the pancreas becomes biologically hypersensitive to recurrent acute pancreatitis.
- Genetic analysis of patients is indicated after their *first* acute pancreatitis event (to guide prevention of RAP and CP).
- Acute pancreatitis is an infrequent and unpredictable event, so proactive preventative interventions guided by demographics or genetics alone are not recommended.
- Prevention of recurrent acute and chronic pancreatitis focuses on identifying the relevant risk factors in individual patients, including genetic susceptibility to gallstones, hypertriglyceridemia, and trypsin-regulating genes.
- Prevention of recurrent acute pancreatitis is etiology-specific and may include cholecystectomy, triglyceride management, or other management based on genetically or mechanistically informed risk models.
- Progression to chronic pancreatitis is strongly affected by recurrent acute pancreatitis, alcohol, and smoking, with additional genetic risk factors in other specialized cells affecting the likelihood of diabetes, pancreatic exocrine insufficiency, chronic pain syndromes, and cancer.
- Acceptance of new technologies allowing rapid access to genetic data, rapid analysis of variant combinations within the patient's clin-

D. C. Whitcomb (✉)
Division of Gastroenterology, Hepatology and Nutrition, Departments of Medicine, Cell Biology and Molecular Physiology, and Human Genetics, University of Pittsburgh and UPMC; and Ariel Precision Medicine, Pittsburgh, PA, USA
e-mail: Whitcomb@pancreas.org

© The Author(s), under exclusive license to Springer Nature Singapore Pte Ltd. 2024
J. A. Windsor et al. (eds.), *Acute Pancreatitis*, https://doi.org/10.1007/978-981-97-3132-9_2

ical context, and clear clinical decision support tools are needed to advance the success in caring for people with pancreatic diseases.

1 Introduction

Acute pancreatitis (AP) describes the inflammatory response of the pancreas after it is stressed or injured above a threshold level. In animal models of AP, the type and amount of injury or stress required to trigger AP and the subsequent responses can be accurately determined, because many key variables can be controlled, including the breed (genetic background), age, sex, diet, and environment. In humans, all of these key variables may be hidden or differ to known and unknown degrees, making accurate *predictions* about the triggering threshold, the magnitude of the inflammatory response, and the subsequent outcomes challenging and *inaccurate*. Thus, treatments of AP in humans tend to be *reactive* and *supportive*.

Many prognostic scores have been developed to anticipate the severity of AP once it has been triggered and the process is rapidly evolving [1–4]. Beginning with Ranson scores [5, 6], numerous models have been built that account for some measurable variables, such as age, sex, body mass index (BMI), and alcohol use, which are then combined with biomarkers of the inflammation such as the systemic inflammatory response syndrome (SIRS) and measures of organ dysfunction [7, 8]. These have some value but none are highly accurate. They are not better than a clinical assessment by a trained physician and so are most useful as post hoc classification tools for categorical population research studies.

Genetic variants remain a key set of missing determinates of AP susceptibility, inflammatory response, end-organ resilience, and subsequent complications [9]. Although genetic variants are of central importance, the traditional models of interpreting genetic data (e.g., Mendelian genet-

ics) and classifying risk variants (based on differences in population frequency between cases and controls) cannot be applied to complex systems analysis. This chapter presents a new approach that segregates genetic variants by the cells and/or systems that they influence and is coupled with a progressive disease model that allows these factors to be organized and interpreted within the context of the other key variables of age, sex, BMI, alcohol, and others. Finally, it presents the construct for a partial solution that could be implemented today—using information sciences, modern health information technology, and low-cost genetic screening tools.

2 Acute, Recurrent Acute, and Chronic Pancreatitis

The sentinel acute pancreatitis event (SAPE) is the *first* clinically recognized episode of acute pancreatitis [10–12]. Mechanistically, the SAPE concept is important because the first episode of AP permanently changes the characteristics of the pancreas through immunological [11] and possibly epigenetic factors. The pancreas becomes hypersensitive to subsequent injury or stress, and this increases the risk of triggering recurrent acute pancreatitis (RAP), as well as that of developing chronic pancreatitis (CP), diabetes mellitus (DM), exocrine pancreatic insufficiency (EPI), chronic pain syndromes, and pancreatic cancer [13–16]. In general, about a third of patients with AP develop RAP, and a third of RAP develop CP, although some patients may go directly from AP to CP or develop CP without known AP [17–20]. The SAPE concept is important in modeling human pancreatitis as it is generally not feasible to anticipate or prevent the first episode of AP, but because of the SAPE-associated hypersensitivity, it is possible to target specific risk factors in humans for further attacks (RAP) and progression to CP and associated disorders.

The clinical course of AP reflects in large part the effects of the innate immune system's inflammatory response to pancreatic injury [21]. Importantly, the inflammatory response to pancreatic injury is far greater than the inflammatory response to an equivalent injury in other organs. The key difference is the activation of trypsinogen to trypsin within the pancreas, which in turn activates the other pancreatic digestive proenzymes, resulting in autodigestion of pancreatic proteins and lipids [22, 23]. The release of these digestive products initiates a robust inflammatory response that can lead to further pancreatic injury and cause systemic inflammation (the cytokine storm) that is recognized clinically as SIRS [21]. Damage to endothelial cells of the pancreas and other organs results in a capillary leak syndrome with extravasation of albumin and large plasma proteins, subsequently leading to multi-organ dysfunction syndrome (MODS) and multi-organ failure (MOF) [24]. The effects of systemic inflammation on gut epithelium also cause barrier breakdown with intraluminal factors entering the submucosa, the lymphatics, and into the circulation to further aggravate SIRS, MODS, and MOF [25].

The challenges to the clinician in undertaking patient management include the following: predicting the threshold level of injury needed to activate trypsin in the pancreas, the mechanisms to control prematurely activated trypsin, the magnitude of the inflammatory response to a given amount of injury, confounding factors that aggravate inflammation such as gut leak and capillary leak syndrome, and the relative resilience of the body to local and systemic inflammation that varies markedly between individual humans. From an observational perspective, the responses of an AP patient to pancreatic injury are therefore unpredictable. Thus, treatment is largely supportive until the clinical course is sufficiently established that severity prediction tools can become of use. There remains significant potential clinical benefit from better and earlier predictive information to guide early and late patient interventions. Over the past 30 years, it has become apparent that the differences in people's innate local and downstream responses to pancreatic injury or stress are determined by *genetic variants* affecting gene expression and gene function.

The 1996 discovery that rare *gain-of-function* mutations in the cationic trypsinogen gene cause hereditary pancreatitis revolutionized our understanding of the possible role of genetic factors in AP, RAP, and CP [26, 27]. Since then, we have learned about more common and less pathogenic genetic factors (i.e., not disease-causing but increasing risks) that can be in exons (changing protein function) or regulatory elements (changing expression). These individual genetic risk factors are neither necessary nor sufficient to cause pancreatitis; just as alcohol alone does not cause pancreatitis, but heavy use is a risk factor for AP, RAP, and CP. Instead, it is the *combination* of genetic and environmental factors that provides the key to understanding the complex syndromes associated with complications in pancreatic diseases. Although more is known about the genetics of CP and RAP, there is value in presenting what is known about the genetics of AP and how genetic testing of patients after their first attack of AP could thus be justified. This thesis postulates that genetic profiling provides strong prognostic information and identifies possible therapeutic targets to prevent RAP, CP, and their complications.

Epidemiologically, a plethora of genetic variants affect the pancreas, with each acting in a specific way in concert with developmental, metabolic, signaling, and stressful factors [9, 21, 28]. Furthermore, each of the 8 billion people in the world today is genetically and physically different than each other—including monozygotic twins [29]. The diversity of physical characteristics and disease susceptibilities between individual people is further determined by epigenetic imprinting, age, body mass, diet, and other factors related to the environment and lifetime histories [21]. Understanding the underlying genomics and pathobiology of each of the components of a complex system is required to solve mechanistic and modeling problems. A more complete conceptual transition is needed to make use of genetic data. Specifically, we know that particular genetic variant effects are localized in specialized cells that express the corresponding genes and proteins that are required to perform specific tasks. The proper function of specialized cells requires the expression of the right gene at the right amount and at the right time (e.g., during cell activation or stress). Thus, a systematic scan of all relevant genetic variants at the time of acute pancreatitis in an individual person has the potential of identifying which specialized cells are most likely to dysfunction and which subcellular systems are likely affected, leading to downstream damage.

The integrated sum of these diverse inputs determines the final response of the individual to acute pancreatitis, its severity, and eventual outcomes [1, 30]. The interplay of these factors also influences a variety of RAP and CP complications, such as the development of exocrine pancreatic insufficiency (EPI), diabetes mellitus (Types 1, 2, 3c), chronic pain syndromes, pancreatic ductal adenocarcinoma (PDAC), and other outcomes [31–35]. Thus, understanding the innate (genetic) features of the individual patient must become an integral part of future advances in effective clinical management.

3   Conceptual Framework

The conceptual framework of this chapter is highlighted in Fig. 1. The current paradigm for acute pancreatitis management (Fig. 1a) focuses on providing comfort to the patient during an acute attack, supporting organ systems that are failing, and then considering preventing RAP. In the case of the commonest etiologies, this is by either removing the gallbladder or counseling the alcoholic patient to stop drinking. Of note, other risk factors are either unknown or not consistently considered, the determinants of severity are often ignored, and the outcomes are generally only addressed symptomatically as they present themselves.

A new paradigm can be considered (Fig. 1b) where each of the major determinates of "AP risk," "AP severity," and "AP outcomes" is determined using a combination of innate genetic signatures, patient characteristics, and supportive biomarkers. In this paradigm, the genetic variants are linked with specific cell types and processes with predictable effects. The advantage of this new paradigm is that insights into disease risks and mechanisms also determine the final therapy. Thus, the hidden variables and deterministic progression in Fig. 1a are changed in Fig. 1b, as the hidden variables are subsequently identified and so targeted interventions change the predetermined rates of progression (dashed lines). This process to discover the hidden variables and develop interventions will be discussed below.

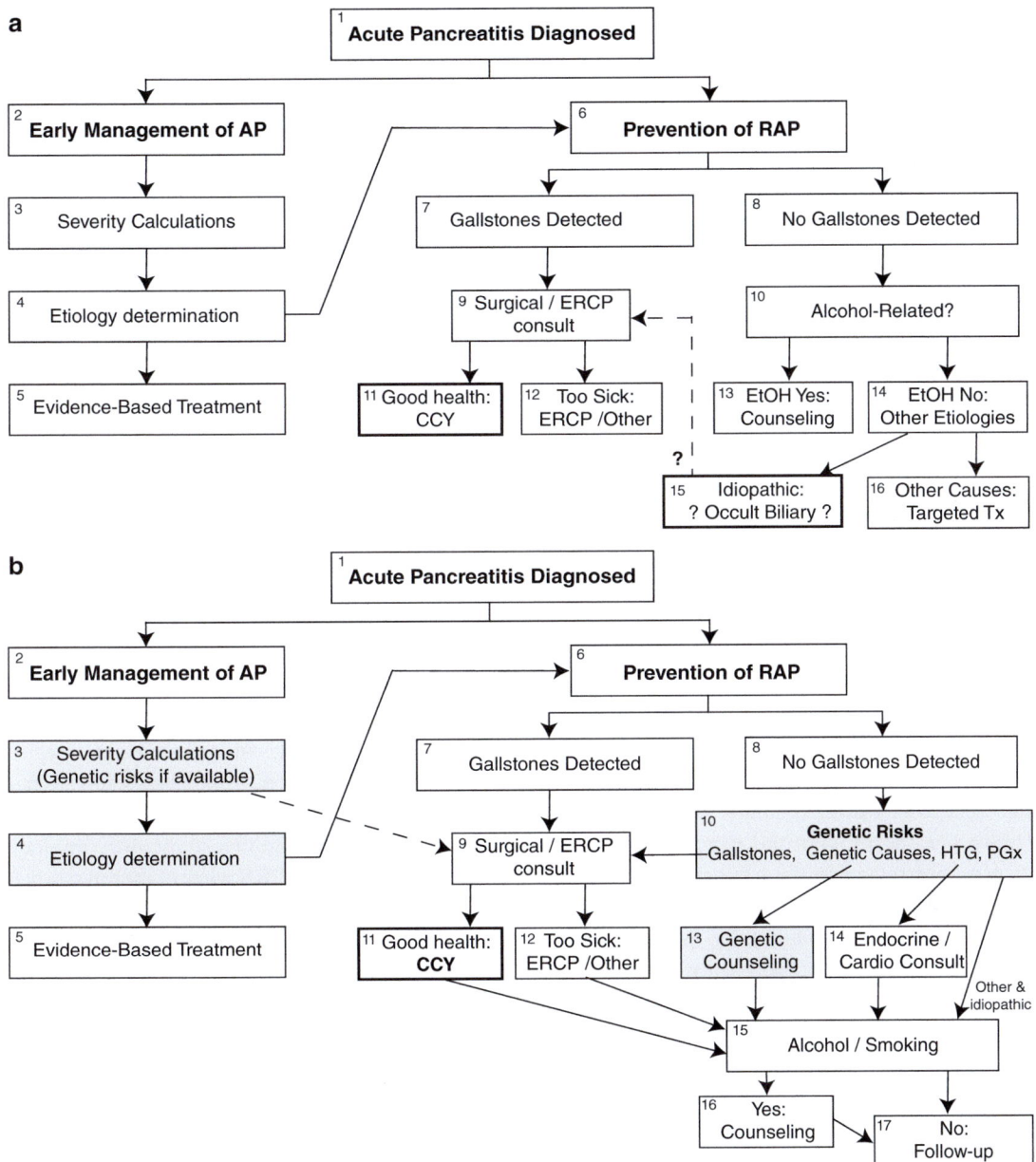

Fig. 1 Algorithm to manage acute pancreatitis and prevent ineffective interventions and disease progression. Steps proceeding from the early diagnosis of acute pancreatitis to prevention of recurrence and chronic pancreatitis. (**a**) Current observational approach with management centering on the detection of gallstones and a recent history of alcoholism. This approach may lead to unnecessary cholecystectomies (CCY) and miss important etiologies with different management approaches. (**b**) A proposed approach integrating genetic variants into the decision-making process. This approach is predicted to reduce unnecessary CCYs and to detect genetically driven etiologies, including many patients diagnosed with alcoholic pancreatitis. This approach should improve care and reduce costs and complications

4 Genetic Factors Related to the Risk and Etiology of AP

The etiology of AP is important to determine because it allows healthcare providers to choose specific established therapies that mitigate RAP. Etiology can however be further divided into the strength of the injury or stress, the susceptibility of the pancreas to trypsinogen activation, and the control status of active trypsin inside the pancreas, as well as the inflammatory response. The most commonly reported etiologies of acute pancreatitis are gallstones, alcohol, hypertriglyceridemia (HTG), drug-induced AP, trauma, genetic factors, and duct obstruction. The relative frequency is affected not only by the patient's age, sex, ancestry, and population characteristics (i.e., environment) but also by the genetic background.

4.1 Gallstones

The best described and understood cause of acute pancreatitis in Western countries is linked to gallstones passing through the pancreatic duct and causing obstruction at the sphincter of Oddi. The "typical" case is a middle-aged, overweight, multigravida woman (traditionally labeled as: fat, fertile, female in their forties) [36]. Smoking is also an important risk for gallstone disease [37]. However, the environmental context is also strongly affected by genetic factors, especially on chromosome 2 at the *ABCG5-ABCG8* locus. *ABCG5* and *ABCG8* form an obligate heterodimer that mediates ATP-dependent sterol transport across the cell membrane. They play an essential role in selective cholesterol and sterol excretion by the liver and gallbladder into bile, the transport of sterols from the distal ileal lumen back into the blood (entero-hepatic circulation). Dysfunction of these transporters results in lithogenic bile and a high risk of gallstone formation.

The strongest genetic effect is with a haplotype linked to rs11887534G > C (*ABCG8* p.D19H), which is considered pathogenic for gallstone disease on ClinVar [38, 39]. This risk haplotype is in about 7% of individuals with European and African ancestry, >9% of some Latin American subpopulations, 4% of South Asians, and 1% of Asian and East Asian ancestries. Likewise, there are additive effects of an intronic variant-tabbed haplotype linked to *ABCG8* rs4245791C > T (with C as the minor allele and risk allele) [36, 39]. Individuals of African-American and Hispanic-American ancestry also have gallstone risk associated with these *ABCG8-ABCG5* haplotypes [39]. Furthermore, in the UK Biobank, the rs11887534 risk haplotype was associated with acute pancreatitis (see supplemental information in this cited publication [38]). Additional genetic variants are associated with gallstone disease (and therefore acute pancreatitis), and polygenic risk scores (PRS) are continually being developed and tested in various populations [36, 40].

Lim et al. recently reported on the interaction between obesity, adiposity, and risk of symptomatic gallstone disease according to genetic susceptibility using a 6 SNP PRS [36]. They confirmed higher risk with increasing age, in women more than men, in subjects with higher BMIs, and in those with higher PRS. The risk effects were additive. In this study, the combined effects of obesity and PRS were higher in women than men, and the reduced risk of normal BMI was greatest in women with a high PRS. The overall risk of gallstone disease (leading to cholecystectomy) was lower in men than women under all conditions. The risk effects of obesity and PGR on symptomatic gallstone diseases were primarily seen in the highest categories.

4.2 Alcohol

Animal and human research over the past 20 years generated new insights into extenuating factors that affect susceptibility, severity, and progression from alcohol-associated AP. First, animal studies demonstrate that high-alcohol diets do not cause pancreatitis [41–43]. Alcohol does however markedly change the immune response to RAP and progression to CP in animal models [41, 44] and accelerates progression from

AP to CP in humans [45, 46]. New data also suggests that the risk of progression to alcohol-associated RAP and CP is associated with a genetic change in the T cell receptor beta (*TRB*) repertoire at the *PRSS1-PRSS2* locus [47], further implicating an altered immune response to drive a more aggressive and destructive inflammatory process, resulting in the rapid development of CP after AP.

If alcohol alone does not cause pancreatitis, what is the trigger? Based on our progressive models, one or more additional factors are necessary to trigger the SAPE and initiate the progression to RAP and CP. In many cases, the requisite factors in alcohol-associated pancreatitis are known susceptibility genes. Wang et al. [48, 49] studied 1061 Chinese CP patients classified as classic alcoholic pancreatitis (ACP, drinking >80 g alcohol per day in men, >60 g in women), light-to-moderate alcohol consumption (LMA-CP, drinking <80 g in men and < 60 g in women for at least 2 years), and idiopathic (ICP, nondrinkers). Each patient's DNA was sequenced for *PRSS1, SPINK1, CTRC,* and *CFTR.* Among ICP patients, 56.2% had significant genetic variants in this limited number of genes. But surprisingly, genetic variants were also identified in 38.3% of LMA-CP patients and 39.8% of ACP patients [48]. Furthermore, the clinical features of the LMA-CP and ACP patients were similar to each other.

The findings of Wang et al. [48] are consistent with the systematic review of Chen et al. [50], considering possible interaction of alcohol and genetic variants in *PRSS1, SPINK1, CTRC, CLDN2, CPA1, CEL,* and *CTRB1-CTRB2.* Chen found that seven genetic variants with relatively weak independent risks were more strongly associated with ACP than non-alcohol-associated CP, especially the *PRSS1-PRSS2* haplotype tag-SNP rs10273639T > C [51] and the *CTRC* haplotype tagged by rs497078C > T (p.G60G) [50, 52] These data provide increasingly strong evidence that alcohol increases the risk of AP, RAP, and CP in the context of additional risk factors that are not sufficient to cause AP, RAP, and CP alone [53].

The genetics therefore support that the most effective approach to preventing RAP in patients with alcohol-associated AP is cessation of alcohol [45, 54]. The results are striking, as the fraction of patients progressing from AP to CP with a marked reduction in alcohol drinking dropped from 57.7% to 9.8% over a 13–17 year follow-up, reported by Takeyama [45], and from 33% to 5.8% with a mean follow-up of 42 months in another representative study, by Stilgiano et al. [54]. In both studies, a significant subset of subject progressed to CP without alcohol, indicating additional complex risk factors, including smoking (below). Furthermore, the evaluation of pancreatitis-risk genes in alcohol-associated pancreatitis is now demonstrating marked enrichment, indicating that in many cases, a second hit is necessary to trigger pancreatitis in patients who drink [53], similar to what we previously found in rats [41]. Additional studies are needed to clarify the triggering mechanisms of AP in alcoholics (including gallstone disease) and to determine if the aggressive immune response in alcohol-related AP➔ CP pathway linked to genetic risks can be blocked (Fig. 1b).

4.3 Smoking

Smoking is a strong risk factor for AP, RAP, and CP [31, 55–57], although most people who smoke do NOT have pancreatic disease. In a meta-analysis of studies between *genetic risk* linked specifically to smoking and digestive diseases by Larsson et al. [37], it demonstrated that the "smoking x gene" interactions were associated with gallstone disease (OR 1.25; CI 1.16–1.35), acute pancreatitis (OR 1.56; CI 1.33–1.83), and chronic pancreatitis (OR 1.86; CI 1.43–2.43). The risk of CP appears to be especially high in patients with regulatory element variants in the *CTRC* gene (e.g., *CTRC* p.G60G [52]) and who smokes [52]. Although smoking is an independent risk factor, the common combination of smoking with alcohol confers additive and possibly multiplicative risk [31, 58].

4.4   Hypertriglyceridemia

As with alcohol, HTG alone does not cause pancreatitis, as the prevalence of AP among patients with severe HTG is about 14% [59, 60]. It does, however, increase the risk of AP when increased non-fasting blood levels are present [61] as well as markedly worsens the severity of AP [60, 62] and can lead to CP [33].

Hypertriglyceridemia is another complex condition. There are rare monogenetic causes such as familial chylomicronemia syndrome (FCS) caused by homozygous or biallelic loss-of-function variants in the *LPL, APOC2, APOA5, LMF1,* or *GPIHBP1* genes [63, 64], and secondary HTG, which is typically milder, more common, and associated with dietary factors, obesity, diabetes mellitus, alcohol abuse, and pregnancy [65]. However, the majority of patients with HTG have multifactorial chylomicronemia syndrome (MCS), indicating that genetic risks are more complex than previously recognized. This means that mild or moderately damaging genetic risk factors may potentiate the effects of metabolic and environmental risk factors for MCS such as diabetes and obesity [66–68]. These in turn can modify the risk of AP.

4.5   Drugs

Acute pancreatitis is a common complication in patients with inflammatory bowel disease because of higher rates of gallstones, involvement of the duodenum causing duct obstruction, and, most commonly, drugs [69]. The primary culprits are thiopurines, including azathioprine (AZA) and its active metabolite 6-mercaptopurine, with incidences of AP above 7% [69]. While there are other less common examples, knowledge of the patients' pharmacogenetics may also play a role in the management of triglycerides, as well as pain and glucose intolerance.

Asparaginase-induced acute pancreatitis. An unusual but important condition is asparaginase-induced AP occurring during the treatment of acute lymphoblastic leukemia (ALL) and non-Hodgkin lymphoma (NHL) [70]. Most leukemic cells depend on exogenous asparagine (Asn) for survival, and depletion of Asn by asparaginase results in cell death. The pancreas may be at high risk for asparaginase treatment as Asn is needed for protein synthesis and is depleted [71]. Amino acid deficiency causes endoplasmic reticulum (ER) stress with the pancreatic acinar cells activating the unfolded protein response (UPR) and the amino acid response (AAR) with upregulation of asparagine synthetase to generate Asn from aspartic acid and glutamine (Gln) [71]. Pancreatic digestive enzymes are rich in both Asn and Gln, making a rich upstream supply of these amino acids essential to exocrine function. Although the pancreas has the highest expression of asparagine synthetase of all organs, ongoing depletion of Asn and Gln may be a key factor in triggering pancreatitis, especially with the depletion of antioxidants, such as retinoids and vitamin A [71].

Asparaginase-induced AP develops in 5%–10% or more of ALL patients [72–74], suggesting additional risk factors are required to trigger AP. While higher doses/exposure, age > 10 years, and obesity increase the risk of AP [72, 74–77], multiple studies suggest underlying genetic risk factors are also important [72, 78–82].

The primary challenge in discovering and replicating genetic risk factors in uncommon conditions using genome-wide association studies (GWAS) is the number of cases needed to overcome false discovery (e.g., $n > 1000$), with a second replication cohort needed to confirm risk factors by statistical inference. However, with strong underlying genetic effect sizes or a three-step approach—(1) statistical screening, (2) candidate gene selection based on disease mechanisms, and (3) functional effects of the genetic variant on gene expression with dysfunctional consequences—early insights into pathogenic mechanism are possible. For asparaginase-induced AP, several candidate genes were identified in earlier, underpowered discovery studies, but these candidate genetic variants have not yet been consistently or sufficiently replicated in other populations [78–80, 82].

MYBBP1A is a gene expressed in all cells that plays a key role in the stress response and carcinogenesis [81]. Abaji et al. [81] identified *MYBBP1A*, *SPEF2,* and *IL16* for risk of asparaginase-induced AP in a GWAS using a Quebec cohort of *n* = 302, followed by validation of *n* = 282. The functional effect of the key variant, a missense mutation MYBBP1A rs3809849G > C, p.Gln8Glu (MAF 0.182), was reported to affect the sensitivity of a pancreatic tumor cell line (PANC1) to asparaginase, but not a lymphoblastic leukemia (NALM6) cell line [73]. This data suggests that in Quebec, failure of the stress response linked to reduced *MYBBP1A* expression contributes to asparaginase-induced AP.

In a small study of 51 patients and 1388 controls from Germany, Bartram et al. [82] identified several SNPs associated with the *ABCC4* gene (rs4148513), a channel similar to *CFTR* that is highly expressed in the pancreas and may function as a multidrug resistance pathway [82]. Although this was strongly associated with asparaginase-induced AP in the initial cohort, it was not replicated in another cohort of 54 patients.

Wolthers et al. collected 244 cases from multiple centers for the largest GWAS to date [79]. The strongest association with AP was rs62228256C > T (MAF 0.028) on chromosome 20, near *ATP9A* (linked by eQTL and expressed in blood and spleen [GTEx]), and *NFATC2*, although no plausible disease mechanism was evident. However, other AP disease risk mechanisms were also discovered. For example, trypsin-associated AP risk factors were identified, including the *PRSS1-PRSS2* risk allele [79, 80], a *CTRC* risk allele (rs10436957G > A [a different haplotype than p.G60G]), with risk signals also seen for *SPINK1*, *CFTR*, and *CLDN2* [79, 80, 82].

Nielsen et al. [80] applied machine learning tools in an effort to develop a model that could predict asparaginase-induced AP. The most predictive genetic factors were SNPs linked to the known *PRSS1-PRSS2* haplotype, the *CTRC* haplotype linked to rs10436957_A, *GALNTL6*, and *EPHB2* in children ages 1–7 years (ROC-AUC:

0.62). The predictive accuracy was increased to ROC-AUC: 0.80 by using the top hits in the Wolthers GWAS [79]. However, the model has not been tested in populations outside the training set, so the clinical utility remains speculative [80].

These studies collectively indicate that risk assessment for drug-induced AP is complex. Furthermore, as in asparaginase-induced AP, different mechanisms may contribute to the genetic risks in different individuals and different populations.

5 Genetic Factors Related to the Severity and Complications of Acute Pancreatitis

The severity of AP is determined by the magnitude of the injury, susceptibility of the pancreas to uncontrolled trypsin activation, the trajectory of the inflammatory response, and resilience of the host to the effects of systemic inflammation. Well-established risk factors for a more severe course include the etiology of acute pancreatitis and host features, such as age, sex, obesity, and serum triglyceride levels [21, 30, 83]. These demographic and physiologic factors alone do not determine severity or outcome, indicating the importance of innate genetic risks that contribute to trajectory and outcome [21, 84].

Genetic risk factors that increase *susceptibility* to acute pancreatitis were discussed above. These factors are key to RAP and CP rather than the severity of an initial attack. The severity of acute pancreatitis is highlighted in Fig. 1a box 3 (current) and 1B box 3(future).

As an inflammatory syndrome, the trajectory and regulation of the immune system after injury plays a critical role in determining the severity and complications, as illustrated by the host genetic risks in SARS-CoV-2 infection (COVID-19) [85–88]. The effect of host genetic variations on the magnitude and effects of SIRS in AP and COVID-19 likely overlap to a large degree, although the mechanisms of injury and activation of the inflammatory response likely differ significantly. In severe AP, there is dysregulated cytokine release manifest by early release TNF-alpha, INF-gamma, IL-IRa, IL-2, IL-6, IL-8, IL-10, IL-18, eNAMPT (visfatin) [89], and other cytokines [21]. There are several factors linked to robust cytokine release (cytokine storm) including obesity [89–92] and genetic variants.

Genetic variants in several key immune genes alter gene expression and are associated with the severity of acute pancreatitis, including MCP1 [93], *TNFA* [94–96], *IL6* [95], *IL8* [97, 98], and *IL10* [99]. A meta-analysis of existing data supported effects in *IL1B* and *IL6* [83]. These early candidate gene studies support the prediction that changes in the expression of key elements of the innate immune system alter the risk of disease course severity, but agnostic, high-quality studies in large cohorts of well-phenotyped and stratified subjects are still lacking [21, 84].

6   The Timing and Emerging Role of Genetic Testing

Clinical use of genetic data requires (a) the availability of the patient's genetic data, (b) interpretation of genetic data within the context of the patient's condition, and (c) application of data to patient management plans using evidence-based guidance. The complexity of genetic data makes it practically impossible for physicians to accurately interpret these data quickly in individual patients. Thus, new tools are needed before the benefits of genetic testing can be realized. As new technologies deliver these new tools to the physician and evidence of effectiveness emerges, the management of AP will likely change dramatically.

It takes time and money to genotype a patient. Currently, the severity of AP in a cohort of patients is calculated post hoc [7, 100], with prospective predictions of progression to multiorgan failure from systemic inflammation being very poor [101]. In an ideal world, the optimal approach is to genotype every person's DNA prior to the development of AP (and other acute disorders). Indeed, accurate prediction models using genetics require that the patient's genetic information is available upon their presentation

to an emergency facility, whether it be a major medical center or a rural clinic. Unlike biomarkers, genetic information does not change over time. But like biomarkers, the genetic data needs to be available at the point of care and in real time to tailor acute phase interventions. Thus, having genetic testing completed in advance, being accessible and available, with interpretation and clinical decision support text, on-demand is needed. While this is not a practical reality (yet), this is the way forward.

7   Genetic Factors Related to Preventing Recurrent AP

Since the index episodes of AP within a large population are uncommon and stochastic, it is not practical to attempt to prevent initial attacks, with the possible exception of symptomatic gallstone disease or hereditary pancreatitis. Thus, most of the focus regarding the use of genetic information in the foreseeable future is on preventing RAP and CP [102–104].

Physicians already know that a patient with AP is likely to develop RAP [12]. The typical clinical response is to immediately focus on two common modifiable etiologic factors: gallstones and alcoholism. Detection of gallstones in the gallbladder and/or common bile duct triggers a cholecystectomy, preferably at the time of the initial diagnosis of AP [105]. Suspicion of alcohol-related AP triggers counseling to stop drinking. Other etiologies and risks may be overlooked or ignored until RAP occurs.

Two approaches to the management of AP are illustrated (Fig. 1) to highlight the benefit of genetic information (Fig. 1b).

7.1   The Standard Approach to Management of AP *without* Genetic Information (Fig. 1a)

The primary treatment for preventing RAP is cholecystectomy (CCY). If no gallstones are detected, then most patients are diagnosed with alcohol-related or idiopathic pancreatitis (Fig. 1a, box A8), the third most common classification of acute pancreatitis. In this case, some experts recommend patients for a CCY [54, 106, 107], even if no biliary disease is detected! [108] An important question is whether or not a person with idiopathic pancreatitis should have a CCY (Fig. 1a, box A15), with the negative decision resulting in the expectant waiting for the second attack, then returning to box A15. The current view is supported by several studies, including a recent systematic review and meta-analysis by the Dutch Pancreatitis Study Group predicting the CCY will reduce idiopathic RAP (IRAP) from about 35–40% down to about 11% [108]. This indicates that about 24–29% of IRAP patients will benefit from a CCY. But it also indicates that 71–76% of IRAP patients would undergo a CCY that they did not require, adding cost and morbidity related to surgical complications, bile leaks, dyspepsia, food intolerance, diarrhea, and other post-CCY symptoms [109, 110]. Furthermore, the idiopathic patients who did not benefit from a CCY still do not have a diagnosis or treatment plan. Another related question is whether some patients with alcohol-associated AP should also have a CCY (especially if they smoke [37]). The decision comes down to the probability that they have occult biliary pancreatitis and the risk-benefit ratio of a CCY, noting the procedure-associated risk, the probability of post-CCY digestive problems, and the cost associated with surgery and rates of unintended and costly outcomes as noted above.

7.2 The Management of AP *with* Genetic Information (Fig. 1b)

An *alternative approach* is proposed in Fig. 1b that includes additional information provided by genetic risk assessment. If genetic information is available to the physician at the point of care and if clear decision support tools are available (grey boxes), then decisions can be made with higher accuracy and, we suspect, better outcomes. For preventing RAP, genetic information is useful for (1) the risk of gallstone disease and AP, (2) a variety of less obvious genetic conditions (e.g.,

hereditary pancreatitis, CFTR-related disorders), (3) disease modifiers such as hypertriglyceridemia, and (4) other etiologies such as drug toxicity (PGx, e.g., azathioprine) (box B10). The key decision point is now box B10 with genetic information informing the decision-maker about the risk of multiple etiologies that are otherwise hidden. Based on the patient's innate genetic risk and information on age, sex, BMI, alcohol use, etc., the probability of a biliary etiology can be determined. Other etiologies may not be corrected with a CCY. Furthermore, if there is a moderate risk of a biliary etiology, mixed with other treatable etiologies, the risk of severe (rather than mild) RAP should be considered (i.e., the host genetic risk of a severe inflammatory response; calculated in box B3). Having genetic information available with relevant probability calculations should be the next step in improving care for patients when CCY is being considered. Specifically, this information will enable the selection of individuals who will most likely benefit from CCY, while, conversely, avoiding unnecessary CCY. Thus, in patients with no clear etiology, high genetic risk of gallstones, and low risk of other etiologies, CCY should be considered. In equivocal cases of biliary risk in subjects without identifiable gallstone on imaging, the decision to proceed to either CCY or to observation can be further strengthened by prior knowledge of the risk of severe AP (box B3 → B9, dashed line). Note that alcohol and smoking are additive risk factors but are rarely the primary cause of AP or RAP and should be considered in all patients (box B15).

Note that Fig. 1b differs from 1A in terms of patient management associated with alcohol consumption and smoking in patients to prevent RAP. Since alcohol and smoking appear to increase the risk of AP (possibly linked to another trigger) and also drive the process of AP→CP, these factors should be eliminated in all AP patients as the other cofactors are identified and managed (box B15).

Patients with HTG-AP are often very difficult to manage. This problem is another example of trying to treat a complex, multigene, multimechanism syndrome with a "one-size-fits-all" approach (Fig. 1b box B10 ➔ 14). Future randomized controlled studies of anti-HTG therapies are needed that are properly stratified for underlying mechanisms.

8   Summary and Conclusions

Our understanding of the genetic factors in AP is relatively nascent. Insights into the innate immune response (and development of systemic inflammation and organ dysfunction) can be inferred from studies in critical illness, multi-trauma, COVID-19, and other conditions. Translation of these insights into AP genetic studies will provide stronger statistical advantages through candidate gene/loci analysis by reducing the statistical penalties for multiple testing.

A deep understanding of genetic risk for RAP and CP has evolved over the past 30 years. The barrier to widespread utilization of this knowledge includes the cost of genotyping, the interpretation of complex genetic combinations, and clinical decision support tools for clinicians. The use of inexpensive SNP arrays, where key variants are included and variants of unknown significance (VUS) are avoided, is a practical first step.

Evidence-based genetic data reveal a number of key opportunities for better management of AP and prevention of RAP including the following: (a) avoiding cholecystectomies in patients with idiopathic acute pancreatitis and low risk of gallstone formation, (b) identifying biliary and genetic etiologies as a triggers for RAP in patients with a history of alcohol-associated pancreatitis, (c) aggressively reducing triglyceride levels in patients with combined gene-environment risk for hypertriglyceridemic (HTG) AP with higher severity of RAP episodes in HTG patients, (d) identifying patients with CFTR-related disorders that may be eligible for gene-specific treatment, (e) identifying pancreatitis risk factors such as hereditary pancreatitis (e.g., *PRSS1* gain of function mutations), (f) identifying complex risk genetic syndromes that may respond to novel therapies, (g) identifying high risk factors for progression to CP (e.g., risk haplotypes linked to

CLDN2 and *PRSS1-PRSS2* loci), (h) identifying individuals at high risk for PDAC and prioritizing screening and early detection (including determining if CA19–9 is expressed and normal levels based on *FUT2* and *FUT3* genetics), and others (not shown).

References

1. Mounzer R, Langmead CJ, Wu BU, Evans AC, Bishehsari F, Muddana V, et al. Comparison of existing clinical scoring systems to predict persistent organ failure in patients with acute pancreatitis. Gastroenterology. 2012;142(7):1476–82.
2. Pavlidis TE, Pavlidis ET, Sakantamis AK. Advances in prognostic factors in acute pancreatitis: a mini-review. Hepatobiliary Pancreat Dis Int. 2010;9(5):482–6.
3. Harshit Kumar A, Singh GM. A comparison of APACHE II, BISAP, Ranson's score and modified CTSI in predicting the severity of acute pancreatitis based on the 2012 revised Atlanta classification. Gastroenterol Rep (Oxf). 2018;6(2):127–31.
4. Langmead C, Lee PJ, Paragomi P, Greer P, Stello K, Hart PA, et al. A novel 5-cytokine panel outperforms conventional predictive markers of persistent organ failure in acute pancreatitis. Clin Transl Gastroenterol. 2021;12(5):e00351.
5. Ranson JH, Rifkind KM, Roses DF, Fink SD, Eng K, Spencer FC. Prognostic signs and the role of operative management in acute pancreatitis. Surg Gynecol Obstet. 1974;139(1):69–81.
6. Ranson JH, Pasternack BS. Statistical methods for quantifying the severity of clinical acute pancreatitis. J Surg Res. 1977;22(2):79–91.
7. Banks PA, Bollen TL, Dervenis C, Gooszen HG, Johnson CD, Sarr MG, et al. Classification of acute pancreatitis--2012: revision of the Atlanta classification and definitions by international consensus. Gut. 2013;62(1):102–11.
8. Working Group IAPAPAAPG. IAP/APA evidence-based guidelines for the management of acute pancreatitis. Pancreatology. 2013;13(4 Suppl 2):e1–15.
9. Zator Z, Whitcomb DC. Insights into the genetic risk factors for the development of pancreatic disease. Ther Adv Gastroenterol. 2017;10(3):323–36.
10. Whitcomb DC. Hereditary pancreatitis: new insights into acute and chronic pancreatitis. Gut. 1999;45:317–22.
11. Geisz A, Sahin-Toth M. Sentinel acute pancreatitis event increases severity of subsequent episodes in mice. Gastroenterology. 2021;161(5):1692–4.
12. Whitcomb DC. Central role of the sentinel acute pancreatitis event (SAPE) model in understanding recurrent acute pancreatitis (RAP): implications for precision medicine. Front Pediatr. 2022;10:941852.

13. Cho J, Scragg R, Petrov MS. Postpancreatitis diabetes confers higher risk for pancreatic cancer than type 2 diabetes: results from a Nationwide cancer registry. Diabetes Care. 2020;43(9):2106–12.

14. Bharmal SH, Cho J, Alarcon Ramos GC, Ko J, Stuart CE, Modesto AE, et al. Trajectories of glycaemia following acute pancreatitis: a prospective longitudinal cohort study with 24 months follow-up. J Gastroenterol. 2020;55(8):775–88.

15. Das SL, Singh PP, Phillips AR, Murphy R, Windsor JA, Petrov MS. Newly diagnosed diabetes mellitus after acute pancreatitis: a systematic review and meta-analysis. Gut. 2014;63(5):818–31.

16. Kirkegard J, Cronin-Fenton D, Heide-Jorgensen U, Mortensen FV. Acute pancreatitis and pancreatic cancer risk: a Nationwide matched-cohort study in Denmark. Gastroenterology. 2018;154(6):1729–36.

17. Sankaran SJ, Xiao AY, Wu LM, Windsor JA, Forsmark CE, Petrov MS. Frequency of progression from acute to chronic pancreatitis and risk factors: a meta-analysis. Gastroenterology. 2015;149(6):1490–500 e1.

18. Machicado JD, Yadav D. Epidemiology of recurrent acute and chronic pancreatitis: similarities and differences. Dig Dis Sci. 2017;62(7):1683–91.

19. Singh VK, Whitcomb DC, Banks PA, AlKaade S, Anderson MA, Amann ST, et al. Acute pancreatitis precedes chronic pancreatitis in the majority of patients: results from the NAPS2 consortium. Pancreatology. 2022;22(8):1091–8.

20. Tao H, Chang H, Li N, Zhu S, Duan L. Clinical characteristics of patients with chronic pancreatitis with or without prior acute pancreatitis are different. Pancreas. 2022;51(8):950–6.

21. Venkatesh K, Glenn H, Delaney A, Andersen CR, Sasson SC. Fire in the belly: a scoping review of the immunopathological mechanisms of acute pancreatitis. Front Immunol. 2022;13:1077414.

22. Geisz A, Sahin-Toth M. A preclinical model of chronic pancreatitis driven by trypsinogen autoactivation. Nat Commun. 2018;9(1):5033.

23. Patel K, Trivedi RN, Durgampudi C, Noel P, Cline RA, DeLany JP, et al. Lipolysis of visceral adipocyte triglyceride by pancreatic lipases converts mild acute pancreatitis to severe pancreatitis independent of necrosis and inflammation. Am J Pathol. 2015;185(3):808–19.

24. Komara NL, Paragomi P, Greer PJ, Wilson AS, Breze C, Papachristou GI, et al. Severe acute pancreatitis: capillary permeability model linking systemic inflammation to multiorgan failure. Am J Physiol Gastrointest Liver Physiol. 2020;319(5): G573–G83.

25. Russell PS, Nachkebia S, Maldonado-Zimbron VE, Chuklin S, Gimel'farb G, Hong J, et al. Therapeutic thoracic duct drainage: a systematic review of the eastern European experience and future potential. Lymphology. 2022;55(3):86–109.

26. Whitcomb DC, Gorry MC, Preston RA, Furey W, Sossenheimer MJ, Ulrich CD, et al. Hereditary pancreatitis is caused by a mutation in the cationic trypsinogen gene. Nat Genet. 1996;14(2):141–5.

27. Gorry MC, Gabbaizedeh D, Furey W, Gates LK Jr, Preston RA, Aston CE, et al. Mutations in the cationic trypsinogen gene are associated with recurrent acute and chronic pancreatitis. Gastroenterology. 1997;113(4):1063–8.

28. Shelton CA, Whitcomb DC. Precision medicine for pancreatic diseases. Curr Opin Gastroenterol. 2020;36(5):428–36.

29. Weber-Lehmann J, Schilling E, Gradl G, Richter DC, Wiehler J, Rolf B. Finding the needle in the haystack: differentiating "identical" twins in paternity testing and forensics by ultra-deep next generation sequencing. Forensic Sci Int Genet. 2014;9:42–6.

30. Juhasz MF, Sipos Z, Ocskay K, Hegyi P, Nagy A, Parniczky A. Admission risk factors and predictors of moderate or severe pediatric acute pancreatitis: a systematic review and meta-analysis. Front Pediatr. 2022;10:947545.

31. Yadav D, Hawes RH, Brand RE, Anderson MA, Money ME, Banks PA, et al. Alcohol consumption, cigarette smoking, and the risk of recurrent acute and chronic pancreatitis. Arch Intern Med. 2009;169(11):1035–45.

32. Mullady DK, Yadav D, Amann ST, O'Connell MR, Barmada MM, Elta GH, et al. Type of pain, pain-associated complications, quality of life, disability and resource utilisation in chronic pancreatitis: a prospective cohort study. Gut. 2011;60(1):77–84.

33. Conwell DL, Banks PA, Sandhu BS, Sherman S, Al-Kaade S, Gardner TB, et al. Validation of demographics, etiology, and risk factors for chronic pancreatitis in the USA: a report of the north American pancreas study (NAPS) group. Dig Dis Sci. 2017;62(8):2133–40.

34. Bellin MD, Whitcomb DC, Abberbock J, Sherman S, Sandhu BS, Gardner TB, et al. Patient and disease characteristics associated with the presence of diabetes mellitus in adults with chronic pancreatitis in the United States. Am J Gastroenterol. 2017;112(9):1457–65.

35. Goodarzi MO, Nagpal T, Greer P, Cui J, Chen YI, Guo X, et al. Genetic risk score in diabetes associated with chronic pancreatitis versus type 2 diabetes mellitus. Clin Transl Gastroenterol. 2019;10(7):e00057.

36. Lim J, Wirth J, Wu K, Giovannucci E, Kraft P, Turman C, et al. Obesity, adiposity, and risk of symptomatic gallstone disease according to genetic susceptibility. Clin Gastroenterol Hepatol. 2022;20(5):e1083–e120.

37. Larsson SC, Burgess S. Appraising the causal role of smoking in multiple diseases: a systematic review and meta-analysis of Mendelian randomization studies. EBioMedicine. 2022;82:104154.

38. Ferkingstad E, Oddsson A, Gretarsdottir S, Benonisdottir S, Thorleifsson G, Deaton AM, et al. Genome-wide association meta-analysis yields 20 loci associated with gallstone disease. Nat Commun. 2018;9(1):5101.

39. Joshi AD, Andersson C, Buch S, Stender S, Noordam R, Weng LC, et al. Four susceptibility loci for gallstone disease identified in a meta-analysis of genome-wide association studies. Gastroenterology. 2016;151(2):351–63 e28.

40. Fairfield CJ, Drake TM, Pius R, Bretherick AD, Campbell A, Clark DW, et al. Genome-wide analysis identifies gallstone-susceptibility loci including genes regulating gastrointestinal motility. Hepatology. 2022;75(5):1081–94.

41. Deng X, Wang L, Elm MS, Gabazadeh D, Diorio GJ, Eagon PK, et al. Chronic alcohol consumption accelerates fibrosis in response to cerulein-induced pancreatitis in rats. Am J Pathol. 2005;166(1):93–106.

42. Li HS, Zhang JY, Thompson BS, Deng XY, Ford ME, Wood PG, et al. Rat mitochondrial ATP synthase ATP5G3: cloning and upregulation in pancreas after chronic ethanol feeding. Physiol Genomics. 2001;6(2):91–8.

43. Yadav D, Whitcomb DC. The role of alcohol and smoking in pancreatitis. Nat Rev Gastroenterol Hepatol. 2010;7(3):131–45.

44. Gukovsky I, Lugea A, Shahsahebi M, Cheng JH, Hong PP, Jung YJ, et al. A rat model reproducing key pathological responses of alcoholic chronic pancreatitis. Am J Physiol Gastrointest Liver Physiol. 2008;294(1):G68–79.

45. Takeyama Y. Long-term prognosis of acute pancreatitis in Japan. Clin Gastroenterol Hepatol. 2009;7(11 Suppl):S15–7.

46. Yadav D, O'Connell M, Papachristou GI. Natural history following the first attack of acute pancreatitis. Am J Gastroenterol. 2012;107(7):1096–103.

47. Fu D, Blobner BM, Greer PJ, Lafyatis R, Bellin MD, Whitcomb DC, et al. Pancreatitis-associated PRSS1-PRSS2 haplotype alters T cell receptor beta (TRB) repertoire more strongly than PRSS1 expression. Gastroenterology. 2022;164(2):289–292.e4.

48. Wang Y-C, Zou W-B, Tang D-A, Wang L, Hu L-H, Quian Y-Y, et al. High clinical and genetic similarity between chronic pancreatitis associated with light-to-moderate alcohol consumption and classical alcoholic chronic pancreatitis. Gastro Hep. Advances. 2023;2:186–95.

49. Whitcomb D. High clinical and genetic similarity between chronic pancreatitis associated with light-to-moderate alcohol consumption and classical alcoholic chronic pancreatitis—rethinking alcohol-associated pancreatitis (editorial). Gastro Hep Advances. 2023;2:281–2.

50. Chen JM, Herzig AF, Genin E, Masson E, Cooper DN, Ferec C. Scale and scope of gene-alcohol interactions in chronic pancreatitis. A Systematic Review Genes (Basel). 2021;12(4):471.

51. Whitcomb DC, Larusch J, Krasinskas AM, Klei L, Smith JP, Brand RE, et al. Common genetic variants in the CLDN2 and PRSS1-PRSS2 loci alter risk for alcohol-related and sporadic pancreatitis. Nat Genet. 2012;44(12):1349–54.

52. LaRusch J, Lozano-Leon A, Stello K, Moore A, Muddana V, O'Connell M, et al. The Common Chymotrypsinogen C (CTRC) Variant G60G (C.180T) Increases Risk of Chronic Pancreatitis But Not Recurrent Acute Pancreatitis in a North American Population. Clin Transl Gastroenterol. 2015;6:e68.

53. Ru N, Xu XN, Cao Y, Zhu JH, Hu LH, Wu SY, et al. The impacts of genetic and environmental factors on the progression of chronic pancreatitis. Clin Gastroenterol Hepatol. 2022;20(6):e1378–e87.

54. Stigliano S, Belisario F, Piciucchi M, Signoretti M, Delle Fave G, Capurso G. Recurrent biliary acute pancreatitis is frequent in a real-world setting. Dig Liver Dis. 2018;50(3):277–82.

55. Lin Y, Tamakoshi A, Hayakawa T, Ogawa M, Ohno Y. Cigarette smoking as a risk factor for chronic pancreatitis: a case-control study in Japan. Research committee on intractable pancreatic diseases. Pancreas. 2000;21(2):109–14.

56. Talamini G, Bassi C, Falconi M, Sartori N, Vaona B, Bovo P, et al. Smoking cessation at the clinical onset of chronic pancreatitis and risk of pancreatic calcifications. Pancreas. 2007;35(4):320–6.

57. Ahmed Ali U, Issa Y, Hagenaars JC, Bakker OJ, van Goor H, Nieuwenhuijs VB, et al. Risk of recurrent pancreatitis and progression to chronic pancreatitis after a first episode of acute pancreatitis. Clin Gastroenterol Hepatol. 2016;14(5):738–46.

58. Cote GA, Yadav D, Slivka A, Hawes RH, Anderson MA, Burton FR, et al. Alcohol and smoking as risk factors in an epidemiology study of patients with chronic pancreatitis. Clin Gastroenterol Hepatol. 2010;9(3):266–73.

59. Carr RA, Rejowski BJ, Cote GA, Pitt HA, Zyromski NJ. Systematic review of hypertriglyceridemia-induced acute pancreatitis: a more virulent etiology? Pancreatology. 2016;16(4):469–76.

60. Nawaz H, Koutroumpakis E, Easler J, Slivka A, Whitcomb DC, Singh VP, et al. Elevated serum triglycerides are independently associated with persistent organ failure in acute pancreatitis. Am J Gastroenterol. 2015;110(10):1497–503.

61. Pedersen SB, Langsted A, Nordestgaard BG. Nonfasting mild-to-moderate hypertriglyceridemia and risk of acute pancreatitis. JAMA Intern Med. 2016;176(12):1834–42.

62. Vipperla K, Somerville C, Furlan A, Koutrompakis E, Saul M, Chennat J, et al. Clinical profile and natural course in a large cohort of patients with hypertriglyceridemia and pancreatitis. J Clin Gastroenterol. 2016;51(1):77–85.

63. Dron JS, Hegele RA. Genetics of hypertriglyceridemia. Front Endocrinol (Lausanne). 2020;11:455.

64. Chyzhyk V, Kozmic S, Brown AS, Hudgins LC, Starc TJ, Davila AD, et al. Extreme hypertriglyceridemia: genetic diversity, pancreatitis, pregnancy, and prevalence. J Clin Lipidol. 2019;13(1):89–99.

65. Pejic RN, Lee DT. Hypertriglyceridemia. J Am Board Fam Med. 2006;19(3):310–6.

66. Schaefer EJ, Geller AS, Endress G. The biochemical and genetic diagnosis of lipid disorders. Curr Opin Lipidol. 2019;30(2):56–62.

67. Dron JS, Wang J, Cao H, McIntyre AD, Iacocca MA, Menard JR, et al. Severe hypertriglyceridemia is primarily polygenic. J Clin Lipidol. 2019;13(1):80–8.

68. Johansen CT, Wang J, Lanktree MB, McIntyre AD, Ban MR, Martins RA, et al. An increased burden of common and rare lipid-associated risk alleles contributes to the phenotypic spectrum of hypertriglyceridemia. Arterioscler Thromb Vasc Biol. 2011;31(8):1916–26.

69. Massironi S, Fanetti I, Vigano C, Pirola L, Fichera M, Cristoferi L, et al. Systematic review-pancreatic involvement in inflammatory bowel disease. Aliment Pharmacol Ther. 2022;55(12):1478–91.

70. Raja RA, Schmiegelow K, Frandsen TL. Asparaginase-associated pancreatitis in children. Br J Haematol. 2012;159(1):18–27.

71. Tsai CY, Kilberg MS, Husain SZ. The role of asparagine synthetase on nutrient metabolism in pancreatic disease. Pancreatology. 2020;20(6):1029–34.

72. Kuo SH, Chen JS, Cheng CN, Lo HY, Chen WC, Lai FP, et al. The characteristics and risk factors of Asparaginase-associated pancreatitis in pediatric acute lymphoblastic leukemia. Pancreas. 2022;51(4):366–71.

73. Abaji R, Roux V, Yssaad IR, Kalegari P, Gagne V, Gioia R, et al. Characterization of the impact of the MYBBP1A gene and rs3809849 on asparaginase sensitivity and cellular functions. Pharmacogenomics. 2022;23(7):415–30.

74. Dharia P, Swartz MD, Bernhardt MB, Chen H, Gramatges MM, Lupo PJ, et al. Clinical and demographic factors contributing to asparaginase-associated toxicities in children with acute lymphoblastic leukemia. Leuk Lymphoma. 2022;63(12):2948–54.

75. Egnell C, Heyman M, Jonsson OG, Raja RA, Niinimaki R, Albertsen BK, et al. Obesity as a predictor of treatment-related toxicity in children with acute lymphoblastic leukaemia. Br J Haematol. 2022;196(5):1239–47.

76. Chen CB, Chang HH, Chou SW, Yang YL, Lu MY, Jou ST, et al. Acute pancreatitis in children with acute lymphoblastic leukemia correlates with L-asparaginase dose intensity. Pediatr Res. 2022;92(2):459–65.

77. Oparaji JA, Rose F, Okafor D, Howard A, Turner RL, Orabi AI, et al. Risk factors for Asparaginase-associated pancreatitis: a systematic review. J Clin Gastroenterol. 2017;51(10):907–13.

78. Liu C, Yang W, Devidas M, Cheng C, Pei D, Smith C, et al. Clinical and genetic risk factors for acute pancreatitis in patients with acute lymphoblastic leukemia. J Clin Oncol. 2016;34(18):2133–40.

79. Wolthers BO, Frandsen TL, Patel CJ, Abaji R, Attarbaschi A, Barzilai S, et al. Trypsin-encoding PRSS1-PRSS2 variations influence the risk of asparaginase-associated pancreatitis in children with acute lymphoblastic leukemia: a Ponte di Legno toxicity working group report. Haematologica. 2019;104(3):556–63.

80. Nielsen RL, Wolthers BO, Helenius M, Albertsen BK, Clemmensen L, Nielsen K, et al. Can machine learning models predict Asparaginase-associated pancreatitis in childhood acute lymphoblastic leukemia. J Pediatr Hematol Oncol. 2022;44(3):e628–e36.

81. Abaji R, Gagne V, Xu CJ, Spinella JF, Ceppi F, Laverdiere C, et al. Whole-exome sequencing identified genetic risk factors for asparaginase-related complications in childhood ALL patients. Oncotarget. 2017;8(27):43752–67.

82. Bartram T, Schutte P, Moricke A, Houlston RS, Ellinghaus E, Zimmermann M, et al. Genetic variation in ABCC4 and CFTR and acute pancreatitis during treatment of pediatric acute lymphoblastic leukemia. J Clin Med. 2021;10(21):4815.

83. van den Berg FF, Kempeneers MA, van Santvoort HC, Zwinderman AH, Issa Y, Boermeester MA. Meta-analysis and field synopsis of genetic variants associated with the risk and severity of acute pancreatitis. BJS Open. 2020;4(1):3–15.

84. Weiss FU, Laemmerhirt F, Lerch MM. Acute pancreatitis: genetic risk and clinical implications. J Clin Med. 2021;10(2):190.

85. Pairo-Castineira E, Clohisey S, Klaric L, Bretherick AD, Rawlik K, Pasko D, et al. Genetic mechanisms of critical illness in Covid-19. Nature. 2020;591(7848):92–8.

86. Chen HH, Shaw DM, Petty LE, Graff M, Bohlender RJ, Polikowsky HG, et al. Host genetic effects in pneumonia. Am J Hum Genet. 2021;108(1):194–201.

87. Russell CD, Lone NI, Baillie JK. Comorbidities, multimorbidity and COVID-19. Nat Med. 2023;29(2):334–43.

88. van der Made CI, Netea MG, van der Veerdonk FL, Hoischen A. Clinical implications of host genetic variation and susceptibility to severe or critical COVID-19. Genome Med. 2022;14(1):96.

89. Bime C, Casanova NG, Camp SM, Oita RC, Ndukum J, Hernon VR, et al. Circulating eNAMPT as a biomarker in the critically ill: acute pancreatitis, sepsis, trauma, and acute respiratory distress syndrome. BMC Anesthesiol. 2022;22(1):182.

90. Evans AC, Papachristou GI, Whitcomb DC. Obesity and the risk of severe acute pancreatitis. Minerva Gastroenterol Dietol. 2010;56(2):169–79.

91. Papachristou GI, Papachristou DJ, Avula H, Slivka A, Whitcomb DC. Obesity increases the severity of acute pancreatitis: performance of APACHE-O score and correlation with the inflammatory response. Pancreatology. 2006;6(4):279–85.

92. Sennello JA, Fayad R, Pini M, Gove ME, Ponemone V, Cabay RJ, et al. Interleukin-18, together with interleukin-12, induces severe acute pancreatitis in obese but not in nonobese leptin-deficient mice. Proc Natl Acad Sci USA. 2008;105(23):8085–90.

93. Sass DA, Papachristou GI, Lamb J, Barmada MM, Brand RE, Money ME, et al. The MCP-1 -2518 a/G polymorphism is not a susceptibility factor for chronic pancreatitis. Pancreatology. 2006;6(4):297–300.

94. Bishehsari F, Sharma A, Stello K, Toth C, O'Connell MR, Evans AC, et al. TNF-alpha gene (TNFA) variants increase risk for multi-organ dysfunction syndrome (MODS) in acute pancreatitis. Pancreatology: official journal of the international association of. Pancreatology. 2012;12(2):113–8.

95. de Madaria E, Martinez J, Sempere L, Lozano B, Sanchez-Paya J, Uceda F, et al. Cytokine genotypes in acute pancreatitis: association with etiology, severity, and cytokine levels in blood. Pancreas. 2008;37(3):295–301.

96. Balog A, Gyulai Z, Boros LG, Farkas G, Takacs T, Lonovics J, et al. Polymorphism of the TNF-alpha, HSP70-2, and CD14 genes increases susceptibility to severe acute pancreatitis. Pancreas. 2005;30(2):e46–50.

97. Bishu S, Koutroumpakis E, Mounzer R, Stello K, Pollock N, Evans A, et al. The −251 a/T polymorphism in the IL8 promoter is a risk factor for acute pancreatitis. Pancreas. 2018;47(1):87–91.

98. Hofner P, Balog A, Gyulai Z, Farkas G, Rakonczay Z, Takacs T, et al. Polymorphism in the IL-8 gene, but not in the TLR4 gene, increases the severity of acute pancreatitis. Pancreatology. 2006;6(6):542–8.

99. Zhang DL, Zheng HM, Yu BJ, Jiang ZW, Li JS. Association of polymorphisms of IL and CD14 genes with acute severe pancreatitis and septic shock. World J Gastroenterol. 2005;11(28):4409–13.

100. Dellinger EP, Forsmark CE, Layer P, Levy P, Maravi-Poma E, Petrov MS, et al. Determinant-based classification of acute pancreatitis severity: an international multidisciplinary consultation. Ann Surg. 2012;256(6):875–80.

101. Paragomi P, Spagnolo D, Breze C, Gougol A, Haupt M, Whitcomb DC, et al. Dynamic analysis of patients with acute pancreatitis: validation of a new predictive tool for severity assessment in a large prospective cohort. Gastroenterol. 2019;156(6):S122–S3.

102. Guda NM, Muddana V, Whitcomb DC, Levy P, Garg P, Cote G, et al. Recurrent acute pancreatitis: international state-of-the-science conference with recommendations. Pancreas. 2018;47(6):653–66.

103. Whitcomb DC, Frulloni L, Garg P, Greer JB, Schneider A, Yadav D, et al. Chronic pancreatitis: an international draft consensus proposal for a new mechanistic definition. Pancreatology. 2016;16:218–24.

104. Whitcomb DC, Shimosegawa T, Chari ST, Forsmark CE, Frulloni L, Garg P, et al. International consensus statements on early chronic Pancreatitis. Recommendations from the working group for the international consensus guidelines for chronic pancreatitis in collaboration with The International Association of Pancreatology, American Pancreatic Association, Japan Pancreas Society, PancreasFest Working Group and European Pancreatic Club. Pancreatology. 2018;S1424–3903(18):30113.

105. van Baal MC, Besselink MG, Bakker OJ, van Santvoort HC, Schaapherder AF, Nieuwenhuijs VB, et al. Timing of cholecystectomy after mild biliary pancreatitis: a systematic review. Ann Surg. 2012;255(5):860–6.

106. Shmelev A, Axentiev A, Hossain MB, Cunningham SC. Predictors of same-admission cholecystectomy in mild, acute, biliary pancreatitis. HPB (Oxford). 2021;23(11):1674–82.

107. Sandzen B, Rosenmuller M, Haapamaki MM, Nilsson E, Stenlund HC, Oman M. First attack of acute pancreatitis in Sweden 1988–2003: incidence, aetiological classification, procedures and mortality - a register study. BMC Gastroenterol. 2009;9:18.

108. Umans DS, Hallensleben ND, Verdonk RC, Bouwense SAW, Fockens P, van Santvoort HC, et al. Recurrence of idiopathic acute pancreatitis after cholecystectomy: systematic review and meta-analysis. Br J Surg. 2020;107(3):191–9.

109. Zackria R, Lopez RA. Postcholecystectomy syndrome. Treasure Island: StatPearls; (FL)2022.

110. Camilleri M, Carlson P, BouSaba J, McKinzie S, Vijayvargiya P, Magnus Y, et al. Comparison of biochemical, microbial and mucosal mRNA expression in bile acid diarrhoea and irritable bowel syndrome with diarrhoea. Gut. 2022;72(1):54–65.

Acinar Cell Events Initiating Acute Pancreatitis

Anna S. Gukovskaya and Ilya Gukovsky

Abbreviations

AP	Acute pancreatitis
Arg	L-arginine
ATG	Autophagy-related protein(s)
CCK	Cholecystokinin-8
CER	Caerulein
CP	Chronic pancreatitis
CTSB	Cathepsin B
CypD	Cyclophilin D
ER	Endoplasmic reticulum
GNPTAB	Gene encoding α/β subunits of GlcNAc-1-phosphotransferase
MAC	Mitochondrial apoptosis channels
MPTP	Mitochondrial permeability transition pore
NF-κB	Nuclear factor kappa B
SOCs	Store-operated Ca^{2+} channels
TFEB	Transcription factor EB
TUDCA	Tauroursodeoxycholic acid
UPR	Unfolded protein response

The original version of the chapter has been revised. A correction to this chapter can be found at https://doi.org/10.1007/978-981-97-3132-9_18

A. S. Gukovskaya · I. Gukovsky (✉)
Department of Medicine, University of California at Los Angeles, Los Angeles, CA, USA
e-mail: agukovsk@ucla.edu; igukovsk@ucla.edu

Key Points

- Pancreatitis is believed to initiate in injured acinar cells. Elucidating the pathogenic mechanisms of cellular events initiating pancreatitis is essential because persistent acinar cell damage perpetuates inflammation and parenchymal necrosis, creating a vicious cycle that drives the disease.
- Both experimental and human pancreatitis are associated with disordering of acinar cell organelles: mitochondria, the endoplasmic reticulum, lysosomes, and autophagy.
- Studies in experimental and genetic mouse and ex vivo models of pancreatitis indicate that dysfunctions of acinar cell organellar network initiate and drive the disease, mediating trypsinogen activation, inflammation, parenchymal cell death, and other pancreatitis responses.
- Strategies to stabilize lysosomes, enhance autophagic efficiency, and normalize mitochondrial and endoplasmic reticulum functions present new therapeutic approaches for pancreatitis treatment and prevention.

Pancreatitis is a potentially fatal disease of the exocrine pancreas and one of the most common reasons for hospital admissions for those with GI disease [1–5]. The etiology of human pancreatitis includes gallstones, alcohol abuse, and the effect of various genetic abnormalities. There are two major forms of the disease, acute and chronic [1–11]. Signature responses of acute pancreatitis

© The Author(s), under exclusive license to Springer Nature Singapore Pte Ltd. 2024, corrected publication 2024
J. A. Windsor et al. (eds.), *Acute Pancreatitis*, https://doi.org/10.1007/978-981-97-3132-9_3

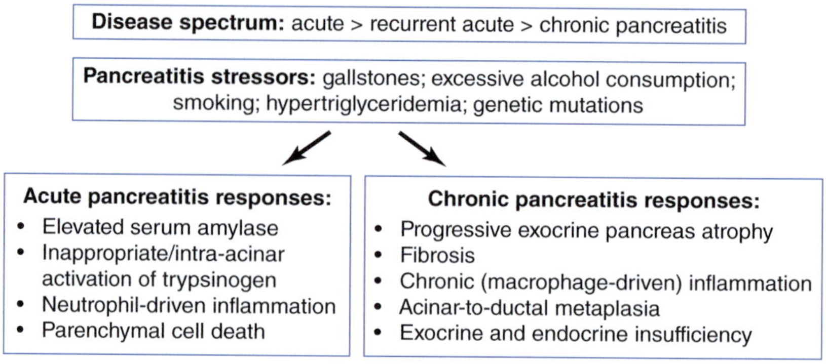

Fig. 1 Responses of acute and chronic pancreatitis

> **Disease spectrum:** acute > recurrent acute > chronic pancreatitis

> **Pancreatitis stressors:** gallstones; excessive alcohol consumption; smoking; hypertriglyceridemia; genetic mutations

Acute pancreatitis responses:
- Elevated serum amylase
- Inappropriate/intra-acinar activation of trypsinogen
- Neutrophil-driven inflammation
- Parenchymal cell death

Chronic pancreatitis responses:
- Progressive exocrine pancreas atrophy
- Fibrosis
- Chronic (macrophage-driven) inflammation
- Acinar-to-ductal metaplasia
- Exocrine and endocrine insufficiency

(AP) include (Fig. 1) the following: increased serum amylase, the inappropriate/premature activation of digestive enzymes within acinar cells (in particular, trypsinogen conversion to trypsin), immune cell infiltration into the pancreas, and acinar cell death [1–3, 6–11]. Recurrent acute pancreatitis is defined as two or more attacks of acute pancreatitis without any evidence of underlying chronic pancreatitis. The key pathologic features of chronic pancreatitis (CP) are progressive loss of acinar tissue, chronic (macrophage-driven) inflammation, and fibrosis [6, 7, 10], ultimately leading to loss of exocrine as well as endocrine pancreatic function (Fig. 1). It is believed that chronic pancreatitis results from repetitive subclinical or clinically evident bouts of AP. Not only is CP associated with poor quality of life, but it is also a major risk factor for pancreatic cancer [12, 13]. Despite decades of intensive research, the pathogenesis of AP remains obscure, and no effective or specific treatment is available [1–5, 10, 11]. This is primarily because of our inadequate knowledge of the molecular and cellular processes initiating and driving the disease.

It is generally held that disordering of pancreatic acinar cell functions mediates both acute and chronic pancreatitis. The central physiological function of acinar cells—to synthesize, store, and secrete digestive enzymes—critically relies on coordinated actions of cytoplasmic organelles, such as the endoplasmic reticulum (ER), mitochondria, lysosomes, and autophagy. Studies of the past decade have revealed a range of functional disorders of these organelles in experimen-

tal and human pancreatitis and, further, provided increasingly compelling evidence that organelle disordering is a key pathogenic mechanism initiating and driving pancreatitis. Although there is still much to be learnt about this mechanism, the findings implicate organellar dysfunctions in mediating key pancreatitis responses, such as the intra-acinar trypsinogen activation, inflammation, and acinar cell death. In this review, we discuss advancements in our understanding of the mechanisms of acinar cell events initiating pancreatitis, with an emphasis on organelle disorders and approaches to alleviate the disease through normalizing organellar functions.

1 Preclinical Animal Models of Pancreatitis

Because of the limited access to human pancreatic tissue, studies addressing pancreatitis disease mechanisms make use of animal models. There are several well-characterized rodent models of pancreatitis, which reproduce pathologies of human disease. These models have greatly advanced our understanding of the cell biology and the molecular factors involved in the disease, which has allowed testing of potential therapeutic approaches. The characteristics of the models and methods of their development are described in detail in various reviews (e.g., Refs. 7, 14). The commonly used mouse AP models are those induced by administering supramaximal doses of caerulein (CER), an ortholog of the hormone cholecystokinin (CCK-

8); by intraductal injection of the bile acid salt taurolithocholic acid-3-sulfate, replicating acute biliary pancreatitis caused by ampullary gallstone obstruction; by intraperitoneal injection of high doses of basic amino acids, such as L-arginine (Arg); or by feeding young female mice choline-deficient, ethionine-supplemented diet [7, 14, 15]. The CER-AP is a milder form of the disease, reproducing features of edematous AP, while the other models develop necrotizing pancreatitis of various severity. Of note, ethanol consumption itself does not cause pancreatitis in rodent models; therefore, alcohol-related AP models have been developed by combining alcohol feeding with other stressors, such as CER or CCK, applied at low doses, which do not induce pancreatitis in control-fed animals [16]. Another model is that induced with ethanol non-oxidative metabolite, palmitoleic acid ethyl ester [17, 18]. Commonly used experimental CP models are developed in mice by repeated episodes of acute pancreatitis induced with CER or Arg injections [19, 20].

2 Early Pathologic Events Leading to Pancreatitis

There is compelling evidence that the disease is initiated by injured acinar cells, the main cell type of the exocrine pancreas, and that the mechanisms mediating pancreatitis are common to all its forms [1–3, 21]. Indeed, rodent and, importantly, human acinar cells subjected to pancreatitis stressors (ex vivo AP models) exhibit early responses of the disease, namely, the inappropriate/premature activation of digestive enzymes, particularly trypsinogen; necrotic and apoptotic cell death; and production and release of cytokines and other mediators initiating inflammation [21–27]. In the following sections, we discuss these acinar cell pathologic events and the mechanisms through which they drive the disease.

3 Trypsinogen Activation

Trypsinogen is one of the major secretory products of the exocrine pancreas [28–33]. Under physiologic conditions, trypsinogen remains inactive during its synthesis, intracellular transport, and secretion—the same as for most other digestive enzymes produced by acinar cells as inactive precursors (zymogens). Physiologically, trypsinogen is only activated when it reaches the intestine where the duodenal brush-border serine protease enteropeptidase (termed enterokinase) cleaves off its N-terminal oligopeptide to convert trypsinogen into trypsin, a potent protease. The significance of this event is that trypsin then proceeds to cleave several other digestive proteases, such as chymotrypsinogen, proelastase, and procarboxypeptidase B1, to generate active enzymes performing digestion of the meal.

Inappropriate (premature) trypsinogen activation within acinar cells is a common early event in experimental and human AP [29–34]. Mutations in the gene encoding human cationic trypsinogen are associated with autosomal dominant hereditary pancreatitis and sporadic nonalcoholic chronic pancreatitis [33–35]. Loss-of-function variants in genes that code for endogenous trypsin inhibitors also increase susceptibility to pancreatitis [34–36]. These findings suggest that intra-acinar trypsinogen activation plays a critical role in pancreatitis development.

Recent studies in mouse genetic models [30, 31, 34, 37–42], however, point to a more nuanced assessment of trypsin's role in pancreatitis. On one hand, CER-AP was indeed worsened in mice expressing mutated (R122H) human trypsinogen [37] or in mice in which the major cationic trypsinogen T7 gene was engineered to generate active trypsin more rapidly [38]. On the other hand, T7 genetic ablation did not lessen the inflammatory response in CER-AP (although it reduced acinar cell injury and necrosis) [30, 31]. Furthermore, spontaneous pancreatitis only developed in transgenic mice engineered to achieve very high levels of trypsinogen activation [38, 39]. The studies [40–42] also shed light on the relative significance of the two known biochemical mechanisms of trypsinogen conversion to trypsin in acinar cells, namely, its' cleavage by the lysosomal protease cathepsin B (CTSB) versus "autoactivation," in which trypsin itself cleaves and thus activates trypsinogen. The latter is believed to mediate hereditary pancreatitis [33–39], whereas the former has been shown to solely operate in CER-AP [40–42]. Interestingly, varying up or down the extent of intra-acinar trypsin activity by genetically modulating CTSB had no effect on parameters of CER-AP, such as parenchymal necrosis, serum amylase, and cytokine levels [40–42].

More work is obviously needed to elucidate the pathologic consequences of intra-acinar trypsinogen activation, but the above-discussed findings, particularly in genetically modified mice [40–42], question the centrality of trypsin in the pathogenic mechanism of pancreatitis.

4 Cell Death

4.1 Types of Eukaryotic Cell Death

The main types of eukaryotic cell death are apoptosis and necrosis; the latter can be nonregulated or genetically controlled [43]. The key feature of both forms of necrosis is loss of the plasma membrane integrity resulting in a leakage of cell content into the interstitial spaces, which can trigger inflammation [43]. A typical cause of nonregulated necrosis is reduction in cellular ATP, which results in the loss of cell's ability to maintain ion gradients across organellar (e.g., lysosomal) and plasma membranes. This leads to collapse of critical intracellular functions and cell death. Genetically programmed forms of necrosis (the major forms being necroptosis, pyroptosis, and ferroptosis) are mediated through specific signaling pathways causing pore formation in the plasma membrane [43–46]. For example, necroptosis is mediated via the formation of a protein complex termed the "necrosome" that involves receptor-interacting protein kinases RIPK1 and RIPK3. Their recruitment to the necrosome causes phosphorylation of the mixed-lineage kinase domain-like pseudokinase (MLKL) followed by its oligomerization, which results in plasma membrane rupture and lytic cell death [44].

During apoptosis, the cell also undergoes a cascade of genetically programmed but distinct molecular events. In contrast to necrosis, the early morphologic events in apoptosis are shrinkage of the cell and condensation of its nuclear chromatin [43]. The shrunken apoptotic cells are recognized and phagocytosed by macrophages. Different from necrosis, apoptotic cell dismantling occurs without rupture of plasma membrane and leakage of cellular contents and thus does not elicit the inflammatory response [43].

4.2 Acinar Cell Death in Pancreatitis

Acinar cells in pancreatitis die through both necrosis and apoptosis. However, morphologic analysis indicates that in all pancreatitis models and in human disease, necrosis is the predominant mechanism of acinar cell death, and the contribution of apoptosis is much less [47–50]. In rodent models of milder pancreatitis, the tissue necrosis/apoptosis ratio is ~3, whereas in models of severe disease, it reaches ~300 [50]. Because necrosis, but not apoptosis, stimulates inflammation, the severity of pancreatitis in AP models correlates directly with the rate of necrosis and inversely with apoptosis [47, 48, 50–53]. In humans, pancreatitis with a high percentage of parenchymal cell death (necrotizing pancreatitis) occurs in 20–30% of AP patients and is associated with high rates of morbidity (up to 95%) and mortality (2–39%) [54].

Nonregulated necrosis caused by a drop in cellular ATP is the major type of acinar cell death in experimental pancreatitis [55–57]. Programmed necrosis, i.e., necroptosis, is also activated in pancreatitis, as evidenced by necrosome formation and MLKL phosphorylation [58–63]. However, its role in pancreatitis remains unclear, with contradictory reports of both a mediatory role of necroptosis in disease severity [59] and of its protective effect [62]. The contribution of pyroptosis and ferroptosis in necrotic cell death in pancreatitis is less studied and has not yet been established [64–67].

Acinar cell death in pancreatitis is discussed in more detail below, in conjunction with mitochondrial dysfunction.

5 Acinar Cell Events Initiating the Inflammatory Response

5.1 Mechanisms Triggering Inflammation

Inflammation is a major defense mechanism that functions to eliminate cells damaged from the original insult and initiate tissue repair [68–70]. Efficient development and resolution of the inflammatory response and restoration of tissue homeostasis depend on the coordinated actions of neutrophils, macrophages, and other types of immune cells, which are controlled by secreted inflammatory mediators. The major class of those are cytokines [71], which include chemokines (cytokines with chemotactic activities), interferons, interleukins, and tumor necrosis factor (TNFα). Production of cytokines and other proinflammatory mediators is stimulated via activation of the proinflammatory transcription factors, such as NF-κB, AP-1, and STAT3 [72, 73]. Another key mechanism of the inflammatory response is through activation of the inflammasome pathway. This results in formation of a multiprotein complex (predominantly in macrophages) that serves as a platform for processing/activation of caspase-1, which in turn

mediates proteolytic maturation and secretion of major cytokines IL-1β and IL-18 [74].

5.2 The Inflammatory Response of Pancreatitis

Inflammation is a critical and universal component of pancreatitis [8, 53, 73, 75, 76]. In most patients, the acute inflammatory response and pancreas damage ultimately resolve. However, in severe cases, the unremitting inflammatory response results in a "cytokine storm," development of the systemic inflammatory response syndrome, and ultimately multiple organ failure (especially the lung and kidney), a major cause of mortality among patients with AP [1, 8, 73, 77]. A key event initiating the inflammatory response of pancreatitis is activation in the injured acinar cells of the proinflammatory transcription factor NF-κB [22, 23, 73, 78, 79], which triggers mRNA expression of major proinflammatory cytokines, including TNFα, IL-6, CCL2, CCL5, and others [24, 80–83]. These mediators recruit into the pancreas neutrophils, monocytes, and macrophages, which secrete large amounts of proinflammatory mediators, perpetuating acinar cell injury and thus creating a vicious circle of more tissue damage and more inflammation [8, 53, 73, 76, 83–87]. In addition, damage-associated molecular pattern molecules (DAMPs) released from necrotic acinar cells cause inflammasome activation and the resultant secretion of IL-1β and IL-18 by macrophages infiltrating the pancreas [75, 88–90].

Experimental studies clearly indicate that downregulation of the inflammatory response of pancreatitis has beneficial effects [8, 49, 73, 76, 85–87, 90]. However, therapeutic approaches to reduce inflammation in human disease have encountered multiple challenges and have not been successful so far [3, 8, 53, 73, 86, 87]. There are several likely reasons for this failure: the therapeutic window for patients with AP is narrow; the effects of inflammatory mediators overlap; and major cytokines, such as TNFα or IL-6, have diverse roles at different phases of the inflammatory response [73, 76, 84]. Manipulating a master regulatory pathway, in particular NF-κB, can have both beneficial and deleterious effects because NF-κB regulates not only inflammation but also cell survival and other processes in pancreatitis [91–96].

Interestingly, infiltrating immune cells contribute to increased intrapancreatic trypsin activity in pancreatitis [49, 97–99], which for a long time was considered an autonomous acinar cell event. Although mechanistic details remain to be elucidated, the data show that mediators produced by inflammatory cells, such as reactive oxygen species (ROS) generated by neutrophils [49] or TNFα [98], promote trypsinogen activation in experimental pancreatitis. Trypsinogen activation can even occur in macrophages, which ingest zymogen-containing vesicles released by damaged acinar cells or endocytose trypsinogen converting it to trypsin in a CTSB-dependent manner [99]. These effects exemplify the mechanisms, whereby inflammation perpetuates acinar cell injury in pancreatitis.

6   Acinar Cell Organellar Dysfunctions Initiate and Drive Pancreatitis

A major reason for why therapeutic approaches to ameliorate pancreatitis by reducing inflammation failed is that persistent acinar cell damage perpetuates both inflammation and parenchymal cell death, continuously creating a vicious cycle that drives the disease. Thus, elucidating the mechanisms mediating acinar cell damage and developing approaches to reduce it are each essential for preventing or alleviating pancreatitis pathologies.

Recent studies have revealed profound dysfunctions of acinar cell organelles, the endoplasmic reticulum (ER), mitochondria, and lysosomes—as well as the autophagy pathway—in experimental and human pancreatitis. This evidence, detailed below, now strongly implicates organellar network disorders in initiating and driving the disease [21]. The main functions of these organelles are summarized in Fig. 2.

Fig. 2 Main functions of intracellular organelles disorders of which mediate pancreatitis. *ER* the endoplasmic reticulum, *ROS* reactive oxygen species

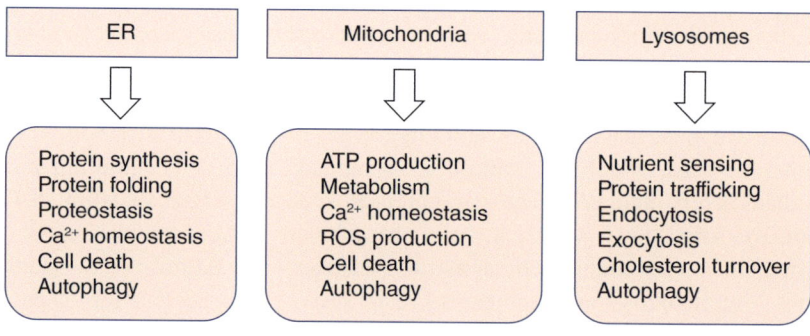

7 ER Dysfunction and Aberrant Ca²⁺ Signaling in Pancreatitis

7.1 Role of Endoplasmic Reticulum in Protein Folding

ER is the principal cellular site of protein and lipid synthesis; it also regulates and monitors the folding of nascent proteins, thus protecting the cell from toxic aggregates of misfolded proteins [100–102]. When ER capacity to perform the folding of nascent proteins is overwhelmed, misfolded (or unfolded) proteins accumulate. In response to this, cells activate the adaptive/protective "unfolded protein response" (UPR), which temporarily reduces general translation and simultaneously upregulates the levels of ER/Golgi chaperones and foldases that mediate protein folding. If the UPR fails to sufficiently increase ER folding capacity, the cell activates the ER-stress signaling programs that subsequently lead to its demise [100–102].

7.2 Role of Endoplasmic Reticulum in Ca²⁺ Transport

Maintaining Ca^{2+} homeostasis is another important ER function (Fig. 2). Cytosolic Ca^{2+} concentration is approximately 100 nM, which is ~10,000-fold lower than that in blood. This gradient is maintained by intracellular Ca^{2+} storage compartments that are primarily the ER and mitochondria [103]. To activate various Ca^{2+}-dependent functions, particularly exocytosis, the cell stimulates increase in cytosolic Ca^{2+} through activating Ca^{2+} release from ER and influx from extracellular milieu. In non-excitable cells, calcium influx is mediated through so-called store-operated channels (SOCs) in the plasma membrane, which are activated by the ER Ca^{2+} depletion [104]. In physiologic conditions, Ca^{2+} pumps return the elevated cytosolic Ca^{2+} back to the ER and/or remove it from the cell [103]. ER can also directly transport Ca^{2+} to mitochondria through specific mitochondria-associated ER membranes [105, 106].

7.3 ER Stress in Pancreatitis

Pancreatic acinar cells, as the primary producers of digestive enzymes, have highly developed ER and demonstrate the greatest basal rate of protein synthesis among mature cells in the human body [107]. Because of this high volume of protein synthesis and processing, acinar cells are particularly vulnerable to ER stress [108, 109]. Indeed, experimental pancreatitis is reported to be associated with persistent ER stress, indicating the failure of homeostatic protein folding machinery [20, 108–111]. The ER failure to perform proper folding of mutated proteins is also thought to play a role in hereditary pancreatitis [111–113].

The harmful effect of ER stress on the pancreas is experimentally supported by the findings that a decrease in ER folding capacity with genetic haplo-ablation ($Xbp1^{+/-}$) of its key mediator, the transcription factor XBP1 (X-box binding protein 1), dramatically worsens pancreas damage in ethanol-fed mice [101, 110]. Conversely, the chemical chaperones 4-phenolbutyrate and tauroursodeoxycholic acid (TUDCA), which assist protein folding and protect against CER-AP [114, 115]. It is of note that TUDCA is now in clinical trials for treatments of other diseases, for example, amyotrophic lateral sclerosis [116] and biliary cholangitis [117], and is reported to be well tolerated, with no reported adverse effects. The alleviating effect of TUDCA on pancreatitis is promising and worth further investigation.

7.4 Dysregulation of Ca²⁺ Signaling in Pancreatitis

Cytosolic Ca^{2+} is a key mediator of exocrine pancreas physiologic secretion [103]. In response to acinar cell stimulation with hormones or neurotransmitters, Ca^{2+} is released from ER into the cytosol and then is rapidly taken back to the ER by Ca^{2+} pumps (or extruded from the cell). This results in repetitive cytosolic Ca^{2+} spikes, which are associated with bursts of acinar cell exocytotic secretion. The oscillatory pattern of Ca^{2+}

signal protects acinar cells from aberrant activation of various calcium-dependent processes that could create profound cellular dysfunction [103]. Pancreatitis is associated with loss of cytosolic Ca^{2+} oscillations, which are replaced by a sustained increase in cytosolic Ca^{2+} ("peak-and-plateau" response) [103, 118]. This occurs because pancreatitis stressors completely deplete the ER of calcium, which in turn promotes massive Ca^{2+} entry into the acinar cell through SOC channels ORAI1 or TRVP4 [118–121]. The resultant abnormal (global and sustained) increase in cytosolic Ca^{2+} is deleterious for acinar cells, as evidenced by the findings that preventing this increase with Ca^{2+} chelators or specific pharmacologic inhibitors of SOCs or by overexpression of a protein inhibitor of Ca^{2+} influx, all abolished intra-acinar trypsinogen activation in experimental pancreatitis [121–124]. SOCs inhibitors also ameliorated necrosis, inflammation, and serum hyperamylasemia in pancreatitis models [121, 123]. Some of the harmful effects of Ca^{2+} are mediated by Ca^{2+}-activated phosphatase calcineurin; the underlying mechanism involves calcineurin-mediated activation of the transcription factor NF-AT [125–128]. Calcineurin's inhibition by genetic or pharmacologic means ameliorated pancreatitis pathologies, in particular inflammation and trypsinogen activation [125–128].

Although the mechanisms linking sustained increases in cytosolic Ca^{2+} to pancreatitis responses are not fully understood, the results strongly indicate that pharmacologic inhibitors of SOCs and calcineurin have great potential for pancreatitis treatment.

8 Mitochondrial Dysfunction in Pancreatitis

8.1 Mitochondria-Mediated Mechanisms of Cell Death

Mitochondria are responsible for a range of cellular functions (Fig. 2), the major ones being energy (ATP) production and cell survival [129–131]. In particular, mitochondrial mem-

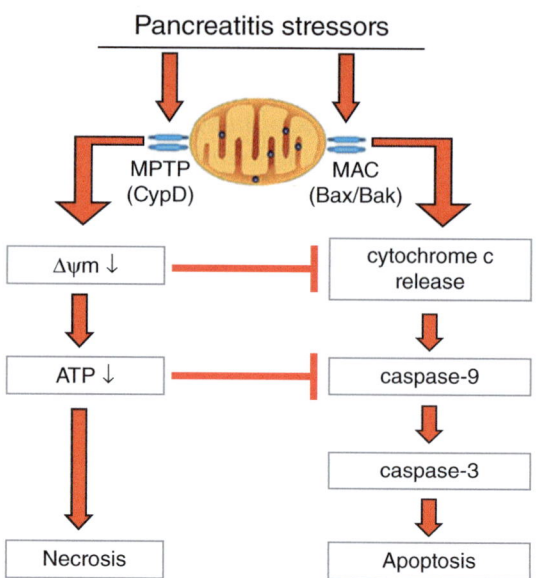

Fig. 3 Mitochondria-mediated pathways of necrosis and apoptosis. $\Delta\Psi m$ mitochondrial membrane potential, *CypD* cyclophilin D, *MAC* mitochondrial apoptosis channels, *MPTP* mitochondrial permeability transition pore

brane permeabilization [132] is a universal trigger of both necrosis and apoptosis (Fig. 3). The mitochondrial permeability transition pore (MPTP), a multiprotein nonspecific channel traversing both the inner and outer mitochondrial membranes, is a key mediator of nonregulated necrosis [132–134]. In its "open" conformation, MPTP allows entry of solutes with molecular mass less than 1500 Da (in particular water) into the matrix, resulting in mitochondrial depolarization and inhibition of its ability to synthesize ATP and ultimately leading to necrosis. Various factors increase the likelihood of MPTP remaining persistently open, the major one being mitochondrial Ca^{2+} overload [135]. MPTP is also activated by fatty acids, phosphate, altered NAD^+/NADH ratio, and defects in electron-transport chain [134, 135]. MPTP backbone is organized around the mitochondrial resident protein cyclophilin D (CypD); genetic, molecular, or pharmacologic inactivation of CypD blocks MPTP opening [135–137].

In contrast, apoptotic stimuli do not stimulate MPTP opening but instead trigger formation in the outer mitochondrial membrane of a specific ion channel termed MAC (mitochondrial apoptosis channel; Fig. 3) [138]. The release through these channels of the mitochondrial resident protein cytochrome c into the cytosol is a central event in apoptosis. Once in the cytosol, cytochrome c causes activation of specific cysteine protease, caspase-9, which in turn cleaves and activates effector caspases (e.g., caspase-3), mediating the downstream apoptotic events [139, 140]. Proteins of the Bcl-2 family tightly control the formation and activation of MACs. Proapoptotic members of this family, Bax and Bak, form MACs, whereas the antiapoptotic Bcl-2 and Bcl-XL prevent their formation and activation [141, 142]. Apoptosis is also limited downstream of cytochrome c release by the inhibitor of apoptosis proteins (IAPs), which reduce caspase activity [139, 140].

8.2 Mitochondrial Dysfunction Mediates Acinar Cell Death in Pancreatitis

Persistent MPTP opening is a common early event in various models of pancreatitis, which manifests itself by mitochondrial depolarization, followed by loss of ATP and necrosis (Fig. 3) [21, 55–57]. Mechanisms of MPTP activation differ between AP models: for example, in AP induced by caerulein or bile acids, the global and sustained increases in cytosolic Ca^{2+} result in mitochondrial Ca^{2+} overload that triggers MPTP opening; in alcohol-mediated AP model, MPTP is activated by a decrease in $NAD^+/NADH$ ratio; and in Arg-AP, by increased complex formation between CypD and mitochondrial F-ATP synthase [55–57].

Acinar cell apoptosis is also activated in pancreatitis [26, 51] as manifested by the release of cytochrome c into the cytosol, followed by caspase activation (Fig. 3). Recent studies [143, 144] showed that apoptosis in AP models is initiated by CTSB, which is released from damaged lysosomes and promotes proteolytic activation of the protein Bax necessary for the formation of MAC channels. The involvement of CTSB in acinar cell apoptosis is supported by the finding that its

genetic ablation prevents apoptosis in AP models induced by caerulein or duct ligation [143]. However, the pro-apoptosis signaling in pancreatitis is counteracted by inhibitory mechanisms on several levels (Fig. 3). In the pancreas, MAC channels are mitochondrial potential-dependent, and therefore depolarization caused by MPTP opening inhibits cytochrome c release in pancreatitis. Moreover, the decrease in cellular ATP caused by mitochondrial depolarization limits caspase activation, which is ATP-dependent [51, 145, 146]. In other words, there is an antagonistic relationship between necrosis and apoptosis in pancreatitis (Fig. 3) [50, 51]. Apoptosis is further limited at the level of caspase activity by IAPs, which are highly expressed in the pancreas [50, 51]. These factors acting together result in much greater acinar tissue necrosis than apoptosis in pancreatitis [50].

8.3 MPTP Inactivation Markedly Improves Experimental Pancreatitis

Despite the difference in the mechanisms of MPTP activation, CypD blockade by genetic, molecular, or pharmacologic means inhibited MPTP opening in all pancreatitis models examined [55–57]. The studies further found that persistent MPTP opening plays a critical role in mediating not only acinar cell death but also other AP responses. In particular, MPTP blockade through CypD genetic or pharmacologic inactivation improved pancreatic histopathology, decreased or completely abrogated trypsinogen activation, and reduced inflammation in several AP models [55–57].

Although the mechanisms linking MPTP to pancreatitis responses are not yet fully understood, these findings suggest that pharmacologic CypD inhibition could be a new and promising therapeutic approach for pancreatitis treatment. However, so far none of the CypD inhibitors have been introduced into clinical practice, mostly owing to their high toxicity, unfavorable pharmacokinetics, and low selectivity for CypD over other cyclophilins. The focus of current research in this field is therefore on the development of selective and nontoxic CypD small-molecule inhibitors, which can be applied in several types of diseases associated with MPTP opening, including pancreatitis [146–148].

9 Lysosomal/Autophagic Dysfunctions and Their Role in Pancreatitis

9.1 The Lysosome

The lysosome is a membrane-bound organelle, the main function of which (Fig. 2) is to degrade all types of biological material [149, 150]. It contains an array of enzymes capable of breaking down proteins, nucleic acids, carbohydrates, and lipids. Efficient lysosomal degradation requires several key elements. These include acidic pH of the lysosomal lumen, which matches the pH optimum of most of the ~60 lysosomal enzymes (acid hydrolases) and the presence and proper function of ~200 membrane proteins, such as the lysosome-associated membrane proteins LAMP1 and LAMP2 [150–154]. LAMPs are critical for maintaining lysosomal structure, protecting the cytosol (and the lysosomal limiting membrane itself) from the acidic luminal pH, and for key lysosomal functions, such as proteolytic degradation and fusion with autophagosomes [151–154].

Eukaryotic cells also possess a unique mechanism for the sorting and delivery of acid hydrolases to the lysosome that involves covalent addition of mannose 6-phosphate to these enzymes; the tagged hydrolases then bind to one of the two transmembrane mannose-6-phosphate receptors which carry them to the lysosome [155–157]. N-acetylglucosamine-1-phosphotransferase is a key enzyme mediating mannose 6-phosphate addition onto acid hydrolases [156–158]; genetic ablation in mice of its' α/β subunits coded by the *Gnptab* gene blocks catalytic activity of this enzyme [158, 159].

Findings of the last decade [160–162] have changed our view of the lysosome from that of a simple "garbage disposal" to a dynamic multi-functional organelle that regulates major cellular processes (Fig. 2). Lysosomes degrade material from outside taken up by the cell through multiple endocytic pathways and the material from inside through the process of autophagy [149, 150]. In addition to degradation, lysosomes control nutrient sensing, endolysosomal damage response, lysosome-dependent cell death, and lipid metabolism (see recent excellent reviews, e.g., Refs. 163, 164). The discovery that transcription factors belonging to the MiT/TFE family (the major ones are TFEB and TFE3) control multiple lysosomal, as well as autophagy genes, has greatly advanced our understanding of the mechanisms through which the lysosome executes its functions [161–165].

9.2 Autophagy

Autophagy/macroautophagy is the principal cellular catabolic process for degradation and recycling of organelles, lipids, and long-lived proteins [21, 149, 166, 167]. Autophagy can be both non-selective and selective in its targeting of specific cellular organelles for degradation, i.e., mitochondria (mitophagy) or ER (ER-phagy) [167–169].

The autophagy process begins with the formation of an isolation membrane, or phagophore, followed by its elongation and closure to form the mature autophagosome. These steps are mediated by sequentially recruited complexes of evolutionary conserved autophagy-related (ATG) proteins. The final step in autophagosome formation is lipidation of cytosolic LC3-I, the mammalian paralog of yeast ATG8, to become membrane-bound LC3-II, a specific marker of autophagic vacuoles. Autophagosomes then fuse with lysosomes to form autolysosomes where cargo breakdown occurs [21, 149, 166–170]. Defects in each step of this process impair autophagic degradation, resulting in accumulation in cells of damaged/dysfunctional organelles, followed by activation of proinflammatory and death signaling pathways [171, 172].

9.3 Role of Lysosomes in Cholesterol Turnover

Relevant to acinar cell functioning and the pathogenesis of pancreatitis is the lysosome's role in cholesterol turnover [173]. Cholesterol is the principal sterol synthesized by all animals, and its unique structure enables the cell to alter membrane fluidity while preserving membrane integrity so that they remain stable without being rigid [173, 174]. The distribution of cholesterol among cellular membranes is very uneven; for example, high cholesterol content of the plasma membrane is essential to support proper conformation of receptors and ion channels [173, 174]. Zymogen granules of the acinar cell (as well as secretory granules in other cells) are enriched in cholesterol, which is necessary for their fusion with the plasma membrane in exocytosis. On the other hand, mitochondria are cholesterol poor [173].

Mammalian cells mostly obtain cholesterol from the circulation through receptor-mediated endocytosis of cholesterol carrying LDL lipoproteins [173–175]. After reaching the lysosome, LDL undergo lipolysis, yielding free cholesterol that exits the lysosome and is distributed between cellular organelles. Mutations in NPC1 and NPC2 proteins that transport cholesterol through lysosomes cause the fatal Niemann-Pick type C disease manifested by massive accumulation of cholesterol in lysosomes due to its inability to egress from the lysosome [176]. This results in reduced cholesterol availability for the cell's needs, in particular a decrease in the plasma membrane cholesterol content, which is greatly detrimental [173, 175, 176]. The relevance of these pathologic effects to AP is discussed later in this chapter.

9.4 Lysosomal/Autophagic Dysfunctions in Pancreatitis

Accumulation in acinar cells of cytoplasmic vacuoles, often filled with cellular debris, has long been recognized as a hallmark of both human and experimental pancreatitis [166, 177–182]. Our studies showed that these vacuoles are autolysosomes containing poorly degraded material, as a result of defective/inefficient autophagic degradation [166, 182]. In addition to acinar cell vacuolization, the impaired autophagic flux also manifests itself by concomitant increases in pancreatic levels of both the autophagy mediator LC3-II and the autophagy substrate p62/SQSTM1 (sequestosome 1) [57, 183–185]. Furthermore, pancreatitis is associated with multiple defects in lysosomal/autophagic pathways, in particular incomplete processing (maturation) of the major lysosomal proteases, cathepsins, and their reduced enzymatic activity in lysosome-enriched pancreatic subcellular fractions [159, 166, 182, 186]; dramatically decreased levels of LAMP1 and LAMP2 [184, 187]; loss of TFEB, the master transcriptional regulator of lysosomal biogenesis and autophagy [185, 188, 189]; and impaired GNPTAB-mediated hydrolase delivery to lysosomes [159].

Studies of mice with genetic modifications targeting different steps in lysosomal/autophagic pathways revealed the essential role of these pathways in acinar cell homeostasis. Specifically, genetic ablation of *Lamp2* or *Gnptab*, which impairs lysosomal proteolytic activity [159, 184]; double knockout of *Tfeb and Tfe3* in acinar cells [188, 189]; and pancreas-specific ablation of *Atg5, Atg7,* or *Vmp1*, key mediators of autophagosome formation [190–192], all cause spontaneous pancreatitis characterized by trypsinogen activation, macrophage-driven inflammation, and parenchymal necrosis. These findings convincingly demonstrate critical role of lysosomal/autophagic dysfunctions in initiating and driving pancreatitis [21, 76] and suggest that pharmacologic approaches to stabilize lysosomal functions and/or increase autophagic efficiency should alleviate the disease.

One promising drug is the natural disaccharide trehalose, which increases lysosomal degradative capacity and enhances autophagic efficiency by upregulating/activating TFEB [193]. We found [57] that trehalose enhanced autophagic degradation and alleviated essentially all pancreatitis responses in dissimilar AP models, Arg-AP and CER-AP. Trehalose was recently approved by FDA for amyotrophic lateral sclerosis platform trials (NCT05136885) and is also in a clinical trial for treatment of Alzheimer's (NCT05332678). Its safety and tolerability have been tested in a clinical trial in patients with spinocerebellar ataxia type 3 (NCT04426149), with no serious adverse events identified. Thus, trehalose is a strong candidate to move rapidly into clinical trials for pancreatitis.

The analysis of the pancreas of mice with genetic ablation of *Gnptab* or *Lamp2* indicates that lysosomal dysfunction, with its concomitant disrupting of cholesterol transport through the lysosome, causes cholesterol accumulation in lysosomes and thus decreases cholesterol availability for acinar cell needs [159], similar to what occurs in NPC disease [176]. Moreover, and also similar to NPC disease, these defects stimulate cholesterol synthesis (likely, as a compensatory response), thus further exacerbating acinar cell cholesterol overload. Consequently, we showed that normalizing acinar cell cholesterol homeostasis with the inhibitor of cholesterol synthesis simvastatin alleviated responses of experimental pancreatitis, including trypsinogen activation, necrosis, and inflammation [159]. The findings that simvastatin, as well as other cholesterol-lowering drugs, alleviate pancreatitis in preclinical (mouse and ex vivo) AP models [159] begin to unravel the role of acinar cell cholesterol dyshomeostasis in pancreatitis pathogenesis. More studies of the effects of cholesterol-lowering drugs with different action mechanisms are needed in various pancreatitis models to establish cholesterol synthesis pathway as a therapeutic target amenable to pharmacologic intervention in pancreatitis and select the best candidate(s) and regimens for clinical trials. Of note, there is ongoing clinical trial (NCT02743364) on the effects of simvastatin in pancreatitis. For years, there were reports, often controversial, on the links between statins and pancreatitis severity in patients. Although early studies implicated statins in drug-induced pancreatitis, subsequent case-control studies, meta-analysis of randomized controlled trials, and population and cohort studies indicated that statin use is independently associated with lower incidence of AP, milder disease course, and decreased mortality

[194–200]. However, until the recent study [159], there was no consideration of statins' effects on acinar cell cholesterol metabolism as a potential therapeutic mechanism.

9.5 Links between Lysosomal/Autophagic Dysfunctions and Pancreatitis Responses

Findings in the above genetic mouse models have uncovered distinct mechanisms, whereby disordering of lysosomal/autophagic pathways leads to "classic" pancreatitis responses. Pancreas of these mice accumulates mitochondria with low membrane potential, reduced activities of respiratory complexes, and diminished ATP production [159, 188, 190, 191], leading to parenchymal necrosis. Damaged mitochondria and toxic aggregates of misfolded proteins that accumulate in autophagy-deficient acinar cells overproduce ROS, thus promoting NF-κB activation, initiating the inflammatory response [22, 23, 79]. ER stress in autophagy-deficient acinar cells manifests, in particular, by upregulation of the transcription factor CHOP, a major ER stress marker and mediator of cell death [190, 191].

Loss or impairment of autophagy also markedly increases intra-acinar trypsin activity [159, 182–184, 188, 190, 191, 201–204], suggesting that autophagy is necessary for efficient elimination of trypsin-containing organelles that accumulate in pancreatitis. Indeed, we and others found that during pancreatitis, trypsin accumulates in autophagic vacuoles [182, 201–204]. Conversely, increasing autophagic efficiency with trehalose reduces intra-acinar trypsin activity in experimental AP models [57].

10 Acinar Cell Organelle Disordering in Human Pancreatitis

Analysis of pancreatic tissue specimens from patients with pancreatitis revealed that human disease exhibit manifestations of lysosomal/autophagic dysfunctions similar to those observed in rodent models, namely, the dramatic decreases in LAMP1 and LAMP2 [184, 187], loss of TFEB [188, 189], and reduction in GNPTAB level [159]. Autophagy impairment in human pancreatitis is evidenced by accumulation of abnormally large autophagic vacuoles in acinar cells, especially striking on electron micrographs [166, 177, 178, 181, 182], and by increased levels of both LC3-II, a marker of autophagic vacuoles, and p62/SQSTM1 (sequestosome 1), an autophagy substrate [57, 183]. Mitochondrial dysfunction and ER stress in human disease manifest themselves on electron microscopy images of the pancreas, by the appearance of swollen mitochondria, characteristic of MPTP opening, and dilated ER [205], and cholesterol dysregulation, by the increased level of HMG-CoA reductase [159].

11 Potential Pharmacologic Approaches to Restore the Function of Acinar Cell Organelles for Pancreatitis Treatment or Prevention

The focus of this review is on the mechanisms of acinar cell organellar dysfunctions and their role in initiating and driving pancreatitis (Fig. 4). In particular, we emphasize the role of lysosomal/autophagic dysfunctions, resulting in an autophagy failure that is unable to normally eliminate damaged mitochondria and ER. Buildup of damaged/dysfunctional organelles and dysregulation of cholesterol homeostasis causes accumulation of trypsin in acinar cells, activates proinflammatory signaling, and promotes parenchymal necrosis, all key responses of AP. Thus, approaches to

Fig. 4 Acinar cell events initiating acute pancreatitis. DAMPs, damage-associated molecular patterns

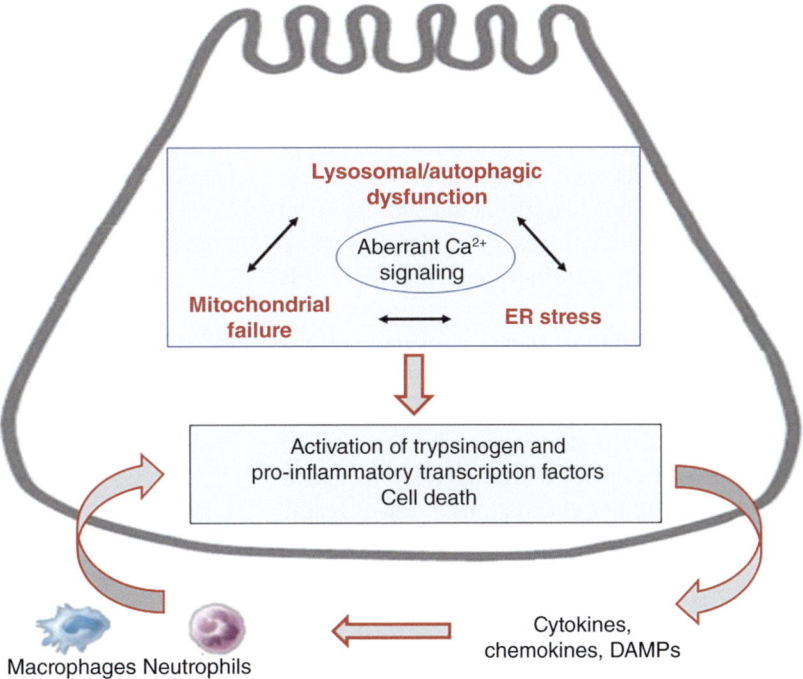

Table 1 Potential therapeutic approaches to mitigate acinar cell dysfunctions initiating and driving pancreatitis

Agent	Action	Targeted pathway	Form of pancreatitis	Status
CM-4620	Inhibition of Orai1 store-operated Ca^{2+} channel	Ca^{2+} signaling	Acute pancreatitis	NCT04681066 phase 2
			Pancreatitis due to asparaginase	NCT04195347 phase 1/2
Indomethacin + tacrolimus	Combination of cyclooxygenase and calcineurin inhibitors	Inflammation and Ca^{2+} signaling	Post-ERCP pancreatitis	NCT05252754 phase 3
TUDCA	Chemical chaperone, promoting protein folding	ER stress	Acute pancreatitis	Preclinical models (Ref. 115)
TRO40303	Inhibitor of mitochondrial permeability transition pore	Mitochondrial dysfunction	Acute pancreatitis	Preclinical models (Ref. 146)
Trehalose	TFEB activator	Lysosomal/ autophagic dysfunction	Acute pancreatitis	Preclinical models (Ref. 57)
Simvastatin	Inhibitor of HMG-CoA reductase, key enzyme in cholesterol biosynthesis	Cholesterol homeostasis	Recurrent, acute, or chronic pancreatitis	NCT02743364 phase 2

ER endoplasmic reticulum, *ERCP* endoscopic retrograde cholangiopancreatography, *HMG-CoA* 3-hydroxy-3-methylglutaryl-CoA, *TFEB* transcription factor EB, *TUDCA* tauroursodeoxycholic acid

stabilize lysosomes, enhance autophagic efficiency, improve mitochondrial and ER functions, or normalize cholesterol homeostasis should be considered for pancreatitis treatment or prevention (Table 1). As we discussed above, candidate drugs for such clinical trials include the chemical chaperone TUDCA, blockers of the mitochondrial permeability transition pore, and the TFEB activator trehalose.

The goal of future studies is to uncover the "upstream" mechanisms, whereby factors predisposing to pancreatitis (such as alcohol consumption, bile acids, and smoking) cause aberrant Ca^{2+} signaling and organellar dysfunctions in acinar cells, and to further elucidate the "downstream" mechanisms linking organelle disordering and classic pancreatitis pathologies. As stated in Ref. 21, a key question is whether there is a critical pathologic defect common to various forms of pancreatitis and leading to failure of the whole organellar network or whether distinct organellar dysfunctions are mediated through different mechanisms so that more than one organelle function has to be restored, for example, by normalizing both autophagy and mitochondrial function. The most promising approach could be to simultaneously restore the organellar network homeostasis (to alleviate acinar cell damage) and resolve or reduce the inflammatory response. These approaches should certainly be further evaluated in preclinical models, but some of them (Table 1) have "ripened" enough for clinical trials or are already being tested.

References

1. Pandol SJ, Saluja AK, Imrie CW, Banks PA. Acute pancreatitis: bench to the bedside. Gastroenterology. 2007;132(3):1127–51. Erratum: *ibid*, 133:1056.
2. Lee PJ, Papachristou GI. New insights into acute pancreatitis. Nat Rev Gastroenterol Hepatol. 2019;16(8):479–96.
3. Habtezion A, Gukovskaya AS, Pandol SJ. Acute pancreatitis: a multi-faceted set of organellar, cellular and organ interactions. Gastroenterology. 2019;156(7):1941–50.
4. Peery AF, Crockett SD, Murphy CC, Jensen ET, Kim HP, Egberg MD, et al. Burden and cost of gastrointestinal, liver, and pancreatic diseases in the United States: update 2021. Gastroenterology. 2022;162(2):621–44.
5. Szatmary P, Grammatikopoulos T, Cai W, Huang W, Mukherjee R, Halloran C, et al. Acute pancreatitis: diagnosis and treatment. Drugs. 2022;82(12):1251–76.

6. Vonlaufen A, Wilson JS, Apte MV. Molecular mechanisms of pancreatitis: current opinion. J Gastroenterol Hepatol. 2008;23(9):1339–48.

7. Lerch MM, Gorelick FS. Models of acute and chronic pancreatitis. Gastroenterology. 2013;144(6):1180–93.

8. Habtezion A. Inflammation in acute and chronic pancreatitis. Curr Opin Gastroenterol. 2015;31(5):395–9.

9. Saluja A, Dudeja V, Dawra R, Sah RP. Early intra-acinar events in pathogenesis of pancreatitis. Gastroenterology. 2019;156(7):1979–93.

10. Beyer G, Habtezion A, Werner J, Lerch MM, Mayerle J. Chronic pancreatitis. Lancet. 2020;396(10249):499–512.

11. Barreto SG, Habtezion A, Gukovskaya A, Lugea A, Jeon C, Yadav D, et al. Critical thresholds: key to unlocking the door to the prevention and specific treatments for acute pancreatitis. Gut. 2021;70(1):194–203.

12. Kirkegard J, Mortensen FV, Cronin-Fenton D. Chronic pancreatitis and pancreatic cancer risk: a systematic review and meta-analysis. Am J Gastroenterol. 2017;112(9):1366–72.

13. Kandikattu HK, Venkateshaiah SU, Mishra A. Chronic pancreatitis and the development of pancreatic cancer. Endocr Metab Immune Disord Drug Targets. 2020;20(8):1182–210.

14. Gorelick FS, Lerch MM. Do animal models of acute pancreatitis reproduce human disease? Cell Mol Gastroenterol Hepatol. 2017;4(2):251–62.

15. Perides G, van Acker GJ, Laukkarinen JM, Steer ML. Experimental acute biliary pancreatitis induced by retrograde infusion of bile acids into the mouse pancreatic duct. Nat Protoc. 2010;5(2):335–41.

16. Pandol SJ, Periskic S, Gukovsky I, Zaninovic V, Jung Y, Zong Y, et al. Ethanol diet increases the sensitivity of rats to pancreatitis induced by cholecystokinin octapeptide. Gastroenterology. 1999;117(3):706–16.

17. Huang W, Booth DM, Cane MC, Chvanov M, Javed MA, Elliott VL, et al. Fatty acid ethyl ester synthase inhibition ameliorates ethanol-induced Ca2+−dependent mitochondrial dysfunction and acute pancreatitis. Gut. 2014;63(8):1313–24.

18. Criddle DN. The role of fat and alcohol in acute pancreatitis: a dangerous liaison. Pancreatology. 2015;15(4 Suppl):S6–S12.

19. Ulmasov B, Oshima K, Rodriguez MG, Cox RD, Neuschwander-Tetri BA. Differences in the degree of cerulein-induced chronic pancreatitis in C57BL/6 mouse substrains lead to new insights in identification of potential risk factors in the development of chronic pancreatitis. Am J Pathol. 2013;183(3):692–708.

20. Sah RP, Garg SK, Dixit AK, Dudeja V, Dawra RK, Saluja AK. Endoplasmic reticulum stress is chronically activated in chronic pancreatitis. J Biol Chem. 2014;289(40):27551–61.

21. Gukovskaya AS, Gorelick F, Groblewski GE, Mareninova O, Lugea A, Antonucci L, et al. Recent insights into the pathogenic mechanism of pancreatitis: role of acinar cell organelle disorders. Pancreas. 2019;48(4):459–70.

22. Gukovsky I, Gukovskaya AS, Blinman TA, Zaninovic V, Pandol SJ. Early NF-kappaB activation is associated with hormone-induced pancreatitis. Am J Phys. 1998;275(6):G1402–14.

23. Steinle AU, Weidenbach H, Wagner M, Adler G, Schmid RM. NF-kappaB/Rel activation in cerulein pancreatitis. Gastroenterology. 1999;116(2):420–30.

24. Han B, Logsdon CD. Cholecystokinin induction of mob-1 chemokine expression in pancreatic acinar cells requires NF-kappaB activation. Am J Phys. 1999;277(1):C74–82.

25. Saluja AK, Bhagat L, Lee HS, Bhatia M, Frossard JL, Steer ML. Secretagogue-induced digestive enzyme activation and cell injury in rat pancreatic acini. Am J Phys. 1999;276(4):G835–42.

26. Gukovskaya AS, Gukovsky I, Jung Y, Mouria M, Pandol SJ. Cholecystokinin induces caspase activation and mitochondrial dysfunction in pancreatic acinar cells. Roles in cell injury processes of pancreatitis. J Biol Chem. 2002;277(25):22595–604.

27. Lugea A, Waldron RT, Mareninova OA, Shalbueva N, Deng N, Su HY, et al. Human pancreatic acinar cells: proteomic characterization, physiologic responses, and organellar disorders in ex vivo pancreatitis. Am J Pathol. 2017;187(12):2726–43.

28. Jamieson JD, Palade GE. Synthesis, intracellular transport, and discharge of secretory proteins in stimulated pancreatic exocrine cells. J Cell Biol. 1971;50(1):135–58.

29. Go VLW, DiMagno EP, Gardner JD, Lebenthal E, Reber WA, Scheele GA. The pancreas: biology, pathobiology, and disease. 2nd ed. New York: Raven Press; 1993.

30. Dawra R, Sah RP, Dudeja V, Rishi L, Talukdar R, Garg P, et al. Intra-acinar trypsinogen activation mediates early stages of pancreatic injury but not inflammation in mice with acute pancreatitis. Gastroenterology. 2011;141(6):2210–7 e2.

31. Ji B, Logsdon CD. Digesting new information about the role of trypsin in pancreatitis. Gastroenterology. 2011;141(6):1972–5.

32. Saluja AK, Lerch MM, Phillips PA, Dudeja V. Why does pancreatic overstimulation cause pancreatitis? Annu Rev Physiol. 2007;69:249–69.

33. Whitcomb DC, Gorry MC, Preston RA, Furey W, Sossenheimer MJ, Ulrich CD, et al. Hereditary pancreatitis is caused by a mutation in the cationic trypsinogen gene. Nat Genet. 1996;14(2):141–5.

34. Hegyi E, Sahin-Toth M. Genetic risk in chronic pancreatitis: the trypsin-dependent pathway. Dig Dis Sci. 2017;62(7):1692–701.

35. Witt H, Luck W, Hennies HC, Classen M, Kage A, Lass U, et al. Mutations in the gene encoding the serine protease inhibitor, Kazal type 1 are associated with chronic pancreatitis. Nat Genet. 2000;25(2):213–6.

36. Rosendahl J, Witt H, Szmola R, Bhatia E, Ozsvari B, Landt O, et al. Chymotrypsin C (CTRC) variants that diminish activity or secretion are associated with chronic pancreatitis. Nat Genet. 2008;40(1):78–82.

37. Huang H, Swidnicka-Siergiejko AK, Daniluk J, Gaiser S, Yao Y, Peng L, et al. Transgenic expression of PRSS1(R122H) sensitizes mice to pancreatitis. Gastroenterology. 2020;158(4):1072–82 e7.

38. Demczak A, Sahin-Toth M. Rate of autoactivation determines pancreatitis phenotype in trypsinogen mutant mice. Gastroenterology. 2022;163(3):761–3.

39. Wang J, Wan J, Wang L, Pandol SJ, Bi Y, Ji B. Wild-type human PRSS2 and PRSS1(R122H) cooperatively initiate spontaneous hereditary pancreatitis in transgenic mice. Gastroenterology. 2022;163(1):313–315 e4.

40. Geisz A, Tran T, Orekhova A, Sahin-Tóth M. Trypsin activity in secretagogue-induced murine pancreatitis is solely elicited by Cathepsin B and does not mediate key pathologic responses. Gastroenterology. 2023;164(4):684–687 e4.

41. Chen W, Imasaka M, Iwama H, Nishiura H, Ohmuraya M. Double deficiency of cathepsin B and L in the mouse pancreas alters trypsin activity without affecting acute pancreatitis severity. Pancreatology. 2022;22:880–6.

42. Lee B, Husain SZ, Gukovsky I. Genetically engineered mouse models shine new light on decades-old story of trypsin in pancreatitis. Gastroenterology. 2023;164(4):524–6.

43. Green DR. The coming decade of cell death research: five riddles. Cell. 2019;177(5):1094–107.

44. Weinlich R, Oberst A, Beere HM, Green DR. Necroptosis in development, inflammation and disease. Nat Rev Mol Cell Biol. 2017;18(2):127–36.

45. Chen X, Kang R, Kroemer G, Tang D. Ferroptosis in infection, inflammation, and immunity. J Exp Med. 2021;218(6):e20210518.

46. Coll RC, Schroder K, Pelegrin P. NLRP3 and pyroptosis blockers for treating inflammatory diseases. Trends Pharmacol Sci. 2022;43(8):653–68.

47. Kaiser AM, Saluja AK, Sengupta A, Saluja M, Steer ML. Relationship between severity, necrosis, and apoptosis in five models of experimental acute pancreatitis. Am J Phys. 1995;269(5 Pt 1):C1295–304.

48. Gukovskaya AS, Perkins P, Zaninovic V, Sandoval D, Rutherford R, Fitzsimmons T, et al. Mechanisms of cell death after pancreatic duct obstruction in the opossum and the rat. Gastroenterology. 1996;110(3):875–84.

49. Gukovskaya AS, Vaquero E, Zaninovic V, Gorelick FS, Lusis AJ, Brennan ML, et al. Neutrophils and NADPH oxidase mediate intrapancreatic trypsin activation in murine experimental acute pancreatitis. Gastroenterology. 2002;122(4):974–84.

50. Sung KF, Odinokova IV, Mareninova OA, Rakonczay Z Jr, Hegyi P, Pandol SJ, et al. Prosurvival Bcl-2 proteins stabilize pancreatic mitochondria and protect against necrosis in experimental pancreatitis. Exp Cell Res. 2009;315(11):1975–89.

51. Mareninova OA, Sung KF, Hong P, Lugea A, Pandol SJ, Gukovsky I, et al. Cell death in pancreatitis: caspases protect from necrotizing pancreatitis. J Biol Chem. 2006;281(6):3370–81.

52. Sendler M, Mayerle J, Lerch MM. Necrosis, apoptosis, necroptosis, pyroptosis: it matters how acinar cells die during pancreatitis. Cell Mol Gastroenterol Hepatol. 2016;2(4):407–8.

53. Mayerle J, Sendler M, Hegyi E, Beyer G, Lerch MM, Sahin-Toth M. Genetics, cell biology, and pathophysiology of pancreatitis. Gastroenterology. 2019;156(7):1951–68 e1.

54. Bugiantella W, Rondelli F, Boni M, Stella P, Polistena A, Sanguinetti A, et al. Necrotizing pancreatitis: a review of the interventions. Int J Surg. 2016;28(Suppl 1):S163–71.

55. Shalbueva N, Mareninova OA, Gerloff A, Yuan J, Waldron RT, Pandol SJ, et al. Effects of oxidative alcohol metabolism on the mitochondrial permeability transition pore and necrosis in a mouse model of alcoholic pancreatitis. Gastroenterology. 2013;144(2):437–46 e6.

56. Mukherjee R, Mareninova OA, Odinokova IV, Huang W, Murphy J, Chvanov M, et al. Mechanism of mitochondrial permeability transition pore induction and damage in the pancreas: inhibition prevents acute pancreatitis by protecting production of ATP. Gut. 2016;65(8):1333–46.

57. Biczo G, Vegh ET, Shalbueva N, Mareninova OA, Elperin J, Lotshaw E, et al. Mitochondrial dysfunction, through impaired autophagy, leads to endoplasmic reticulum stress, deregulated lipid metabolism, and pancreatitis in animal models. Gastroenterology. 2018;154(3):689–703.

58. Linkermann A, Brasen JH, De Zen F, Weinlich R, Schwendener RA, Green DR, et al. Dichotomy between RIP1- and RIP3-mediated necroptosis in tumor necrosis factor-alpha-induced shock. Mol Med. 2012;18:577–86.

59. Louhimo J, Steer ML, Perides G. Necroptosis is an important severity determinant and potential therapeutic target in experimental severe pancreatitis. Cell Mol Gastroenterol Hepatol. 2016;2(4):519–35.

60. Newton K, Dugger DL, Maltzman A, Greve JM, Hedehus M, Martin-McNulty B, et al. RIPK3 deficiency or catalytically inactive RIPK1 provides greater benefit than MLKL deficiency in mouse models of inflammation and tissue injury. Cell Death Differ. 2016;23(9):1565–76.

61. Wu J, Mulatibieke T, Ni J, Han X, Li B, Zeng Y, et al. Dichotomy between receptor-interacting protein 1- and receptor-interacting protein 3-mediated necroptosis in experimental pancreatitis. Am J Pathol. 2017;187(5):1035–48.

62. Boonchan M, Arimochi H, Otsuka K, Kobayashi T, Uehara H, Jaroonwitchawan T, et al. Necroptosis protects against exacerbation of acute pancreatitis. Cell Death Dis. 2021;12(6):601.

63. Ouyang Y, Wen L, Armstrong JA, Chvanov M, Latawiec D, Cai W, et al. Protective effects of

Necrostatin-1 in acute pancreatitis: partial involvement of receptor interacting protein kinase 1. Cells. 2021;10(5):1035.

64. Fan R, Sui J, Dong X, Jing B, Gao Z. Wedelolactone alleviates acute pancreatitis and associated lung injury via GPX4 mediated suppression of pyroptosis and ferroptosis. Free Radic Biol Med. 2021;173:29–40.

65. Gao L, Dong X, Gong W, Huang W, Xue J, Zhu Q, et al. Acinar cell NLRP3 inflammasome and gasdermin D (GSDMD) activation mediates pyroptosis and systemic inflammation in acute pancreatitis. Br J Pharmacol. 2021;178(17):3533–52.

66. Lin T, Song J, Pan X, Wan Y, Wu Z, Lv S, et al. Downregulating Gasdermin D reduces severe acute pancreatitis associated with pyroptosis. Med Sci Monit. 2021;27:e927968.

67. Liu K, Liu J, Zou B, Li C, Zeh HJ, Kang R, et al. Trypsin-mediated sensitization to ferroptosis increases the severity of pancreatitis in mice. Cell Mol Gastroenterol Hepatol. 2022;13(2):483–500.

68. Chen L, Deng H, Cui H, Fang J, Zuo Z, Deng J, et al. Inflammatory responses and inflammation-associated diseases in organs. Oncotarget. 2018;9(6):7204–18.

69. Medzhitov R. The spectrum of inflammatory responses. Science. 2021;374(6571):1070–5.

70. Nathan C. Nonresolving inflammation redux. Immunity. 2022;55(4):592–605.

71. Turner MD, Nedjai B, Hurst T, Pennington DJ. Cytokines and chemokines: at the crossroads of cell signalling and inflammatory disease. Biochim Biophys Acta. 2014;1843(11):2563–82.

72. Fan Y, Mao R, Yang J. NF-kappaB and STAT3 signaling pathways collaboratively link inflammation to cancer. Protein Cell. 2013;4(3):176–85.

73. Gukovsky I, Li N, Todoric J, Gukovskaya A, Karin M. Inflammation, autophagy, and obesity: common features in the pathogenesis of pancreatitis and pancreatic cancer. Gastroenterology. 2013;144(6):1199–209 e4.

74. Broz P, Dixit VM. Inflammasomes: mechanism of assembly, regulation and signalling. Nat Rev Immunol. 2016;16(7):407–20.

75. Hoque R, Sohail M, Malik A, Sarwar S, Luo Y, Shah A, et al. TLR9 and the NLRP3 inflammasome link acinar cell death with inflammation in acute pancreatitis. Gastroenterology. 2011;141(1):358–69.

76. Gukovskaya AS, Gukovsky I, Algul H, Habtezion A. Autophagy, inflammation, and immune dysfunction in the pathogenesis of pancreatitis. Gastroenterology. 2017;153(5):1212–26.

77. Singh VK, Wu BU, Bollen TL, Repas K, Maurer R, Mortele KJ, et al. Early systemic inflammatory response syndrome is associated with severe acute pancreatitis. Clin Gastroenterol Hepatol. 2009;7(11):1247–51.

78. Vaquero E, Gukovsky I, Zaninovic V, Gukovskaya AS, Pandol SJ. Localized pancreatic NF-kappaB activation and inflammatory response in taurocholate-induced pancreatitis. Am J Physiol Gastrointest Liver Physiol. 2001;280(6):G1197–208.

79. Rakonczay Z Jr, Hegyi P, Takacs T, McCarroll J, Saluja AK. The role of NF-kappaB activation in the pathogenesis of acute pancreatitis. Gut. 2008;57(2):259–67.

80. Grady T, Liang P, Ernst SA, Logsdon CD. Chemokine gene expression in rat pancreatic acinar cells is an early event associated with acute pancreatitis. Gastroenterology. 1997;113(6):1966–75.

81. Gukovskaya AS, Gukovsky I, Zaninovic V, Song M, Sandoval D, Gukovsky S, et al. Pancreatic acinar cells produce, release, and respond to tumor necrosis factor-alpha. Role in regulating cell death and pancreatitis. J Clin Invest. 1997;100(7):1853–62.

82. Blinman TA, Gukovsky I, Mouria M, Zaninovic V, Livingston E, Pandol SJ, et al. Activation of pancreatic acinar cells on isolation from tissue: cytokine upregulation via p38 MAP kinase. Am J Physiol Cell Physiol. 2000;279(6):C1993–2003.

83. Orlichenko LS, Behari J, Yeh TH, Liu S, Stolz DB, Saluja AK, et al. Transcriptional regulation of CXC-ELR chemokines KC and MIP-2 in mouse pancreatic acini. Am J Physiol Gastrointest Liver Physiol. 2010;299(4):G867–76.

84. Norman J. The role of cytokines in the pathogenesis of acute pancreatitis. Am J Surg. 1998;175(1):76–83.

85. Bhatia M, Brady M, Shokuhi S, Christmas S, Neoptolemos JP, Slavin J. Inflammatory mediators in acute pancreatitis. J Pathol. 2000;190(2): 117–25.

86. Shamoon M, Deng Y, Chen YQ, Bhatia M, Sun J. Therapeutic implications of innate immune system in acute pancreatitis. Expert Opin Ther Targets. 2016;20(1):73–87.

87. Szatmary P, Gukovsky I. The role of cytokines and inflammation in the genesis of experimental pancreatitis. In: Williams JA, editor. Pancreatitis. Mountain View: CA. Michigan Publishing; 2016. p. 42–52.

88. Hoque R, Mehal WZ. Inflammasomes in pancreatic physiology and disease. Am J Physiol Gastrointest Liver Physiol. 2015;308(8):G643–51.

89. Ferrero-Andres A, Panisello-Rosello A, Rosello-Catafau J, Folch-Puy E. NLRP3 inflammasome-mediated inflammation in acute pancreatitis. Int J Mol Sci. 2020;21(15):5386.

90. Sendler M, van den Brandt C, Glaubitz J, Wilden A, Golchert J, Weiss FU, et al. NLRP3 inflammasome regulates development of systemic inflammatory response and compensatory anti-inflammatory response syndromes in mice with acute pancreatitis. Gastroenterology. 2020;158(1):253–69 e14.

91. Chen X, Ji B, Han B, Ernst SA, Simeone D, Logsdon CD. NF-kappaB activation in pancreas induces pancreatic and systemic inflammatory response. Gastroenterology. 2002;122(2):448–57.

92. Baumann B, Wagner M, Aleksic T, von Wichert G, Weber CK, Adler G, et al. Constitutive IKK2 activation in acinar cells is sufficient to induce pancreatitis in vivo. J Clin Invest. 2007;117(6):1502–13.

93. Neuhofer P, Liang S, Einwachter H, Schwerdtfeger C, Wartmann T, Treiber M, et al. Deletion of IkappaBalpha activates RelA to reduce acute pancreatitis in mice through up-regulation of Spi2A. Gastroenterology. 2013;144(1):192–201.

94. Huang H, Liu Y, Daniluk J, Gaiser S, Chu J, Wang H, et al. Activation of nuclear factor-kappaB in acinar cells increases the severity of pancreatitis in mice. Gastroenterology. 2013;144(1):202–10.

95. Gukovsky I, Gukovskaya A. Nuclear factor-kappaB in pancreatitis: Jack-of-all-trades, but which one is more important? Gastroenterology. 2013;144(1):26–9.

96. Chan LK, Gerstenlauer M, Konukiewitz B, Steiger K, Weichert W, Wirth T, et al. Epithelial NEMO/IKKγ limits fibrosis and promotes regeneration during pancreatitis. Gut. 2017;66(11):1995–2007.

97. Abdulla A, Awla D, Thorlacius H, Regner S. Role of neutrophils in the activation of trypsinogen in severe acute pancreatitis. J Leukoc Biol. 2011;90(5):975–82.

98. Sendler M, Dummer A, Weiss FU, Kruger B, Wartmann T, Scharffetter-Kochanek K, et al. Tumour necrosis factor alpha secretion induces protease activation and acinar cell necrosis in acute experimental pancreatitis in mice. Gut. 2013;62(3):430–9.

99. Sendler M, Weiss FU, Golchert J, Homuth G, van den Brandt C, Mahajan UM, et al. Cathepsin B-mediated activation of trypsinogen in endocytosing macrophages increases severity of pancreatitis in mice. Gastroenterology. 2018;154(3):704–18 e10.

100. Wang M, Kaufman RJ. Protein misfolding in the endoplasmic reticulum as a conduit to human disease. Nature. 2016;529(7586):326–35.

101. Waldron J, Pandol S, Lugea A, Groblewski GE. Endoplasmic reticulum stress and the unfolded protein response in exocrine pancreas physiology and pancreatitis. In: Williams JA, editor. Pancreatitis. Mountain view. CA: Michigan Publishing; 2016. p. 88–96.

102. Hetz C, Zhang K, Kaufman RJ. Mechanisms, regulation and functions of the unfolded protein response. Nat Rev Mol Cell Biol. 2020;21(8):421–38.

103. Petersen OH, Gerasimenko JV, Gerasimenko OV, Gryshchenko O, Peng S. The roles of calcium and ATP in the physiology and pathology of the exocrine pancreas. Physiol Rev. 2021;101(4):1691–744.

104. Lopez JJ, Jardin I, Albarran L, Sanchez-Collado J, Cantonero C, Salido GM, et al. Molecular basis and regulation of store-operated calcium entry. Adv Exp Med Biol. 2020;1131:445–69.

105. Rizzuto R, Pinton P, Carrington W, Fay FS, Fogarty KE, Lifshitz LM, et al. Close contacts with the endoplasmic reticulum as determinants of mitochondrial Ca2+ responses. Science. 1998;280(5370):1763–6.

106. Fan Y, Simmen T. Mechanistic connections between endoplasmic reticulum (ER) redox control and mitochondrial metabolism. Cells. 2019;8(9):1071.

107. Case RM. Synthesis, intracellular transport and discharge of exportable proteins in the pancreatic acinar cell and other cells. Biol Rev Camb Philos Soc. 1978;53(2):211–354.

108. Kubisch CH, Sans MD, Arumugam T, Ernst SA, Williams JA, Logsdon CD. Early activation of endoplasmic reticulum stress is associated with arginine-induced acute pancreatitis American journal of physiology Gastrointestinal and liver physiology. 2006;291(2):G238–45.

109. Kubisch CH, Logsdon CD. Endoplasmic reticulum stress and the pancreatic acinar cell. Expert Rev Gastroenterol Hepatol. 2008;2(2):249–60.

110. Lugea A, Tischler D, Nguyen J, Gong J, Gukovsky I, French SW, et al. Adaptive unfolded protein response attenuates alcohol-induced pancreatic damage. Gastroenterology. 2011;140(3):987–97.

111. Sahin-Toth M. Genetic risk in chronic pancreatitis: the misfolding-dependent pathway. Curr Opin Gastroenterol. 2017;33(5):390–5.

112. Hegyi E, Sahin-Toth M. Human CPA1 mutation causes digestive enzyme misfolding and chronic pancreatitis in mice. Gut. 2019;68(2):301–12.

113. Mounzer R, Whitcomb DC. Genetics of acute and chronic pancreatitis. Curr Opin Gastroenterol. 2013;29(5):544–51.

114. Ye R, Mareninova OA, Barron E, Wang M, Hinton DR, Pandol SJ, et al. Grp78 heterozygosity regulates chaperone balance in exocrine pancreas with differential response to cerulein-induced acute pancreatitis. Am J Pathol. 2010;177(6):2827–36.

115. Seyhun E, Malo A, Schafer C, Moskaluk CA, Hoffmann RT, Goke B, et al. Tauroursodeoxycholic acid reduces endoplasmic reticulum stress, acinar cell damage, and systemic inflammation in acute pancreatitis. Am J Physiol Gastrointest Liver Physiol. 2011;301(5):G773–82.

116. Elia AE, Lalli S, Monsurro MR, Sagnelli A, Taiello AC, Reggiori B, et al. Tauroursodeoxycholic acid in the treatment of patients with amyotrophic lateral sclerosis. Eur J Neurol. 2016;23(1):45–52.

117. Ma H, Zeng M, Han Y, Yan H, Tang H, Sheng J, et al. A multicenter, randomized, double-blind trial comparing the efficacy and safety of TUDCA and UDCA in Chinese patients with primary biliary cholangitis. Medicine. 2016;95(47):e5391.

118. Gerasimenko JV, Gerasimenko OV, Petersen OH. The role of Ca2+ in the pathophysiology of pancreatitis. J Physiol. 2014;592(2):269–80.

119. Son A, Park S, Shin DM, Muallem S. Orai1 and STIM1 in ER/PM junctions: roles in pancreatic cell function and dysfunction. Am J Physiol Cell Physiol. 2016;310(6):C414–22.

120. Liu H, Kabrah A, Ahuja M, Muallem S. CRAC channels in secretory epithelial cell function and disease. Cell Calcium. 2019;78:48–55.

121. Wen L, Voronina S, Javed MA, Awais M, Szatmary P, Latawiec D, et al. Inhibitors of ORAI1 prevent cytosolic calcium-associated injury of human pancreatic acinar cells and acute pancreatitis in 3 mouse models. Gastroenterology. 2015;149(2):481–92 e7.

122. Son A, Ahuja M, Schwartz DM, Varga A, Swaim W, Kang N, et al. Ca(2+) influx channel inhibitor SARAF protects mice from acute pancreatitis. Gastroenterology. 2019;157(6):1660–72 e2.

123. Waldron RT, Chen Y, Pham H, Go A, Su HY, Hu C, et al. The Orai ca(2+) channel inhibitor CM4620 targets both parenchymal and immune cells to reduce inflammation in experimental acute pancreatitis. J Physiol. 2019;597(12):3085–105.

124. Swain SM, Romac JM, Shahid RA, Pandol SJ, Liedtke W, Vigna SR, et al. TRPV4 channel opening mediates pressure-induced pancreatitis initiated by Piezo1 activation. J Clin Invest. 2020;130(5):2527–41.

125. Husain SZ, Grant WM, Gorelick FS, Nathanson MH, Shah AU. Caerulein-induced intracellular pancreatic zymogen activation is dependent on calcineurin. Am J Physiol Gastrointest Liver Physiol. 2007;292(6):G1594–9.

126. Awla D, Zetterqvist AV, Abdulla A, Camello C, Berglund LM, Spegel P, et al. NFATc3 regulates trypsinogen activation, neutrophil recruitment, and tissue damage in acute pancreatitis in mice. Gastroenterology. 2012;143(5):1352–60 e7.

127. Muili KA, Ahmad M, Orabi AI, Mahmood SM, Shah AU, Molkentin JD, et al. Pharmacological and genetic inhibition of calcineurin protects against carbachol-induced pathological zymogen activation and acinar cell injury. Am J Physiol Gastrointest Liver Physiol. 2012;302(8):G898–905.

128. Wen L, Javed TA, Dobbs AK, Brown R, Niu M, Li L, et al. The protective effects of calcineurin on pancreatitis in mice depend on the cellular source. Gastroenterology. 2020;159(3):1036–50 e8.

129. Galluzzi L, Kepp O, Trojel-Hansen C, Kroemer G. Mitochondrial control of cellular life, stress, and death. Circ Res. 2012;111(9):1198–207.

130. Nunnari J, Suomalainen A. Mitochondria: in sickness and in health. Cell. 2012;148(6):1145–59.

131. Spinelli JB, Haigis MC. The multifaceted contributions of mitochondria to cellular metabolism. Nat Cell Biol. 2018;20(7):745–54.

132. Galluzzi L, Blomgren K, Kroemer G. Mitochondrial membrane permeabilization in neuronal injury. Nat Rev Neurosci. 2009;10(7):481–94.

133. Bernardi P, Rasola A, Forte M, Lippe G. The mitochondrial permeability transition pore: channel formation by F-ATP synthase, integration in signal transduction, and role in pathophysiology. Physiol Rev. 2015;95(4):1111–55.

134. Bonora M, Giorgi C, Pinton P. Molecular mechanisms and consequences of mitochondrial permeability transition. Nat Rev Mol Cell Biol. 2022;23(4):266–85.

135. Bernardi P, Carraro M, Lippe G. The mitochondrial permeability transition: recent progress and open questions. FEBS J. 2022;289(22):7051–74.

136. Baines CP, Kaiser RA, Purcell NH, Blair NS, Osinska H, Hambleton MA, et al. Loss of cyclophilin D reveals a critical role for mitochondrial permeability transition in cell death. Nature. 2005;434(7033):658–62.

137. Giorgio V, Soriano ME, Basso E, Bisetto E, Lippe G, Forte MA, et al. Cyclophilin D in mitochondrial pathophysiology. Biochim Biophys Acta. 2010;1797(6-7):1113–8.

138. Kinnally KW, Antonsson B. A tale of two mitochondrial channels, MAC and PTP, in apoptosis. Apoptosis: an international journal on programmed cell death. 2007;12(5):857–68.

139. Shi Y. Mechanisms of caspase activation and inhibition during apoptosis. Mol Cell. 2002;9(3): 459–70.

140. Fan TJ, Han LH, Cong RS, Liang J. Caspase family proteases and apoptosis. Acta Biochim Biophys Sin. 2005;37(11):719–27.

141. Dejean LM, Ryu SY, Martinez-Caballero S, Teijido O, Peixoto PM, Kinnally KW. MAC and Bcl-2 family proteins conspire in a deadly plot. Biochim Biophys Acta. 2010;1797(6-7):1231–8.

142. Wolf P, Schoeniger A, Edlich F. Pro-apoptotic complexes of BAX and BAK on the outer mitochondrial membrane. Biochim Biophys Acta, Mol Cell Res. 2022;1869(10):119317.

143. Sendler M, Maertin S, John D, Persike M, Weiss FU, Kruger B, et al. Cathepsin B activity initiates apoptosis via digestive protease activation in pancreatic acinar cells and experimental pancreatitis. J Biol Chem. 2016;291(28):14717–31.

144. Talukdar R, Sareen A, Zhu H, Yuan Z, Dixit A, Cheema H, et al. Release of cathepsin B in cytosol causes cell death in acute pancreatitis. Gastroenterology. 2016;151(4):747–58 e5.

145. Gukovskaya AS, Pandol SJ. Cell death pathways in pancreatitis and pancreatic cancer. Pancreatology: official journal of the International Association of Pancreatology. 2004;4(6):567–86.

146. Javed MA, Wen L, Awais M, Latawiec D, Huang W, Chvanov M, et al. TRO40303 ameliorates alcohol-induced pancreatitis through reduction of fatty acid ethyl ester-induced mitochondrial injury and necrotic cell death. Pancreas. 2018;47(1):18–24.

147. Shore ER, Awais M, Kershaw NM, Gibson RR, Pandalaneni S, Latawiec D, et al. Small molecule inhibitors of Cyclophilin D to protect mitochondrial function as a potential treatment for acute pancreatitis. J Med Chem. 2016;59(6):2596–611.

148. Haleckova A, Benek O, Zemanova L, Dolezal R, Musilek K. Small-molecule inhibitors of cyclophilin D as potential therapeutics in mitochondria-related diseases. Med Res Rev. 2022;42(5):1822–55.

149. Ohsumi Y. Historical landmarks of autophagy research. Cell Res. 2014;24(1):9–23.

150. Xu H, Ren D. Lysosomal physiology. Annu Rev Physiol. 2015;77:57–80.

151. Saftig P, Klumperman J. Lysosome biogenesis and lysosomal membrane proteins: trafficking meets function. Nat Rev Mol Cell Biol. 2009;10(9):623–35.

152. Mindell JA. Lysosomal acidification mechanisms. Annu Rev Physiol. 2012;74:69–86.

153. Schwake M, Schroder B, Saftig P. Lysosomal membrane proteins and their central role in physiology. Traffic. 2013;14(7):739–48.

154. Saftig P, Haas A. Turn up the lysosome. Nat Cell Biol. 2016;18(10):1025–7.

155. Ghosh P, Dahms NM, Kornfeld S. Mannose 6-phosphate receptors: new twists in the tale. Nat Rev Mol Cell Biol. 2003;4(3):202–12.

156. Braulke T, Bonifacino JS. Sorting of lysosomal proteins. Biochim Biophys Acta. 2009;1793(4):605–14.

157. Coutinho MF, Prata MJ, Alves S. Mannose-6-phosphate pathway: a review on its role in lysosomal function and dysfunction. Mol Genet Metab. 2012;105(4):542–50.

158. Tiede S, Storch S, Lubke T, Henrissat B, Bargal R, Raas-Rothschild A, et al. Mucolipidosis II is caused by mutations in GNPTA encoding the alpha/beta GlcNAc-1-phosphotransferase. Nat Med. 2005;11(10):1109–12.

159. Mareninova OA, Vegh ET, Shalbueva N, Wightman CJ, Dillon DL, Malla S, et al. Dysregulation of mannose-6-phosphate-dependent cholesterol homeostasis in acinar cells mediates pancreatitis. J Clin Invest. 2021;131(15):e146870. https://doi.org/10.1172/JCI146870.

160. Settembre C, Di Malta C, Polito VA, Garcia Arencibia M, Vetrini F, Erdin S, et al. TFEB links autophagy to lysosomal biogenesis. Science. 2011;332(6036):1429–33.

161. Settembre C, Fraldi A, Medina DL, Ballabio A. Signals from the lysosome: a control Centre for cellular clearance and energy metabolism. Nat Rev Mol Cell Biol. 2013;14(5):283–96.

162. Slade L, Pulinilkunnil T. The MiTF/TFE family of transcription factors: master regulators of organelle signaling, metabolism, and stress adaptation. Molecular cancer research : MCR. 2017;15(12):1637–43.

163. Perera RM, Zoncu R. The lysosome as a regulatory hub. Annu Rev Cell Dev Biol. 2016;32:223–53.

164. Ballabio A, Bonifacino JS. Lysosomes as dynamic regulators of cell and organismal homeostasis. Nat Rev Mol Cell Biol. 2020;21(2):101–18.

165. Sardiello M, Palmieri M, di Ronza A, Medina DL, Valenza M, Gennarino VA, et al. A gene network regulating lysosomal biogenesis and function. Science. 2009;325(5939):473–7.

166. Gukovskaya AS, Gukovsky I. Autophagy and pancreatitis. Am J Physiol Gastrointest Liver Physiol. 2012;303(9):G993–G1003.

167. Morishita H, Mizushima N. Diverse cellular roles of autophagy. Annu Rev Cell Dev Biol. 2019;35:453–75.

168. Kirkin V, Rogov VV. A diversity of selective autophagy receptors determines the specificity of the autophagy pathway. Mol Cell. 2019;76(2):268–85.

169. Trelford CB, Di Guglielmo GM. Molecular mechanisms of mammalian autophagy. Biochem J. 2021;478(18):3395–421.

170. Klionsky DJ, Abdel-Aziz AK, Abdelfatah S, Abdellatif M, Abdoli A, Abel S, et al. Guidelines for the use and interpretation of assays for monitoring autophagy (4th edition). Autophagy. 2021;17(1):1–382.

171. Levine B, Kroemer G. Autophagy in the pathogenesis of disease. Cell. 2008;132(1):27–42.

172. Ichimiya T, Yamakawa T, Hirano T, Yokoyama Y, Hayashi Y, Hirayama D, et al. Autophagy and autophagy-related diseases: a review. Int J Mol Sci. 2020;21(23):8974.

173. Ikonen E. Cellular cholesterol trafficking and compartmentalization. Nat Rev Mol Cell Biol. 2008;9(2):125–38.

174. Korber M, Klein I, Daum G. Steryl ester synthesis, storage and hydrolysis: a contribution to sterol homeostasis. Biochim Biophys Acta Mol Cell Biol Lipids. 2017;1862(12):1534–45.

175. Thelen AM, Zoncu R. Emerging roles for the lysosome in lipid metabolism. Trends Cell Biol. 2017;27(11):833–50.

176. Vanier MT. Complex lipid trafficking in Niemann-pick disease type C. J Inherit Metab Dis. 2015;38(1):187–99.

177. Helin H, Mero M, Markkula H, Helin M. Pancreatic acinar ultrastructure in human acute pancreatitis. Virchows Arch A Pathol Anat Histol. 1980;387(3):259–70.

178. Aho HJ, Nevalainen TJ, Havia VT, Heinonen RJ, Aho AJ. Human acute pancreatitis: a light and electron microscopic study. Acta Pathol Microbiol Immunol Scand A. 1982;90(5):367–73.

179. Koike H, Steer ML, Meldolesi J. Pancreatic effects of ethionine: blockade of exocytosis and appearance of crinophagy and autophagy precede cellular necrosis. Am J Phys. 1982;242(4):G297–307.

180. Niederau C, Grendell JH. Intracellular vacuoles in experimental acute pancreatitis in rats and mice are an acidified compartment. J Clin Invest. 1988;81(1):229–36.

181. Willemer S, Kloppel G, Kern HF, Adler G. Immunocytochemical and morphometric analysis of acinar zymogen granules in human acute pancreatitis. Virchows Arch A Pathol Anat Histopathol. 1989;415(2):115–23.

182. Mareninova OA, Hermann K, French SW, O'Konski MS, Pandol SJ, Webster P, et al. Impaired autophagic flux mediates acinar cell vacuole formation and trypsinogen activation in rodent models of acute pancreatitis. J Clin Invest. 2009;119(11):3340–55.

183. Li N, Wu X, Holzer RG, Lee JH, Todoric J, Park EJ, et al. Loss of acinar cell IKKalpha triggers spontaneous pancreatitis in mice. J Clin Invest. 2013;123(5):2231–43.

184. Mareninova OA, Sendler M, Malla SR, Yakubov I, French SW, Tokhtaeva E, et al. Lysosome associated membrane proteins maintain pancreatic acinar cell homeostasis: LAMP-2 deficient mice develop pancreatitis. Cell Mol Gastroenterol Hepatol. 2015;1(6):678–94.

185. Mareninova OA, Jia W, Gretler SR, Holthaus CL, Thomas DDH, Pimienta M, et al. Transgenic expression of GFP-LC3 perturbs autophagy in exocrine pancreas and acute pancreatitis responses in mice. Autophagy. 2020;16(11):2084–97.

186. Saluja A, Hashimoto S, Saluja M, Powers RE, Meldolesi J, Steer ML. Subcellular redistribution of lysosomal enzymes during caerulein-induced pancreatitis. Am J Phys. 1987;253(4 Pt 1):G508–16.

187. Fortunato F, Burgers H, Bergmann F, Rieger P, Buchler MW, Kroemer G, et al. Impaired autolysosome formation correlates with Lamp-2 depletion: role of apoptosis, autophagy, and necrosis in pancreatitis. Gastroenterology. 2009;137(1):350–60; 60.e1-5.

188. Wang S, Ni HM, Chao X, Wang H, Bridges B, Kumer S, et al. Impaired TFEB-mediated lysosomal biogenesis promotes the development of pancreatitis in mice and is associated with human pancreatitis. Autophagy. 2019;15(11):1954–69.

189. Wang S, Ni HM, Chao X, Ma X, Kolodecik T, De Lisle R, et al. Critical role of TFEB-mediated lysosomal biogenesis in alcohol-induced pancreatitis in mice and humans. Cell Mol Gastroenterol Hepatol. 2020;10(1):59–81.

190. Antonucci L, Fagman JB, Kim JY, Todoric J, Gukovsky I, Mackey M, et al. Basal autophagy maintains pancreatic acinar cell homeostasis and protein synthesis and prevents ER stress. Proc Natl Acad Sci USA. 2015;112(45):E6166–74.

191. Diakopoulos KN, Lesina M, Wormann S, Song L, Aichler M, Schild L, et al. Impaired autophagy induces chronic atrophic pancreatitis in mice via sex- and nutrition-dependent processes. Gastroenterology. 2015;148(3):626–38 e17.

192. Wang S, Chao X, Jiang X, Wang T, Rodriguez Y, Yang L, et al. Loss of acinar cell VMP1 triggers spontaneous pancreatitis in mice. Autophagy. 2022;18(7):1572–82.

193. Jeong SJ, Stitham J, Evans TD, Zhang X, Rodriguez-Velez A, Yeh YS, et al. Trehalose causes low-grade lysosomal stress to activate TFEB and the autophagy-lysosome biogenesis response. Autophagy. 2021;17(11):3740–52.

194. Thisted H, Jacobsen J, Munk EM, Norgaard B, Friis S, McLaughlin JK, et al. Statins and the risk of acute pancreatitis: a population-based case-control study. Aliment Pharmacol Ther. 2006;23(1):185–90.

195. Preiss D, Tikkanen MJ, Welsh P, Ford I, Lovato LC, Elam MB, et al. Lipid-modifying therapies and risk of pancreatitis: a meta-analysis. JAMA. 2012;308(8):804–11.

196. Gornik I, Gasparovic V, Gubarev Vrdoljak N, Haxiu A, Vucelic B. Prior statin therapy is associated with milder course and better outcome in acute pancreatitis--a cohort study. Pancreatology. 2013;13(3):196–200.

197. Wu BU, Pandol SJ, Liu IL. Simvastatin is associated with reduced risk of acute pancreatitis: findings from a regional integrated healthcare system. Gut. 2015;64(1):133–8.

198. Lee PJ, Modha K, Chua T, Chak A, Jang D, Lopez R, et al. Association of statins with decreased acute pancreatitis severity: a propensity score analysis. J Clin Gastroenterol. 2018;52(8):742–6.

199. Poropat G, Archibugi L, Korpela T, Cardenas-Jaen K, de-Madaria E, Capurso G. Statin use is not associated with an increased risk of acute pancreatitis-a meta-analysis of observational studies. United European Gastroenterol J. 2018;6(8):1206–14.

200. Machicado JD, Papachristou GI. Pharmacologic management and prevention of acute pancreatitis. Curr Opin Gastroenterol. 2019;35(5):460–7.

201. Dolai S, Liang T, Orabi AI, Holmyard D, Xie L, Greitzer-Antes D, et al. Pancreatitis-induced depletion of syntaxin 2 promotes autophagy and increases basolateral exocytosis. Gastroenterology. 2018;154(6):1805–21 e5.

202. De Faveri F, Chvanov M, Voronina S, Moore D, Pollock L, Haynes L, et al. LAP-like noncanonical autophagy and evolution of endocytic vacuoles in pancreatic acinar cells. Autophagy. 2020;16(7):1314–31.

203. Malla SR, Krueger B, Wartmann T, Sendler M, Mahajan UM, Weiss FU, et al. Early trypsin activation develops independently of autophagy in caerulein-induced pancreatitis in mice. Cell Mol Life Sci. 2020;77(9):1811–25.

204. Dolai S, Takahashi T, Qin T, Liang T, Xie L, Kang F, et al. Pancreas-specific SNAP23 depletion prevents pancreatitis by attenuating pathological basolateral exocytosis and formation of trypsin-activating autolysosomes. Autophagy. 2021;17(10):3068–81.

205. Lee KT, Ching SP. Effect of gallstones on pancreatic acinar cells. An ultrastructural study. European surgical research/Europaische chirurgische forschung/Recherches chirurgicales europeennes. 1988;20(5-6):341–51.

Pathophysiology of Local Pancreatic Complications

Nicholas J. Zyromski

1 Introduction

About 20% of patients with acute pancreatitis develop a severe course of the disease marked by systemic inflammation, organ failure, and variable necrosis of the pancreatic parenchyma and peripancreatic soft tissue. Both of the widely used contemporary classification systems, the Revised Atlanta Criteria [1] and the Determinant Based Classification [2], recognize local complications as an important factor defining moderately severe, severe, and critical acute pancreatitis.

Local complications are inexorably linked with pancreatic necrosis. A clear definition of local pancreatic complications has been an important advance for diagnosis, management, and research (Fig. 1). The morphology and extent of necrosis have clinical importance and are related to the likelihood of certain local complications, which include both pancreatic and peripancreatic complications. In addition to pancreatic complications, there are important vascular, alimentary, and biliary complications (Fig. 2).

Fig. 1 Local pancreatic complications defined by the Revised Atlanta Classification, based on the content of the collection, duration of collection, and whether it is infected. (Adapted from [3])

Content	Acute (<4 weeks, no defined wall)		Chronic (>4 weeks, defined wall)	
	No infection	Infection	No infection	Infection
Fluid	**Acute pancreatic fluid collection**	Infected APFC	**Pseudocyst**	Infected pseudocyst
Solid fluid	**Acute necrotic collection**	Infected ANC	**Walled off necrosis**	Infected WON

N. J. Zyromski (✉)
Department of Surgery, Indiana University,
Indianapolis, IN, USA
e-mail: nzyromsk@iupui.edu

© The Author(s), under exclusive license to Springer Nature Singapore Pte Ltd. 2024
J. A. Windsor et al. (eds.), *Acute Pancreatitis*, https://doi.org/10.1007/978-981-97-3132-9_4

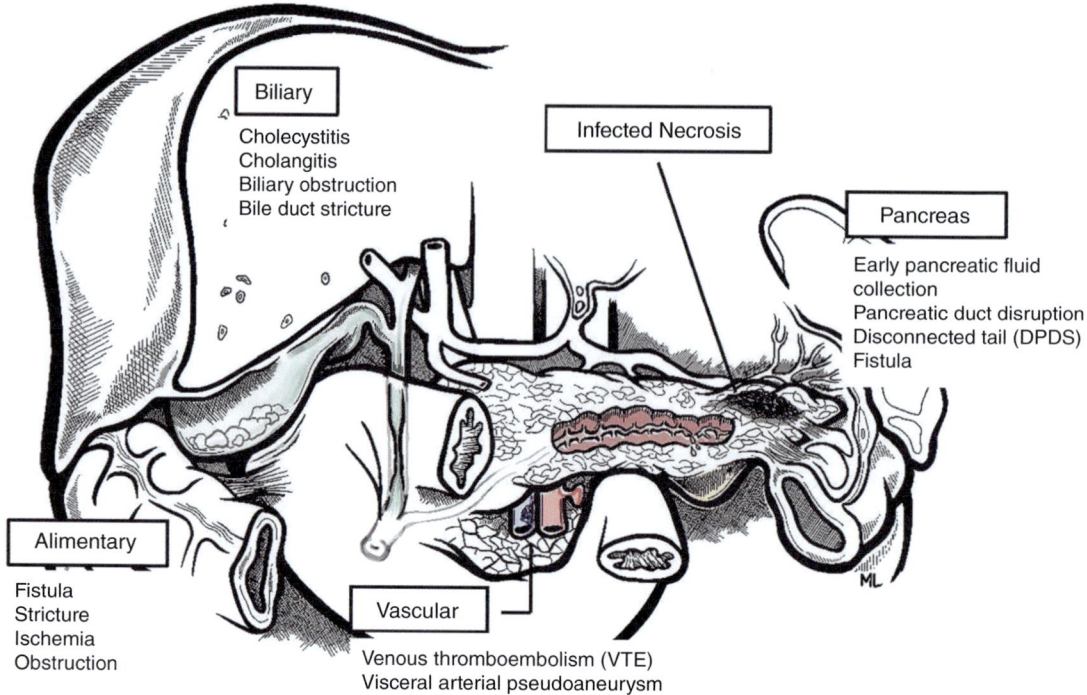

Biliary
Cholecystitis
Cholangitis
Biliary obstruction
Bile duct stricture

Infected Necrosis

Pancreas
Early pancreatic fluid collection
Pancreatic duct disruption
Disconnected tail (DPDS)
Fistula

Alimentary
Fistula
Stricture
Ischemia
Obstruction

Vascular
Venous thromboembolism (VTE)
Visceral arterial pseudoaneurysm

Fig. 2 Sequelae to local complications of pancreatitis including vascular, alimentary, and biliary complications

Local complications can occur at any time point along the typically months-long necrotizing pancreatitis disease course. Specific complications, however, do have more typical times of presentation. For example, infection of pancreatic necrosis typically occurs relatively later (e.g., 4–6 weeks into the disease course), while ischemia of the colon and gallbladder usually presents much earlier. Strictures of alimentary tract organs or bile ducts are nearly always present later. Recent studies on the natural history of pancreatic collections have revealed that pancreatic necrosis becomes largely or fully encapsulated in 43% of patients by 3 weeks and 100% by week 5 [4].

The goal of this chapter is to discuss the pathophysiology of pancreatic and peripancreatic complications with an eye to relevant molecular and cellular mechanisms covered more fully in Chap. 6.

1.1 Cellular Events and Calcium Signaling

Acinar cells, stellate cells, and ductal epithelial cells all play important roles in the cellular pathogenesis of acute pancreatitis and related local complications. The acinar cell is the most common pancreatic cell type and is functionally important for its enzyme production. The secretory demand on the acinar cell, a task that is accomplished by exocytosis, requires enormous energy consumption. Exocytosis is modulated by calcium signaling currents [5]. Cholinergic and cholecystokinin receptors on the basolateral acinar cell membrane trigger an intracellular calcium flux, mostly at the apical zymogen granule region. Further intracellular calcium is released from basolateral endoplasmic reticulum (ER) [6]. In pathologic conditions, complete emptying of the ER calcium stores leads to intracellular calcium overload, necrosis, and cell death. Both ethanol degradation to fatty acid ethyl esters and bile salts lead to strong calcium release from intracellular stores. Sustained increased intracellular calcium concentrations then lead to trypsin activation and ultimately necrotic cell death. Thus, calcium channels are attractive targets for pharmacologic intervention.

An understanding of the role of stellate cells in acute pancreatitis pathogenesis is emerging [7]. Calcium signaling in stellate cells produces inflammatory factors. Interesting recent work has shown that blockade of trypsin by deleting the trypsinogen gene decreased pancreatic necrosis but not the inflammatory response in murine experimental models of AP [5]. These data suggest a possible role of stellate cells directly modulating and promoting acute pancreatitis. And stellate cells may have a role in regeneration after acute pancreatitis [8].

Ductal epithelial cells may have a larger role in acute pancreatitis pathogenesis than previously considered. The decreasing flow of bicarbonate-rich fluid secreted by ductal cells potentially increases cellular exposure to activated enzymes within the pancreas, thereby worsening local autodigestion and subsequent necrosis [9].

Elucidation of these pathophysiologic mechanisms has identified potential therapeutic targets, including calcium cell channels such as the CRAC channel, which is the target in a current clinical trial [10, 11].

1.2 Pancreatic Necrosis and Mechanism of Cell Death

Acinar cell necrosis underlies nearly every local complication associated with severe acute pancreatitis. Although trypsin-mediated cell death leads to pancreatic injury in the early stages of pancreatitis, multiple parallel mechanisms, including activation of inflammatory cascades, endoplasmic reticulum stress, autophagy, and mitochondrial dysfunction in the acinar cells, are now recognized to be important in driving the profound systemic inflammatory response and

extensive pancreatic injury seen in acute pancreatitis [5]. It is known that acinar cells in clinical and experimental acute pancreatitis die apoptosis, nonregulated and programmed necrosis. Apoptosis is programmed cell death biologically necessary to eliminate senescent and unneeded cells. The apoptotic process leads to cellular shrinkage, nuclear fragmentation, and ultimately apoptotic bodies, which are phagocytized. During apoptosis, the cell membrane remains intact, and no leakage of intracellular organelles occurs. Therefore, this process of apoptosis does not lead to inflammation, which is the major difference from necrosis. Not surprisingly, as necrosis causes inflammation, more severe acute pancreatitis is correlated with a higher percentage of necrotic cell death. In fact, the necrosis-to-apoptosis ratio is 10:1 in mild acute pancreatitis and greater than 1000:1 in severe acute pancreatitis. These numbers are consistent in animal experimental models of pancreatitis and analysis of human acute pancreatitis patients [12].

The mechanisms mediating acinar cell necrosis in acute pancreatitis are less well understood. Necrosis may occur from external factors, such as mechanical pressure, chemical, or thermal injury, or from internal factors, such as loss of ATP, leading to the inability to maintain ion gradients through plasma and organelle membranes. The intracellular calcium overload that is a pathological condition in acute pancreatitis leads to mitochondrial overload and opening of the PTP nonselective calcium channel in the mitochondrial membrane [6]. This situation ultimately leads to loss of ATP production and cell necrosis. Other factors are also involved in the pathogenesis of pancreatic necrosis, including Ischemia due to splanchnic vasoconstriction secondary to hypovolemia, microthrombosis in a procoagulant milieu, and cytokine-mediated endothelial injury.

Importantly, necrosis leads to inflammation and is always pathological. Traditionally, cellular necrosis was thought to occur in a nonregulated fashion, but several avenues of programmed or regulated necrosis have been highlighted. These include necroptosis, pyroptosis, and ferroptosis [13, 14]. These three programmed necrosis phenotypes all result in loss of plasma membrane integrity, with an associated cellular inflammatory process. Necroptosis has been established to play a role (although to a lesser extent than unprogrammed necrosis) in acute pancreatitis. Less is known about the other two pathways of programmed necrosis in acute pancreatitis. The mechanisms of each of these three pathways are being unraveled, and each offers potential targets for intervention [12]. These include RIP kinases in necroptosis, caspases in pyroptosis, and peroxidases in ferroptosis.

Our current understanding is that unprogrammed necrosis regulated by PTP represents the major type of cell death in necrotizing pancreatitis. Experimental approaches to reduce necrosis include blocking the proteins mediating PTP channel opening, normalizing cell and mitochondrial calcium signaling, and enhancing the efficiency of autophagy to eliminate damaged mitochondria [15]. Some drugs targeting these mechanisms are currently in clinical trials for autoimmune diseases, psoriasis, Alzheimer's disease, and Covid-19.

1.3 Influence of Fluid Resuscitation on Development of Pancreatic Necrosis

Fluid resuscitation is considered a cornerstone treatment in acute pancreatitis, although there are many unanswered questions [16]. Variables that have been studied in acute pancreatitis are the rate and volume of fluid delivered as well as the type of intravenous fluid. Early clinical studies recognized that hemoconcentration, which reflects decreased intravascular volume (dehydration), is associated with increased pancreatic and peripancreatic necrosis.

The importance of adequate resuscitation to restore intravascular volume has been studied in both preclinical and clinical studies. Preclinical models of acute pancreatitis using in vivo microscopy and relative oxygen tension measurement have documented decreased blood flow to areas of the pancreas that correlate with increased parenchymal ischemia and necrosis. Randomized

animal studies, both in small animal (mice) and large animal (pig) models, have shown the ability to decrease regional hypoperfusion with increasing fluid volume administration [17, 18]. This strategy was found to increase survival but, interestingly, did not routinely change the histologic severity of necrosis. These types of studies in general support the concept that fluid resuscitation increases pancreatic perfusion and decreases the extent of pancreatic necrosis.

Several well-controlled prospective clinical studies have evaluated different resuscitation strategies, but very few of these studies included the development of necrosis as an endpoint. One study of aggressive intravascular volume resuscitation has shown decreased systemic inflammation, early organ failure, and length of hospitalization but did not change the incidence or volume of necrosis [19]. But aggressive fluid resuscitation, including rapid correction of hematocrit [20, 21], has been shown to increase new-onset organ failure and in particular increased rates of respiratory failure [22]. The recently published Waterfall trial randomized 744 patients from a multinational consortium to aggressive versus non-aggressive goal-directed fluid resuscitation in early acute pancreatitis. Interestingly, the development of necrosis development was lower (7.1%) in the moderate resuscitation group compared to the aggressive resuscitation group (13.9%). The trial was closed early as early aggressive fluid resuscitation led to a higher incidence of fluid overload without change in clinical outcome [23]. While fluid resuscitation is a cornerstone treatment, delineating its effect on the development of pancreatic necrosis requires further study, but the evidence appears clear that aggressive fluid resuscitation should be avoided.

1.4 Infection of Pancreatic Necrosis

Infection of established pancreatic necrosis contributes directly to increased systemic inflammation, organ dysfunction, and mortality in AP patients [24]. Most infected necrosis occurs in areas of established necrosis and later in the disease course. The median time to necrosis infection in several large prospective series is between 3 and 4 weeks [4].

The diagnosis of infection in early necrotizing pancreatitis is challenging due to the coincidence of noninfectious systemic inflammation with increased fever, leukocytosis, and tachycardia, which directly overlap with signs of infection. The diagnosis is usually suspected when there is a secondary deterioration in the patient's status after 2 or more weeks, associated with rising inflammatory markers (C-reactive protein, leukocytosis). A CT scan may show speckled gas within the necrotic collection in around 50% of patients with infected necrosis, but this can rarely be due to an associated enteric fistula. There may be a role for measuring procalcitonin to increase diagnostic certainty of infected necrosis [25]. Aspiration of fluid within the acute necrotic collection to confirm infection by percutaneous and endoscopic means is no longer recommended [26].

A gut origin for the majority of infecting organisms has been repeatedly confirmed, but it remains unclear about the relative importance of the different routes of infection, which include translocation, hematogenous, transcoelomic, transmural, and lymphatic pathways [27]. The primary mechanism of bacterial infection in pancreatic necrosis is probably the translocation of bacteria from the gut. For this to occur, the gut needs to be injured and the gut barrier compromised. This injury is thought to be ischemic due to reflex splanchnic vasoconstriction (in response to hypovolemia) and can be exacerbated by nonselective inotropes, aggressive resuscitation (with reperfusion injury), and aggressive early enteral feeding. It has also been shown that activated luminal pancreatic enzymes increase gut injury [28]. To achieve translocation, bacteria need to traverse the mucous layer, glycocalyx intestinal mucosa, and evade the host immune response. Activation of the immune system promotes systemic inflammatory response syndrome (SIRS). The role of the compensatory anti-inflammatory response (CARS)-associated immunosuppression results in a reduced host immune response and increases the likelihood of infection [29].

Specific data suggest a prominent role of regulatory T cells [30], which highlight potential therapeutic targets for intervention.

Contemporary analyses show an increasing proportion of gram-positive organisms infecting pancreatic necrosis compared to historical data [31] in which gram-negative and anaerobic GI flora predominated. Recent data also shows an increasing incidence of fungal infection in necrosis and up to 50% in some series [32]. No established role exists for fungal prophylaxis, but fungal infection should be treated when confirmed.

Another significant and increasing problem is the rise in the incidence of multidrug-resistant organisms in pancreatic necrosis [33]. Antibiotic stewardship is likely the best way to combat this [34]. No role exists for prophylactic antibiotic treatment to prevent infected necrosis, although a low threshold for starting antibiotics when there is a high suspicion of infected necrosis is recommended [35]. While there have been studies of antibiotic penetration of the pancreas, the challenge is obtaining a minimum inhibitory concentration in the necrotic pancreas [36]. Therapy of extra pancreatic infections for a defined period of time is clearly indicated to treat pneumonia, urinary tract, infection, catheter-based infections, and others [37]. Biliary decompression (in addition to systemic antibiotic therapy) is the key to treating acute cholangitis and cholecystitis. Decompression may be accomplished with ERCP, to treat cholangitis, and percutaneous cholecystostomy or cholecystectomy (depending on the clinical situation), to treat cholecystitis [38].

Treatment of established infection in necrotic material is more challenging. Up to 25% of patients with infected necrosis can be treated definitively with antibiotics alone. But patients who do not respond to antibiotic treatment should be treated following the step-up approach, which means either endoscopic or percutaneous drainage [39]. Failure to progress despite adequate drainage will require the removal of infected necrosis. This can be done endoscopically, minimally invasively (laparoscope or nephroscope) [40], and openly (transabdominal or transgastric) [41].

2   Local Vascular Complications

Vascular complications of pancreatitis can affect both splanchnic venous and arterial systems.

2.1   Venous Complications

Venous thrombosis and thromboembolism (VTE) in the setting of necrotizing pancreatitis is a significant and remarkably common problem [42]. Isolated splenic vein thrombosis is the most common, affecting about 50% of patients with splanchnic thrombi. Many patients have a combination of splenic with portal and/or superior mesenteric vein (SMV) thrombosis. VTE is both a local and systemic complication, including systemic inflammation and hypercoagulability. Large retrospective and prospective surveillance studies have documented the risk of VTE in 57% to 65% of necrotizing pancreatitis patients [43]. Not surprisingly, a substantial proportion of venous thrombosis is found locally in the splanchnic circulation (48% to 50% of all thrombi). Extremity deep vein thrombosis (DVT) has an incidence of 16 to 38% and pulmonary emboli 6% of NP patients. The extremity DVT and PE incidence are up to tenfold higher than the incidence observed in a general hospitalized population [42, 44]. A screening strategy is important for early identification of extremity DVT, permitting early treatment. This strategy has been shown to decrease symptomatic pulmonary embolism.

Local splanchnic vein thrombosis is caused by pressure from the pancreatic collection (fluid ± necrosis) as well as the local and systemic hypercoagulable effects of the inflammatory process [45]. The risk factors for developing venous thromboembolism are male gender, history of previous venous thrombosis, and necrosis infection.

Based on evidence from retrospective studies, a prospective screening protocol for DVT has been introduced for necrotizing pancreatitis patients [42, 44]. The patient underwent four extremity duplex ultrasonography on a weekly basis during the acute phase of their disease. An even greater number of extremity DVTs (38%) were diagnosed compared to patients reviewed retrospectively. DVT was diagnosed a mean time of 44 days after disease initiation. Importantly, symptomatic pulmonary emboli were prevented in *all* patients with no contraindication to anticoagulation.

It has been suggested that the measurement of anti-factor Xa concentration could be helpful in the setting of prophylactic anticoagulation [46]. Satisfactory anti-Xa concentration was only achieved in 21% of patients, and no extremity DVT developed in patients who were able to achieve appropriate anti-factor Xa levels. These data suggest that an increased dose of pharmacologic prophylactic antithrombotic medication administration may be necessary for the inflammatory setting of necrotizing pancreatitis and that an individualized dosing strategy based on anti-factor Xa measurement may be an effective way to measure the appropriate dose.

Splanchnic venous thrombosis can be complete or partial and occur without or with mass effect from adjacent necrosis. Early decompression of the necrosis mass effect may prevent some splanchnic venous thrombosis, though this has not been proven. Currently, there are no high-quality evidence-based recommendations to guide the management of anticoagulation in patients with acute pancreatitis [47]. Analysis of a large series of splanchnic venous thrombosis suggests that isolated splenic vein thrombosis has a relatively benign clinical course, and it is not considered essential that anticoagulation should be administered to isolated splenic vein thrombosis. On the other hand, superior mesenteric vein and portal vein thromboses are associated with significant clinical consequences. Complete SMV/PV thrombosis is unlikely to recannulate especially in the clinical setting where necrosis around the pancreatic head remains in situ. The decision as to whether to anticoagulate complete SMV/PV vein thrombosis is debated [48]. These patients have substantial challenges with enteral absorption and often require prolonged parenteral nutritional support. Ultimately, collateral vein development around the pancreatic head (so-called "cavernous transformation")

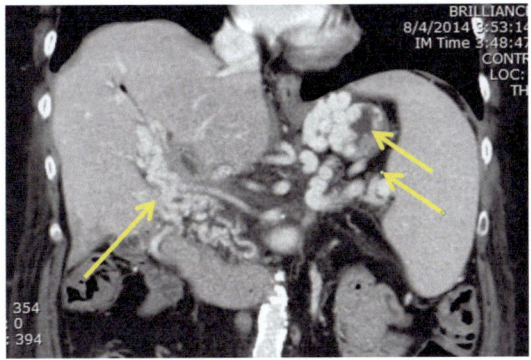

Fig. 3 Coronal CT image of patient whose splanchnic vein thrombosis resolved with collateral vein formation in the porta hepatis ("cavernous transformation"—arrow) and left upper quadrant (left-sided or "sinistral" portal hypertension—double arrow)

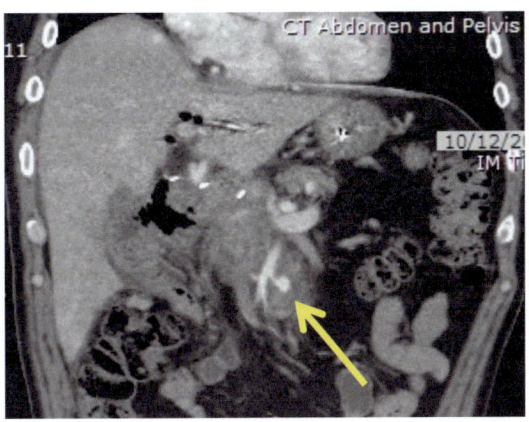

Fig. 4 Pseudoaneurysm arising from the superior mesenteric artery (arrow). Note hematoma mixed with necrosis surrounding the pseudoaneurysm

will allow relatively normal alimentation in many patients, though this process often takes many months (Fig. 3). Patients with nonocclusive SMV/PV thrombosis will usually benefit from systemic anticoagulation to stabilize the clot, prevent progression to complete thrombosis, and allow thrombolysis over time. Future work in this area will help to understand the role of the local and systemic anti-inflammatory response on the hypercoagulable state and ideally identify a strategy to select patients for anticoagulation [48].

2.2 Arterial Complications

Visceral artery pseudoaneurysms (PSA) is a potentially life-threatening local complication of NP. The mortality associated with PSA is 14% and is due to bleeding [49]. Risk factors for the development of PSA include age greater than 50, organ failure, infection of necrosis, and disconnected pancreatic duct syndrome. The clinician's index of suspicion for PSA should be raised in the setting of these clinical findings. The pathophysiology of arterial wall weakening and pseudoaneurysm development is likely due to persistent inflammation and pancreatic enzyme bioactivity [49]. There is a plausible association between infected necrosis and the site of a PSA site. It is likely that the early treatment of infected

pancreatic necrosis will reduce the risk of visceral PSA formation.

In a large series of 647 patients with pancreatic necrosis, there were 28 (4.3%) who developed visceral PSA. The most common arteries involved were the splenic artery (36%) and the gastroduodenal artery (24%). It is important to recognize that virtually any artery in the visceral arterial distribution may develop PSA in the setting of pancreatitis (Fig. 4). Pseudoaneurysms were recognized at a median of 63 days after the initial AP insult, although a broad range of time to diagnosis was seen, including PSA diagnosed more than a year after the patient's hospital admission.

Patients with PSA do not usually have clinical signs or symptoms related to it. There may be an increase in abdominal pain with active bleeding, and this will usually be associated with signs of hypotension. A PSA is sometimes diagnosed incidentally on cross-sectional imaging. This diagnosis of PSA must be considered when blood appears in an abdominal or percutaneous drain. The increasing use of endoscopic transgastric draining does not allow early detection of bleeding from a PSA, and it might be evident with blood in the nasogastric tube or with hematemesis. The "herald" or "index" bleed is important to recognize, because there is often time before a second catastrophic bleed, giving time for diagnosis and treatment.

The early recognition of the presence of a pseudoaneurysm can facilitate expedited care in an expert center of a complex pathology that may require angiographic, percutaneous, endoscopic, or surgical intervention to prevent catastrophic hemorrhage [50]. The preferred approach to treatment is interventional radiology (IR) splanchnic angiography. A combination of coil or glue embolization and occasionally stenting are usually offered [51]. These IR approaches are successful in treating virtually all PSAs, and surgical approaches are almost never indicated.

3 Alimentary Tract Complications

Local complications of necrotizing pancreatitis can affect the stomach and all parts of the alimentary tract distal to it and can include ischemia, perforation, fistula, stricture, or ileus.

3.1 Stomach

Gastric ileus is a well-recognized but poorly studied clinical problem. In the setting of necrotizing pancreatitis, the retrogastric local collections and inflammation are thought to be important in the pathophysiology of gastric ileus. And opioid analgesia may also contribute. In some cases, the mass effect due to the collection can result in extrinsic compression of the stomach gastric outlet obstruction. From a therapeutic standpoint, a cautious trial of oral feeding is reasonable, and feeding tolerance does not correlate well with the CT findings. If the patient does not tolerate oral diet, nasogastric or nasojejunal tube feeding may be warranted. Persistent feeding intolerance will result in the need for parenteral nutrition to achieve nutritional requirements.

3.2 Duodenum

The local complications involving the duodenum include fistula and stricture [52]. Despite its robust blood supply, duodenal fistula is most

likely related to a consequence of ischemia instrumentation, either by percutaneous drain, endoscopic intervention, or operative intervention [53]. Ischemia can lead to perforation of the duodenum, and while this might result in a contained collection, it can cause peritonitis. Duodenal stricture is a later consequence of the disease and is often diagnosed a year or more from the onset of AP. Patients with duodenal stricture most commonly have parenchymal necrosis in the pancreatic head and are due to local inflammation, followed by scarring and fibrotic healing process after resolution of this necrosis.

Risk factors for developing both fistula and stricture include for severe pancreatitis, increased degree of pancreatic necrosis, infected necrosis, organ failure, and disease duration [52]. Both stricture and fistula of the duodenum are difficult problems to manage. Fistula presents the clinician with challenges maintaining fluid and electrolyte balance, which is critically important in the short and intermediate term to nurse the patient to the point where intervention will be possible. Less well appreciated is the fact that losses of foregut secretions including bile causes a large energy deficit to the body. Refeeding of proximal fistula GI loss through the downstream feeding tube, when technically feasible, will facilitate recuperation in patients with high-volume loss. Duodenal fistula is associated with substantially increased mortality with up to a third of NP patients with duodenal fistula dying because of this complication (ref). Stricture of the duodenum can present a significant management challenge [52]. The Strictured duodenal anatomy is very difficult to manage endoscopically. Most patients with duodenal complications require operative correction—itself a substantial undertaking that should be managed at appropriate time in the disease course.

3.3 Small Bowel

Few studies have investigated isolated jejunal and ileal complications in patients with severe acute pancreatitis. Small bowel fistula is relatively common [54] and is associated with local inflammatory response and pancreatic necrosis. Prompt clearance of surrounding infected necrosis is important in treating small bowel fistula. Percutaneous drainage with appropriate drain downsizing and stepwise withdrawal can dissuade cutaneous for internal drainage and may be all that is required in some patients with isolated small bowel fistula. The majority of small bowel fistulae ultimately require surgical treatment. The principles of this are to restore hydration, electrolytes, and nutritional status before surgical resection and anastomosis [55]. Small bowel stricture of the midgut is rarely seen in the context of acute pancreatitis.

Jejunal and ileal ischemia is relatively rare in clinical practice. The pathophysiology of small bowel ischemia is usually due to a vascular catastrophe or shock in a critically ill patient. In the latter setting, splanchnic vasoconstriction in response to hypovolemia can result in nonocclusive mesenteric ischemia, which can be exacerbated by aggressive enteral nutrition and inotropic support [56]. Less commonly, mid-small bowel ischemia may be related to local mesenteric venous thrombosis. Small bowel ileus [57] is reasonably common, especially in the early stages of severe pancreatitis. It is thought to occur as a result of ischemic gut injury as well as narcotics. Though early enteral nutrition is attractive and clearly beneficial to patients who tolerate this treatment, clinicians must be conscious of the potential for enteral feeding intolerance in the setting of ileus. This means that enteral nutrition should be advanced judiciously in these patients.

3.4   Colon

Colonic complications occur in up to 15% of patients with necrotizing pancreatitis and also encompass ischemia, fistula, and stricture [58]. The clinical detection of ischemia and necrosis (usually with peritonitis) is at a median of 25 [1, 2, 4–56] days and colonic strictures (usually with bowel obstruction) at a median of 50 (10–270) days [58]. Ischemia of the colon is commonly related to nonocclusive mesenteric ischemia,

venous thrombosis, and outflow obstruction. This venous obstruction often happens at a local segmental level of the bowel and is related to local inflammation and possibly compression from adjacent acute fluid and necrotic collections. The diagnosis of mesenteric vein thrombosis should also alert clinicians to the potential for colonic ischemia, as ischemia was noted to develop approximately 2 weeks after the diagnosis of mesenteric vein thrombosis.

Ischemic perforation is more common in the colon than in any other location of the GI tract and is more common in the right than left colon. This is a challenge to diagnose in patients with severe acute necrotizing pancreatitis who often have severe abdominal pain and peritonism on top of coincident multiple confounding comorbidities. It can be associated with colonic bleeding. Diagnosis is especially difficult in patients who are ventilated in the intensive care unit, where clinical examination is unhelpful. The diagnosis of pneumatosis intestinalis and free air on CT scanning is diagnostic, and impaired mucosal perfusion may be evident on the arterial contrast phase.

Injury to the colonic flexures and fistulation can occur when these are "taken down" at the time open necrosectomy to allow better access and facilitate insertion of retroperitoneal flank drains. This was also thought to reduce the risk of instrumental colonic injury at the time of necrosectomy and later due to erosion by the drains themselves. More recently colonic fistulae have been reported in relation to the insertion of flank drains by radiologists and by minimally invasive surgical approaches to pancreatic debridement, especially from the left, where the splenic flexure is particularly vulnerable.

Colonic stricture is a much later problem and is probably most often a long-term consequence of ischemia with fibrosis. Colon ischemic strictures are typically quite long, which makes endoscopic stenting more difficult and colectomy more often required [58].

Pseudomembranous colitis from *Clostridioides* (formerly *Clostridium*) *difficile* (*C diff*) infection is an infectious complication unique to the colon. *C. diff* infection can affect up to 10% of necrotizing pancreatitis patients [59]. It is usual to attribute *C. diff* infection to the use of broad-spectrum antibiotic therapy, but other factors such as colonic ischemia, dysbiosis, and protein-calorie malnutrition may be risk factors. It appears that the morbidity and mortality of *C. diff* in patients with severe acute pancreatitis is no higher than in other patients with critical illness. Therapy of *C. diff* is the same as that provided to any other patient population: systemic and enteral antibiotics directed toward the causative organism are the cornerstone of treatment. The role of probiotics and fecal microbiotic transplantation remain to be defined in the NP population. Prevention of *C. diff* by judicious prescription of systemic antibiotics is the best way to minimize this problem in the setting of necrotizing pancreatitis.

4   Biliary Complications

Local biliary complications can involve the gallbladder or the extrahepatic biliary tree.

Patients with necrotizing pancreatitis of biliary etiology are at risk from gallstone-related complications, including acute cholecystitis, choledocholithiasis, and acute cholangitis. It is worth noting that biliary complications, including acalculous cholecystitis, can also arise in patients with other etiologies for acute pancreatitis.

Acute cholecystitis is a challenging diagnosis in the early phase of necrotizing pancreatitis. Symptoms and signs of cholecystitis are easily masked by abdominal pain, distention, nausea, and vomiting that are often present in this phase of severe AP. Indeed, cholecystitis may progress to gallbladder necrosis and perforation. Depending on the clinical circumstance, percutaneous cholecystostomy may be the most appropriate therapy for acute cholecystitis in the early NP course. However, should a patient fail to improve promptly after cholecystostomy, the diagnosis of gangrenous cholecystitis must be considered.

Cholecystectomy is recommended before discharge in patients with mild to moderate acute pancreatitis of biliary etiology [60]. But in patients with severe acute pancreatitis due to gallstones, cholecystectomy is usually delayed until need for intervention for infected pancreatic necrosis is determined. This strategy permitted cholecystectomy to be performed under a single anesthetic along with debridement of infected necrosis. With the widespread application of minimally invasive approaches to pancreatic debridement, this presents a new challenge for timely cholecystectomy and the prevention of recurrence of acute pancreatitis [60].

Acute cholangitis in the acute phase of necrotizing pancreatitis may be a consequence of choledocholithiasis, while later in the disease course, it might also be secondary to biliary stricture or an occluded biliary stent. The early diagnosis of cholangitis is important as it is in indication for decompression of the biliary tree [61]. The diagnosis of cholangitis can be difficult but helped by the clinical recognition of Charcot's triad (obstructive jaundice, biliary-type pain, and fever with rigors) and cholestatic liver dysfunction. The acute treatment is broad-spectrum antibiotics and biliary decompression by either endoscopic sphincterotomy and/or stenting by either the endoscopic or percutaneous transhepatic route [61]. This should only be offered to those with cholangitis and not just for cholestasis alone.

An extrahepatic biliary stricture is a later complication in patients with NP and presents at a median interval of 4.2 months from the onset of pancreatitis [62]. Risk factors for bile duct stricture include pancreatic head necrosis, splanchnic vein thrombosis, and atrial fibrillation. Cholestasis and jaundice are the most common presentations. Patients presented less frequently with abdominal pain and a small proportion (4%) with overt acute cholangitis [62]. Most patients with necrotizing pancreatitis who develop biliary strictures are successfully managed by stenting (endoscopic or less

Fig. 5 Biliary stricture during acute episode of necrotizing pancreatitis (**a**, arrows) resolved after 3 months of biliary stenting (**b**)

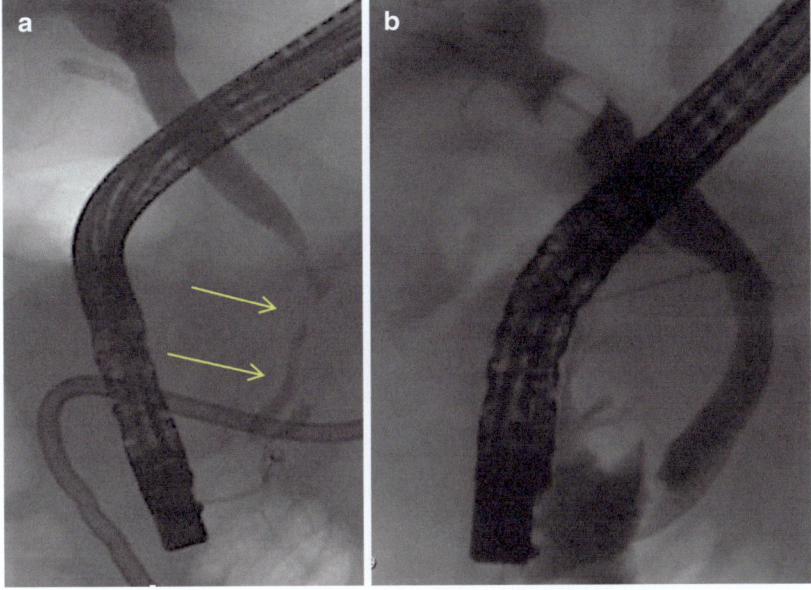

often percutaneous) with surgical hepatico-jejunostomy required in about 20% (Fig. 5) [63].

5 Other Pancreatic Complications

In addition to the obvious pancreatic parenchymal necrosis, pancreas-associated local complications include acute fluid collections (AFC), pancreatic ascites, disconnected pancreatic duct syndrome (DPDS), and peripancreatic necrosis.

5.1 Acute Fluid Collections and Pseudocysts

Acute fluid collections are a common feature with acute pancreatitis (Fig. 1), especially when severe, but they are not a marker of severity [64]. Early percutaneous drainage of pancreatic acute fluid collections does not impact disease progression and can introduce infection [65]. The vast majority reabsorb spontaneously and drainage should be reserved for when there is high suspicion of infection [66]. When they encapsulate, in the absence of necrosis, they are defined as pseu-

docysts and may warrant treatment, either endoscopic or surgical [67]. Absolute size thresholds for intervention are no longer advised, and treatment is usually reserved for those with symptoms related to the mass effect, for instance, gastric or duodenal obstruction and/or early satiety [65].

5.2 Disconnected Pancreatic Duct Syndrome

Disconnected Pancreatic Duct Syndrome (DPDS) is defined as a peripancreatic fluid collection due to leakage of pancreatic secretions from the main pancreatic duct in the setting where there is viable proximal pancreas upstream (toward the spleen) that has lost continuity with the remaining distal pancreas downstream (toward the duodenum) (Fig. 6). This can occur with complete disconnection or with partial disruption of the main pancreatic duct. The pathophysiology of the DPDS in AP is related to pancreatic necrosis causing injury to the main pancreatic duct. This means that the collection is technically not a pseudocyst, because there is underlying necrosis, which means that after 4 weeks, it is defined as walled off necrosis. The collection is often large

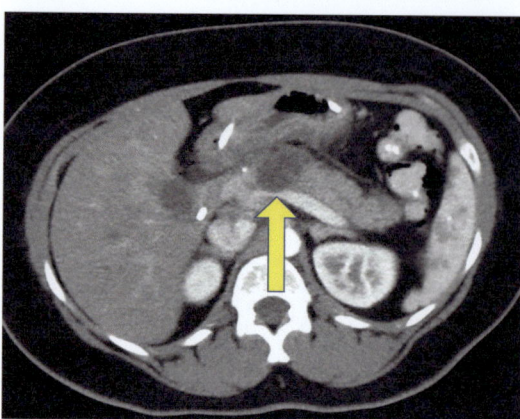

Fig. 6 Axial CT image showing typical example of DPDS—parenchymal necrosis at the pancreatic neck (arrow) with viable gland upstream to the tail

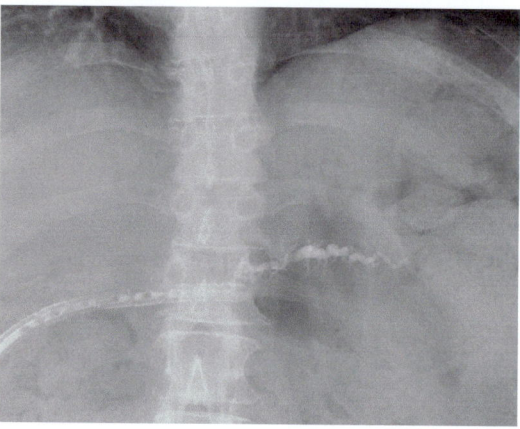

Fig. 7 Contrast sinogram through surgical drain left at the time of pancreatic debridement. The patient had externally controlled pancreatic fistula draining about 150 mL per day and was recovering clinically. Contrast communicates with a large viable pancreatic tail remnant

(10–30 cm in diameter). Review of a large single tertiary center experience of 647 patients with necrotizing pancreatitis identified 299 (46%) who developed DPDS [44]. This review is biased on tertiary referral practice, meaning that the overall incidence of DPDS is a lot lower. DPDS represents a remarkably heterogeneous process and can range from a large volume of viable tail with small neck disruption to nearly complete necrosis of the pancreatic body/tail with just a small "nugget" of viable tail in the splenic hilum. The volume of upstream viable pancreatic tail

impacts treatment decisions (Fig. 7), which can be endoscopic or surgical. Radiological external drainage of the collection is not advised, as this is likely to result in a pancreatic fistula, which will likely persist. For this reason, DPDS should be considered when considering treatment of a persistent fluid collection. Endoscopic treatment entails internal drainage of the collection into the stomach or duodenum with plastic or metal stents [68]. Rarely, pancreas duct disruption in the neck or body of the gland can be treated with endoscopic transpapillary stenting. Disruptions further to the left are best treated operatively [69]. Stenting across the point of leakage from the main pancreatic duct is usually easier if the duct is only partially disrupted. Long-term follow-up of endoscopically treated patients is not available. Surgical treatment involves either drainage or resection. Drainage in this setting means a pancreato-enterostomy, where the jejunum is anastomosed to the side or dependent portion of the mature (encapsulated) collection (i.e., has a thick enough wall to take a suture). Sometimes, this is within the lesser sac and less often through the transverse mesocolon in the infracolic compartment. This approach can also be used for walled off necrosis, with debridement performed before the formation of the anastomosis. Drainage is preferable to resection of the proximal pancreas. Maintaining the patency of the anastomosis requires a sufficient flow of pancreatic secretion, and preserving islet cell mass is important in reducing the risk of diabetes. However, a small-volume residual tail responsible for a persistent collection may be best treated by resection. This is often made substantially more challenging by the presence of splenic vein thrombosis with left-sided (sinistral) portal hypertension.

5.3 Pancreatic Ascites

Pancreatic ascites results from disruption of the pancreatic duct and drainage of pancreatic secretions into the peritoneal cavity [70]. This is usually into the lesser sac but will spread to the whole peritoneal cavity via the foramen of

Winslow. This is sparce evidence in the literature about the incidence, treatment, and outcomes for pancreatic ascites. If the leak from the main pancreatic duct is in the head and neck, it may be possible to treat it by the endoscopic transpapillary route [71]. Persistent symptomatic ascites may require surgery. Pancreatico-jejunostomy is rarely possible, and resection will be necessary but only after an interval when the abdomen is less hostile and the patient's condition has improved and stabilized.

5.4 Peripancreatic Necrosis

The significance of extra- or peripancreatic necrosis has only been appreciated relatively recently [72], is evident on contrast CT scanning, and is an independent risk factor for pancreatitis severity [73], and this probably mediated by increased unsaturated fatty acids [74].

6 Conclusion

Most local complications associated with severe acute pancreatitis are related to the development of pancreatic and peripancreatic necrosis and associated inflammation. Clearly defining and understanding the pathophysiology of the different local complications is helpful in treating the underlying cause. While the expert and expeditious early management of acute pancreatitis may reduce the incidence of local complications, they will continue to present challenges to the treating clinician. Understanding the natural history and prognostic significance of local complications helps in determining the optimal timing and type of intervention to give the best opportunity to reduce their impact on clinical outcome.

References

1. Banks PA, Bollen TL, Dervenis C, Gooszen HG, Johnson CD, Sarr MG, et al. Classification of acute pancreatitis—2012: revision of the Atlanta classification and definitions by international consensus. Gut. 2013;62(1):102–11.

2. Dellinger EP, Forsmark CE, Layer P, Levy P, Maravi-Poma E, Petrov MS, et al. Determinant-based classification of acute pancreatitis severity: an international multidisciplinary consultation. Ann Surg. 2012;256(6):875–80.

3. Windsor JA, Petrov MS. Acute pancreatitis reclassified. Gut. 2013;62(1):4–5.

4. van Grinsven J, van Brunschot S, van Baal MC, Besselink MG, Fockens P, van Goor H, et al. Natural history of gas configurations and encapsulation in necrotic collections during necrotizing pancreatitis. J Gastrointest Surg. 2018;22(9):1557–64.

5. Saluja A, Dudeja V, Dawra R, Sah RP. Early intra-acinar events in pathogenesis of pancreatitis. Gastroenterology. 2019;156(7):1979–93.

6. Petersen OH. The 2022 George E Palade medal lecture: toxic ca(2+) signals in acinar, stellate and endogenous immune cells are important drivers of acute pancreatitis. Pancreatology. 2023;23(1):1–8.

7. Omary MB, Lugea A, Lowe AW, Pandol SJ. The pancreatic stellate cell: a star on the rise in pancreatic diseases. J Clin Invest. 2007;117(1):50–9.

8. Zimmermann A, Gloor B, Kappeler A, Uhl W, Friess H, Buchler MW. Pancreatic stellate cells contribute to regeneration early after acute necrotising pancreatitis in humans. Gut. 2002;51(4):574–8.

9. Hegyi P, Petersen OH. The exocrine pancreas: the acinar-ductal tango in physiology and pathophysiology. Rev Physiol Biochem Pharmacol. 2013;165:1–30.

10. Bruen C, Miller J, Wilburn J, Mackey C, Bollen TL, Stauderman K, et al. Auxora for the treatment of patients with acute pancreatitis and accompanying systemic inflammatory response syndrome: clinical development of a calcium release-activated Calcium Channel inhibitor. Pancreas. 2021;50(4):537–43.

11. Petersen OH, Gerasimenko JV, Gerasimenko OV, Gryshchenko O, Peng S. The roles of calcium and ATP in the physiology and pathology of the exocrine pancreas. Physiol Rev. 2021;101(4):1691–744.

12. Green DR. The cell's dilemma, or the story of cell death: an entertainment in three acts. FEBS J. 2016;283(14):2568–76.

13. Linkermann A, Green DR. Necroptosis. N Engl J Med. 2014;370(5):455–65.

14. Yang WS, Stockwell BR. Ferroptosis: death by lipid peroxidation. Trends Cell Biol. 2016;26(3):165–76.

15. Toth E, Maleth J, Zavogyan N, Fanczal J, Grassalkovich A, Erdos R, et al. Novel mitochondrial transition pore inhibitor N-methyl-4-isoleucine cyclosporin is a new therapeutic option in acute pancreatitis. J Physiol. 2019;597(24):5879–98.

16. Haydock MD, Mittal A, Wilms HR, Phillips A, Petrov MS, Windsor JA. Fluid therapy in acute pancreatitis. Ann Surg. 2013;257(2):182–8.

17. Kusterer K, Enghofer M, Zendler S, Blochle C, Usadel KH. Microcirculatory changes in sodium taurocholate-induced pancreatitis in rats. Am J Phys. 1991;260(2 Pt 1):G346–51.

18. Kinnala PJ, Kuttila KT, Gronroos JM, Havia TV, Nevalainen TJ, Niinikoski JH. Splanchnic and pan-

creatic tissue perfusion in experimental acute pancreatitis. Scand J Gastroenterol. 2002;37(7):845–9.

19. Di Martino M, Van Laarhoven S, Ielpo B, Ramia JM, Manuel-Vazquez A, Martinez-Perez A, et al. Systematic review and meta-analysis of fluid therapy protocols in acute pancreatitis: type, rate and route. HPB (Oxford). 2021;23(11):1629–38.

20. Mao EQ, Tang YQ, Fei J, Qin S, Wu J, Li L, et al. Fluid therapy for severe acute pancreatitis in acute response stage. Chin Med J. 2009;122(2):169–73.

21. Mao EQ, Fei J, Peng YB, Huang J, Tang YQ, Zhang SD. Rapid hemodilution is associated with increased sepsis and mortality among patients with severe acute pancreatitis. Chin Med J. 2010;123(13):1639–44.

22. Jin T, Jiang K, Deng L, Guo J, Wu Y, Wang Z, et al. Response and outcome from fluid resuscitation in acute pancreatitis a prospective cohort study. HPB (Oxford); 2018.

23. de Madaria E, Buxbaum JL, Maisonneuve P, Garcia Garcia de Paredes A, Zapater P, Guilabert L, et al. Aggressive or moderate fluid resuscitation in acute pancreatitis. N Engl J Med. 2022;387(11):989–1000.

24. Besselink MG, van Santvoort HC, Boermeester MA, Nieuwenhuijs VB, van Goor H, Dejong CH, et al. Timing and impact of infections in acute pancreatitis. Br J Surg. 2009;96(3):267–73.

25. Mofidi R, Suttie SA, Patil PV, Ogston S, Parks RW. The value of procalcitonin at predicting the severity of acute pancreatitis and development of infected pancreatic necrosis: systematic review. Surgery. 2009;146(1):72–81.

26. van Baal MC, Bollen TL, Bakker OJ, van Goor H, Boermeester MA, Dejong CH, et al. The role of routine fine-needle aspiration in the diagnosis of infected necrotizing pancreatitis. Surgery. 2014;155(3):442–8.

27. Bakoyiannis A, Delis S, Dervenis C. Pathophysiology of acute and infected pancreatitis. Infect Disord Drug Targets. 2010;10(1):2–4.

28. Schmid-Schonbein GW, Chang M. The autodigestion hypothesis for shock and multi-organ failure. Ann Biomed Eng. 2014;42(2):405–14.

29. Lee PJ, Papachristou GI. New insights into acute pancreatitis. Nat Rev Gastroenterol Hepatol. 2019;16(8):479–96.

30. Glaubitz J, Wilden A, Frost F, Ameling S, Homuth G, Mazloum H, et al. Activated regulatory T-cells promote duodenal bacterial translocation into necrotic areas in severe acute pancreatitis. Gut. 2023;72(7):1355–69.

31. Howard TJ, Temple MB. Prophylactic antibiotics alter the bacteriology of infected necrosis in severe acute pancreatitis. J Am Coll Surg. 2002;195(6):759–67.

32. Singh RR, Mitchell W, David Y, Cheesman A, Dixon RE, Nagula S, et al. Pancreatic fungal infection in patients with necrotizing pancreatitis: a systematic review and meta-analysis. J Clin Gastroenterol. 2021;55(3):218–26.

33. Soulountsi V, Schizodimos T. Use of antibiotics in acute pancreatitis: ten major concerns. Scand J Gastroenterol. 2020;55(10):1211–8.

34. Barrie J, Jamdar S, Smith N, McPherson SJ, Siriwardena AK, O'Reilly DA. Mis-use of antibiotics in acute pancreatitis: insights from the United Kingdom's National Confidential Enquiry into patient outcome and death (NCEPOD) survey of acute pancreatitis. Pancreatology. 2018;18(7):721–6.

35. Dellinger EP, Tellado JM, Soto NE, Ashley SW, Barie PS, Dugernier T, et al. Early antibiotic treatment for severe acute necrotizing pancreatitis: a randomized, double-blind, placebo-controlled study. Ann Surg. 2007;245(5):674–83.

36. Bassi C, Pederzoli P, Vesentini S, Falconi M, Bonora A, Abbas H, et al. Behavior of antibiotics during human necrotizing pancreatitis. Antimicrob Agents Chemother. 1994;38(4):830–6.

37. Brown LA, Hore TA, Phillips AR, Windsor JA, Petrov MS. A systematic review of the extra-pancreatic infectious complications in acute pancreatitis. Pancreatology. 2014;14(6):436–43.

38. Hallensleben ND, Stassen PMC, Schepers NJ, Besselink MG, Anten MGF, Bakker OJ, et al. Patient selection for urgent endoscopic retrograde cholangio-pancreatography by endoscopic ultrasound in predicted severe acute biliary pancreatitis (APEC-2): a multicentre prospective study. Gut. 2023;72(8):1534–42.

39. Besselink MG. The 'step-up approach' to infected necrotizing pancreatitis: delay, drain, debride. Dig Liver Dis. 2011;43(6):421–2.

40. Freeman ML, Werner J, van Santvoort HC, Baron TH, Besselink MG, Windsor JA, et al. Interventions for necrotizing pancreatitis: summary of a multidisciplinary consensus conference. Pancreas. 2012;41(8):1176–94.

41. Driedger M, Zyromski NJ, Visser BC, Jester A, Sutherland FR, Nakeeb A, et al. Surgical Transgastric Necrosectomy for necrotizing pancreatitis: a single-stage procedure for walled-off pancreatic necrosis. Ann Surg. 2020;271(1):163–8.

42. Roch AM, Maatman TK, Carr RA, Colgate CL, Ceppa EP, House MG, et al. Venous thromboembolism in necrotizing pancreatitis: an underappreciated risk. J Gastrointest Surg. 2019;23(12):2430–8.

43. Anis FS, Adiamah A, Lobo DN, Sanyal S. Incidence and treatment of splanchnic vein thrombosis in patients with acute pancreatitis: a systematic review and meta-analysis. J Gastroenterol Hepatol. 2022;37(3):446–54.

44. Maatman TK, Roch AM, Ceppa EP, Easler JJ, Gromski MA, House MG, et al. The continuum of complications in survivors of necrotizing pancreatitis. Surgery. 2020;168(6):1032–40.

45. Oyon D, Marra-Lopez C, Bolado F, Lopez-Lopez S, Ibanez-Beroiz B, Canaval-Zuleta HJ, et al. Determinants and impact of splanchnic vein thrombosis in acute pancreatitis. Dig Liver Dis. 2023;55(11):1480–6.

46. Kramme K, Sarraf P, Munene G. Prophylactic enoxaparin adjusted by anti-factor Xa peak levels compared with recommended Thromboprophylaxis and

rates of clinically evident venous thromboembolism in surgical oncology patients. J Am Coll Surg. 2020;230(3):314–21.

47. Ghazanfar MA, Ke L, Ramsay G, Smith M, Giovinazzo F, Mohamed M, et al. Management of Splanchnic Vein Thrombosis in patients with acute pancreatitis: an international survey of current practice. Pancreas. 2022;51(9):1211–6.

48. Chandan S, Buddam A, Khan SR, Mohan BP, Ramai D, Bilal M, et al. Use of therapeutic anticoagulation in splanchnic vein thrombosis associated with acute pancreatitis: a systematic review and meta-analysis. Ann Gastroenterol. 2021;34(6):862–71.

49. Maatman TK, Heimberger MA, Lewellen KA, Roch AM, Colgate CL, House MG, et al. Visceral artery pseudoaneurysm in necrotizing pancreatitis: incidence and outcomes. Can J Surg. 2020;63(3):E272–E7.

50. Evans RP, Mourad MM, Pall G, Fisher SG, Bramhall SR. Pancreatitis: preventing catastrophic haemorrhage. World J Gastroenterol. 2017;23(30):5460–8.

51. Zabicki B, Limphaibool N, Holstad MJV, Juszkat R. Endovascular management of pancreatitis-related pseudoaneurysms: a review of techniques. PLoS One. 2018;13(1):e0191998.

52. Banter LR, Maatman TK, McGuire SP, Ceppa EP, House MG, Nakeeb A, et al. Duodenal complications in necrotizing pancreatitis: challenges of an overlooked complication. Am J Surg. 2021;221(3):589–93.

53. Tsiotos GG, Smith CD, Sarr MG. Incidence and management of pancreatic and enteric fistulas after surgical management of severe necrotizing pancreatitis. Arch Surg. 1995;130(1):48–52.

54. Kochhar R, Jain K, Gupta V, Singhal M, Kochhar S, Poornachandra KS, et al. Fistulization in the GI tract in acute pancreatitis. Gastrointest Endosc. 2012;75(2):436–40.

55. Ashkenazi I, Turegano-Fuentes F, Olsha O, Alfici R. Treatment options in gastrointestinal cutaneous fistulas. Surg J (N Y). 2017;3(1):e25–31.

56. Al-Diery H, Phillips A, Evennett N, Pandanaboyana S, Gilham M, Windsor JA. The pathogenesis of nonocclusive mesenteric ischemia: implications for research and clinical practice. J Intensive Care Med. 2019;34(10):771–81.

57. Moran RA, Jalaly NY, Kamal A, Rao S, Klapheke R, James TW, et al. Ileus is a predictor of local infection in patients with acute necrotizing pancreatitis. Pancreatology. 2016;16(6):966–72.

58. Mohamed SR, Siriwardena AK. Understanding the colonic complications of pancreatitis. Pancreatology. 2008;8(2):153–8.

59. Maatman TK, Westfall-Snyder JA, Nicolas ME, Yee EJ, Ceppa EP, House MG, et al. The morbidity of C. Difficile in necrotizing pancreatitis. Am J Surg. 2020;219(3):509–12.

60. Di Martino M, Ielpo B, Pata F, Pellino G, Di Saverio S, Catena F, et al. Timing of cholecystectomy after moderate and severe acute biliary pancreatitis. JAMA Surg. 2023;158(10):e233660.

61. Mederos MA, Reber HA, Girgis MD. Acute pancreatitis: a review. JAMA. 2021;325(4):382–90.

62. Maatman TK, Ceppa EP, Fogel EL, Easier JJ, Gromski MA, House MG, et al. Biliary stricture after necrotizing pancreatitis: an underappreciated challenge. Ann Surg. 2022;276(1):167–72.

63. Nakai Y, Isayama H, Wang HP, Rerknimitr R, Khor C, Yasuda I, et al. International consensus statements for endoscopic management of distal biliary stricture. J Gastroenterol Hepatol. 2020;35(6):967–79.

64. Cui ML, Kim KH, Kim HG, Han J, Kim H, Cho KB, et al. Incidence, risk factors and clinical course of pancreatic fluid collections in acute pancreatitis. Dig Dis Sci. 2014;59(5):1055–62.

65. Habashi S, Draganov PV. Pancreatic pseudocyst. World J Gastroenterol. 2009;15(1):38–47.

66. Agalianos C, Passas I, Sideris I, Davides D, Dervenis C. Review of management options for pancreatic pseudocysts. Transl Gastroenterol Hepatol. 2018;3:18.

67. Farias GFA, Bernardo WM, De Moura DTH, Guedes HG, Brunaldi VO, Visconti TAC, et al. Endoscopic versus surgical treatment for pancreatic pseudocysts: systematic review and meta-analysis. Medicine (Baltimore). 2019;98(8):e14255.

68. Verma S, Rana SS. Disconnected pancreatic duct syndrome: updated review on clinical implications and management. Pancreatology. 2020;20(6):1035–44.

69. Maatman TK, Roch AM, Lewellen KA, Heimberger MA, Ceppa EP, House MG, et al. Disconnected pancreatic duct syndrome: Spectrum of operative management. J Surg Res. 2020;247:297–303.

70. Fernandez-Cruz L, Margarona E, Llovera J, Lopez-Boado MA, Saenz H. Pancreatic ascites. Hepato-Gastroenterology. 1993;40(2):150–4.

71. Kozarek RA. Management of pancreatic ascites. Gastroenterol Hepatol (N Y). 2007;3(5):362–4.

72. Bakker OJ, van Santvoort H, Besselink MG, Boermeester MA, van Eijck C, Dejong K, et al. Extrapancreatic necrosis without pancreatic parenchymal necrosis: a separate entity in necrotising pancreatitis? Gut. 2013;62(10):1475–80.

73. Bezmarevic M, van Dijk SM, Voermans RP, van Santvoort HC, Besselink MG. Management of (Peri) pancreatic collections in acute pancreatitis. Visc Med. 2019;35(2):91–6.

74. Noel P, Patel K, Durgampudi C, Trivedi RN, de Oliveira C, Crowell MD, et al. Peripancreatic fat necrosis worsens acute pancreatitis independent of pancreatic necrosis via unsaturated fatty acids increased in human pancreatic necrosis collections. Gut. 2016;65(1):100–11.

Mechanisms in Systemic Inflammation

Julia Mayerle and Matthias Sendler

Key Points

1. Macrophages/monocytes and neutrophils are the first immune cells to migrate into the pancreas, act in a pro-inflammatory manner and are responsible for the cytokine storm and the systemic inflammatory response syndrome (SIRS).
2. In parallel with the pro-inflammation, a systemic counter-regulation is established, which is mainly mediated by regulatory T cells. An excessive anti-inflammatory state can result in immune paralysis and promote the infection of the pancreatic necrosis by commensal intestinal and other bacteria.
3. Establishing the correct balance between pro- and anti-inflammation states is a key challenge for the treatment of inflammation in severe acute pancreatitis.

1   Introduction

Acute pancreatitis is the consequence of proteolytically induced cell death of acinar cells. The resulting damage triggers an immune response, which ultimately spreads and induces a systemic inflammatory response syndrome. The severity of the pancreatic damage is driven by necrotic cell death in the pancreas, but the systemic immune response determines morbidity and mortality. Acute pancreatitis is a primarily a sterile inflammatory response, where immune cells are activated via the release of cytokines as well as DAMPs (damage-associated molecular patterns) and start to amplify the inflammation. Since DAMPs are primarily released by necrotic cell death, there is a direct link between the local damage and the systemic immune response. Life-threatening complications such as multiple organ failure or infected pancreatic necrosis are associated with an increase in morbidity and in mortality of up to 30%. These complications are caused by an excessive immune response, which decouples the severity of pancreatitis from the local processes taking place in the pancreas. The disengaged immune response is one reason why there is no causal treatment strategy for severe acute pancreatitis, but all efforts rely on symptom focussed therapies and preservation of organ function.

The activation of the transcription factor NFκB (nuclear factor "kappa-light-chain-enhancer" of activated B cells) is an initiating event, which occurs early in acinar cells and induces a first localized immune response. Infiltrating and activated cells of the innate immune system, such as macrophages or neutrophils, then enhance this immune response via the release of cytokines and chemokines. Furthermore, both cell types are able

J. Mayerle (✉)
LMU Klinikum, Klinik und Poliklinik für Innere Medizin II, Munich, Germany
e-mail: julia.mayerle@med.uni-muenchen.de

M. Sendler
universitymedicine Greifswald, Greifswald, Germany
e-mail: matthias.sendler@uni-greifswald.de

© The Author(s), under exclusive license to Springer Nature Singapore Pte Ltd. 2024
J. A. Windsor et al. (eds.), *Acute Pancreatitis*, https://doi.org/10.1007/978-981-97-3132-9_5

to amplify the acinar cell damage, which leads to a self-fuelling inflammatory cycle. If this inflammatory cascade reaches a systemic threshold, it is called SIRS (systemic inflammatory response syndrome). SIRS is responsible for early organ failure during severe acute pancreatitis. Infected pancreatic necrosis, a serious complication, usually occurs following SIRS. A compensatory anti-inflammatory response syndrome (CARS) is thought to be responsible for systemic immunosuppression, which facilitates infection of pancreatic necrosis by commensal bacteria.

Balancing this immune response is a likely key to optimal treatment of severe acute pancreatitis. Nevertheless, the actual translation of this is challenging, and a deeper understanding of the involved signaling pathways is needed to identify new therapeutic targets and strategies. The pro-inflammatory immune response is mainly induced by the infiltration of cells belonging to innate immunity, such as macrophages and neutrophils. First and most importantly, macrophages/monocytes and neutrophil granulocytes migrate rapidly into the damaged organ and in turn release further cytokines and chemokines that translate the local immune response into a systemic one. The innate immune system actions are nonspecific and provide a general immune response to the tissue damage or infection. Conversely, the cells of the adaptive immune response can act on specific pathogens. In the overall response of acute pancreatitis, both arms of the immune system communicate with each other to work in a coordinated joint manner. T cells, in addition to B cells, are a key part of the adaptive immune system and in the absence of pathogens, the act as immunoregulators. They are responsible for a systemic counter-regulation to the pro-inflammatory response and attenuate or prevent SIRS.

2 Pancreatic Necrosis, the Origin of the Inflammatory Cascade

Acute pancreatitis starts within the pancreatic acinar cell. Premature intracellular activation of pancreatic proteases [1], increased ER stress [2],

and increased mitochondrial damage [3] result in necrotic cell death of acinar cells and represent the onset of the disease [4]. In parallel, activation of the transcription factor NFκB (nuclear factor "kappa-light-chain-enhancer" of activated B cells) occurs within these damaged cells [5]. NFκB controls the transcription of various inflammatory proteins, such as the cytokines IL1β, IL6, or tumor necrosis factor (TNF), as well as various chemokines, such as monocyte chemoattractant protein 1 (MCP-1). Activation of NFκB is the first step in the inflammatory cascade and is responsible for the induction of the immune response, which is further fuelled by the release of damage-associated molecular patterns (DAMPs) by necrotic acinar cell death [6].

The release of chemokines and cytokines in turn causes mobilization of myeloid cells from the bone marrow. As a consequence, mainly cells of the innate immune system migrate into the damaged organ. Monocytes and neutrophilic granulocytes are the most important leukocytes, which rapidly infiltrate the pancreas. Both cell populations play an important role for the manifestation and severity of acute pancreatitis by directly inducing acinar cell damage and secondary fuelling the inflammatory cascade through the release of cytokines [6–10]. In contrast, lymphoid cells, such as CD4[+] T-helper cells or CD8[+] T cells, are hardly detectable during this early phase of acute pancreatitis; they remain sequestered in the lymphoid organs such as the spleen or the mesenteric lymph nodes, where they affect the systemic immune response [11]. It is in the later phase of disease that they tend to accumulate in the chronically inflamed pancreas and are involved in fibrogenesis [12].

3 Neutrophil Granulocytes

Neutrophil granulocytes are recruited rapidly after onset of disease from the bone marrow and are usually the first immune cells which reach the site of inflammation. They are characterized by a very short half-life of only a few hours and are primarily responsible for neutralizing pathogenic germs. Pathogens are killed by these cells via the massive release of reactive oxygen species

(ROS), in a process called an "oxidative or respiratory burst." Neutrophils can also eject NETs (neutrophil extracellular trap formation) consisting of their own DNA via a "suicide" cell death mechanism in order to stop invading pathogens, a form of cell death called NETosis. However, since acute pancreatitis is a primarily a sterile inflammatory reaction, this repertoire of pathogen control is not required at this early stage and instead becomes another factor contributing to local pancreatic damage. In this regard, it has been shown that neutrophils are the main source of ROS during pancreatitis and increase initial trypsinogen activation and local damage [9]. The formation of extracellular traps can also lead to further organ damage by occluding smaller pancreatic ducts, which results in a blockage of fluid secretion [13]. Intrapancreatic ductal pressure is known to induce pathophysiological Ca^{2+} signaling in acinar cells via PIEZO receptor signaling [14]. In summary, neutrophils do not clear the pancreatic inflammation but rather are responsible for increasing the early local damage.

4 Macrophages/Monocytes

Macrophages represent the most abundant immune cells present in the inflamed pancreas. On the one hand, monocyte-derived macrophages, which are mobilized from the bone marrow similar to neutrophils, are recruited into the pancreas via chemokines such as MCP-1 [10, 15]. Conversely, tissue resident macrophages are already present in the pancreas and do not need to be recruited. These macrophages are the first immune cells able to immediately react to the local tissue damage and the necrotic acinar cell death. Macrophages can be divided into two broad categories: (1) the classically activated macrophages, which display a pro-inflammatory phenotype, and (2) the alternatively activated macrophages, which act rather pro-fibrotic or in a tissue-regenerating manner and do not increase inflammation [12, 16]. However, the polarization of macrophage phenotypes are not strictly demarcated into these two directions, but instead, there is a spectrum of activity exhibited between these two alignments, which allows the cells to react

specifically to the respective surrounding circumstances [6, 11, 16–18]. In the case of acute pancreatitis, different macrophage phenotypes are found, depending on their location in the organ [11]. Macrophages located in necrotic areas polarize to a classically activated proinflammatory phenotype, while macrophages, which are located outside damaged areas of the pancreas, are more likely to differentiate to an alternative activated phenotype. Macrophage activation is not only regulated by cytokines released by acinar cells but to a large extent by DAMPs released by necrotic acinar cells, such as free DNA, free ATP, or mitochondrial DNA. DAMPs activate cells via the Toll-like receptor/MyD88 signaling pathway in a manner similar to pathogenic associated molecular patterns (PAMPs) and induce macrophage polarization toward a classically activated phenotype [11, 19]. These classically activated macrophages represent a double-edged sword. On the one hand, they phagocytose necrotic cells to clear organ damage, and on the other hand, they promote pro-inflammation by secreting cytokines such as IL-6, TNFα, and IL-1β [6]. The fact that macrophages secrete multiple cytokines ranks them as important regulators of the immune response during acute pancreatitis.

4.1 IL-6 Signaling

Interleukin 6 is a pro-inflammatory cytokine that can be released by almost all immune cells but also by pancreatic acinar cells. IL-6 acts either directly via the IL-6 receptor, a heterodimer consisting of the IL-6R chain, and the gp130 chain or indirectly as a complex of IL-6 and the soluble IL-6R on the homodimer of gp130 (IL-6 trans signaling). While the heterodimeric IL-6 receptor is almost exclusively expressed on immune cells, the homodimeric gp130 receptor is present on a large number of different cells. Furthermore, IL-6 signaling or IL-6 trans signaling results in the activation of the transcription factor STAT3, which is responsible for activation of various immune cells as well as the regulation of immune cell migration. It is known that IL-6 trans signaling switches the immune cell recruitment from neutrophilic cells to monocytes via induction of the chemokine MCP-1 [20], which could be responsible for the dominant role of macrophages during pancreatitis. Furthermore IL-6 signaling induces the activation of endothelial cells and enables immune cell migration via increasing the expression of cell adhesion molecules like ICAM-1, VCAM, and E-selectin [21]. During pancreatitis, serum levels of IL-6 have been shown to correlate positively with increased organ damage [22]. In animal models of acute pancreatitis, IL-6 trans-signaling, in particular, has been shown to be directly related to lung damage [23].

4.2 TNFα-Induced Acinar Cell Necroptosis

TNFα, FasL, or TRAIL belong to the cytokines of the TNF-superfamily and are known to have various effects in the inflammatory cascade. All three cytokines act via the TNF-receptor family and the TNF-receptor-associated factor (TRAF), which results in the activation of the transcription factor NFκB. This signaling pathway is the backbone of the pro-inflammatory cascade. However, besides the induction of NFκB, various cell death pathways can be induced via TNF-receptor signaling (TNFR-1). For example, apoptosis is initiated via activation of caspases, and the regulated form of necrosis, known as necroptosis, is induced via the TNF-R1 signaling pathway. TNFα-induced necroptosis is mediated by the formation of the RIP1/RIP3 (receptor-interacting protein kinase) complex, triggering an increase of the intracellular Ca^{2+} concentration. Acinar cells express TNF-R1 and respond to TNFα [24] in two ways: excessive cytosolic Ca^{2+} induces necroptosis [25] and premature protease activation [7]. Acinar cells express TNF-R1 and respond to TNFα by inducing intracellular protease activation and necroptotic cell death, which in turn leads to the release of DAMPs. Thus, this creates a self-fuelling inflammatory cascade that further increases primary acinar cell damage.

4.3 The Cytokines of the IL-1 Family

Another important group of cytokines is the family of IL-1 cytokines, including IL-1β, IL-1α, IL-18, and IL-33, which are mainly released by macrophages and play a crucial role for the innate immunity [26]. IL-1α and IL-33 are considered alarmins, which are present in the cytoplasm and are released during cell lysis, like necrotic or pyroptotic cell death, to initiate an immune response. The situation is somewhat different for the cytokines IL-1β and IL-18; as the expression of both cytokines needs to be induced in a first step; then, in a second step, the pro-forms of both cytokines are proteolytically activated via the inflammasome complex. The final release of mature IL-1β and IL-18 occurs via a gasdermin-pore complex in the cell membrane, which also initiates pyroptotic cell death. IL-1β and IL-18 in pancreatitis are mainly released by classical activated macrophages. These cytokines enhance the pro-inflammatory response and seem to be significantly contribute to the induction of the systemic immune response [11]. The IL-1 receptor signaling pathway ends up in the activation of NFκB via MyD88/IRAK (interleukin-1 receptor-associated kinase/interleukin-1 receptor-associated kinase) pathway. With acute pancreatitis, the IL-1/inflammasome signaling plays a crucial role in enhancing inflammation and inflammation-related pancreatic damage [11, 27, 28]. IL-1 family cytokines, along with IL-12 family cytokines, represent important mediators of the crosstalk between the innate and adaptive immune systems and can induce a T-cell response and differentiation.

5 T Cells and the Role of the Adaptive Immune Response

T cells, especially CD4+ T-helper cells, are subclassified with respect to their differentiation and according to their different functions. During pancreatitis, a T-cell response occurs in a severity-

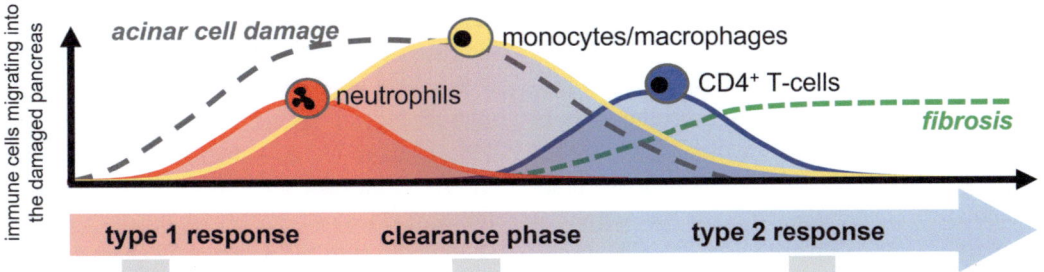

Fig. 1 The local immune response in the pancreas is divided into three phases. (1) The pro-inflammation driven by a type 1 immune response of neutrophils and macrophages/monocytes, which are recruited and activated. (2) The clearance phase, which mainly involves phagocytosing macrophages to remove necrotic cells. (3) The induction of wound healing, which involves type 2 immune cells, such as Th2 cells, alternatively activated macrophages, and innate type 2 lymphoid cells activating stellate cells, resulting in fibrogenesis

dependent manner within the lymphoid tissue and is marked by a prominent activation of T-regulatory cells (T_{regs}) and Th2 cells [11, 29]. T_{regs} represent the anti-inflammatory arm of the immune system, whereas Th2 cells act via secretion of IL-4/IL-13 on macrophage polarization to induce alternative activated macrophages, which in turn activate pancreatic stellate cells and mediate wound healing and scar formation [12, 16, 17]. Besides the type 2 immune response, T_{regs} and Th2 cells counteract the pro-inflammatory signaling via the secretion of IL-10 [11, 30].

The inflammatory cascade starts in the pancreas with a distinct pro-inflammatory response arising from the cells of the innate immune system. The adaptive immune response plays only a minor role locally and is mainly active systemically. Pancreatic macrophages play a crucial role through providing the link between local and sys-

temic immune response and ultimately translating pancreatic damage into a systemic immune response (Fig. 1).

6 The Transformation From Local Inflammation to Systemic Inflammation

Pancreatic macrophages phagocytose necrotic acinar cells and then in response release a variety of cytokines. This results in a cytokine storm that orchestrates the systemic immune response. Thus, the amount of necrotic cells, or the extent of pancreatic damage, determines the intensity of this initial immune response. If this pro-inflammatory cytokine storm then develops into a self-propelling immune response, it will lead to a continuous recruitment of immune cells into the pancreas and, thus, continuous damage of the organ. This is called the systemic inflammatory response syndrome (SIRS). Thus, the pro-inflammatory SIRS originates from the cells of the innate immune system within the damaged pancreas. Parallels could be found in other inflammatory responses such as in sepsis or severe trauma by extensive burns [31–33].

To counteract the excessive hyper-inflammation, immunosuppressive cells such as regulatory T cells or myeloid derived suppressor cells (MDSCs) are activated [32, 34], preventing systemic therapy refractory shock. This counter-regulation can increase in intensity and results ultimately in the inhibition of the immune system to such an extent that immune paralysis can occur. This hypo-inflammation is called compensatory anti-inflammatory response syndrome (CARS) [31–33, 35]. Regulatory T cells expand and become activated during acute pancreatitis. Tregs can suppress the T effector cell response to the point of immune paralysis. This weakens the immunologic arm of the intestinal barrier and allows commensal bacteria from the intestine to infiltrate the pancreatic necrosis [35]. The consequence of immune paralysis is a diminished immunological response to infection or, conversely, the unhindered colonization of pancreatic necrosis by commensal intestinal bacteria. Infected pancreatic necrosis represents a high-risk factor for a severe course of acute pancreatitis and is associated with a significantly increased morbidity and mortality [36].

Persistent SIRS can lead to systemic shock and is associated with early organ failure and early mortality in the course of acute pancreatitis after only a few days [37]. Infection of necrosis usually occurs after 1–2 weeks and represents a second episode in the disease course and significantly contributing to severity. Due to this temporal sequence, it has long been assumed that SIRS and CARS follow each other in time and that CARS is ultimately the consequence of SIRS. However, more recent data show that SIRS and CARS develop in parallel [11]. This has been known for severe trauma states such as burns in which pro- and anti-inflammation arises in parallel [11, 31, 33]. Ultimately, pancreatitis is a pri-

marily sterile inflammation that is triggered by massive cell necrosis and thus has many parallels with severe wound reactions. Therefore, from an immunological point of view, pancreatitis behaves more like a wound reaction with a parallel type 2 immune response that initiates wound closure [11].

In contrast to SIRS, which is characterized by a systemic cytokine storm that can be measured in serum (via IL-6, IL-1β, or TNFα), CARS is not easy to determine. The absence of pro-inflammatory markers has often been interpreted as an indication of CARS, but data from patients clearly show that very early on, during the peak phase of SIRS, significantly elevated serum levels of anti-inflammatory cytokines such as IL-10 can already be measured, and these correlate with the severity of the disease [11, 34]. In diagnostic terms, CARS behaves like an iceberg; usually only the tip is recognized and often, unfortunately, too late. CARS is often accompanied by increased immune cell apoptosis and is exacerbated by the fact that T_{regs} are more resistant to the induction of apoptosis compared to T-effector cells [38]. Cytokines that are released more frequently during SIRS, such as TNFα, FasL, or IL-1β, can drive immune cells into apoptosis and thus promote immunosuppression. TNFα and FasL regulate neutrophil count via induction of apoptosis, which could result in neutropenia [39]. IL-1β has been shown to induce apoptosis of T cells in the intestine, thereby weakening the intestinal barrier and causing secondary infections [40]. This suggests that the extent of CARS is determined by extent of SIRS and does not progress in sequence, but rather in parallel (Fig. 2).

This represents a challenge for clinical management, as treatment of SIRS and any attempts to limit pro-inflammation may result in an increase in immunosuppression. Conversely, treating immunosuppression may result in an uncontrolled increasing hyper-inflammation. Therefore, effective treatment should involve modulating both arms of the immune response to reach a balance of the immune system to prevent SIRS and CARS.

The ubiquitous presence of inflammation in acute pancreatitis therefore has made this coma

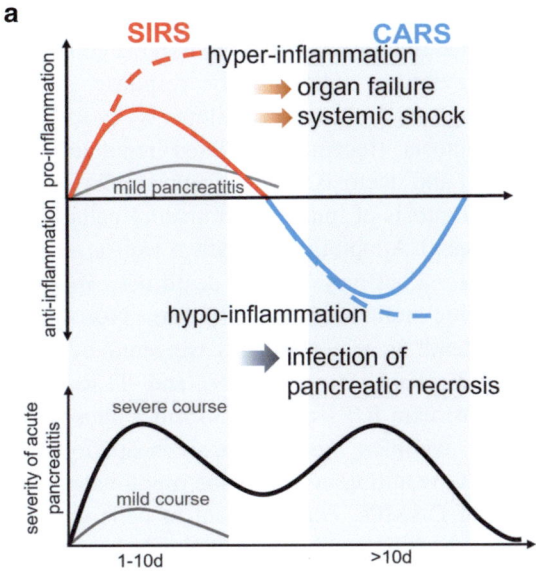

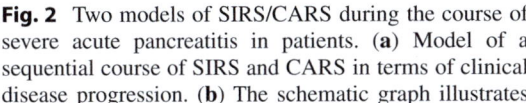

b

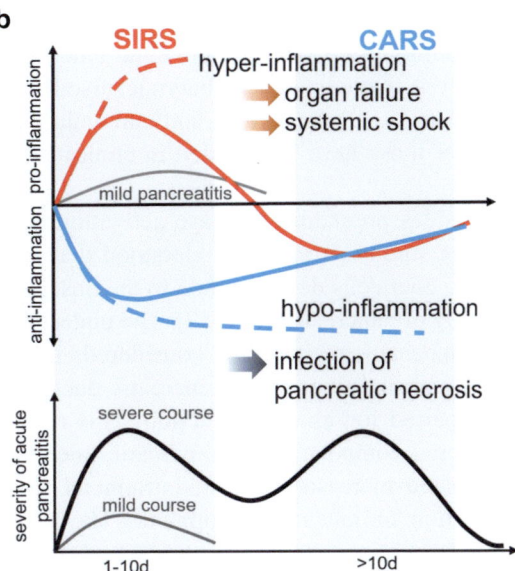

Fig. 2 Two models of SIRS/CARS during the course of severe acute pancreatitis in patients. (**a**) Model of a sequential course of SIRS and CARS in terms of clinical disease progression. (**b**) The schematic graph illustrates the parallel course of SIRS and CARS in terms of disease progression. *SIRS* systemic inflammatory response syndrome, *CARS* compensatory anti-inflammatory response syndrome

plex cluster of pathological mechanisms the subject of several therapeutic attempts to control its severity and therefore modulate the disease.

6.1 Protease/Antiprotease Balance to Prevent and Treat Systemic Inflammation

In 1896, Hans Chiari proposed that pancreatitis is a process of autodigestion of the gland, with activation of pancreatic proteases starts in acinar cells and then the gland is digested by its own proteases. In light of all the mutations detected since 1996 in pancreatic proteases or antiproteases and in line with Chiaris proposal, premature activation of pancreatic proteases, especially of trypsinogen, is suggested to be the cause and start of the disease [4]. Therapeutic targeting of trypsin dependent protease activity has been attempted using gabexate-mesilate but it was only found beneficial to prevent post-ERCP pancreatitis and in some cases of necrotizing pancreatitis if administered as an infusion into the mesenteric artery [41, 42].

Cathepsin B is known to be able to cleave and thereby activate trypsinogen and, as such, is likely the starting point of premature intracellular protease activation, resulting in pancreatic cell death and evoking a systemic inflammatory response syndrome [6, 43–45]. However, whether cathepsin B inhibition is more beneficial than gabexate-mesilate needs to be resolved in future studies [46]. One obvious treatment strategy would be to use a protease inhibitor to enhance the antiprotease response. One of the crucial endogenous inhibitors of trypsin activity is SPINK1 (serine peptidase inhibitor Kazal type 1). Mutations in SPINK1 are known to increase the risk of idiopathic chronic pancreatitis 15 fold in homozygous subjects, and thus, SPINK appears to be an interesting drug target. However, as we do not yet understand the mode of action and how the susceptibility to chronic pancreatitis is mediated for the most common point mutation in the SPINK1 gene, (the N34S mutation) its current targeting remains impossible [47–49].

Another interesting treatment concept is targeting the damage mechanism of mutated pancreatic proteases which induces pancreatitis by

ER-stress due to misfolded proteins. Several interesting agents are available to ameliorate ER-stress, (including phenylbutyrate, ursodeoxycholic acid, BiP inducer X, and curcumin), but none of those have been tested in clinical trials [50].

Besides premature protease activation from genetic studies, it is well understood that pancreatic duct cells do contribute to the onset and severity of pancreatitis [51, 52]. The underlying pathomechanism here is considered to be mainly obstruction of the pancreatic ducts due to impaired ion channel function. This results in altered composition of pancreatic juice and associated increased risks of intraductal stone formation or mucus development. The major culprits here are the CFTR channel as well as the calcium channels involving SOCE channels (store-operated calcium entry, STIM-Orai1) and the calcium-sensing receptors (CASR) [53]. If restoring of genetically impaired ductal cell function is the goal, then CFTR (cystic fibrosis conductance regulator) channel modulators, such as ivacaftor (Kalydeco®, CFTR-G551D), lumacaftor/ivacaftor (Orkambi®, CFTR-ΔF508), tezacaftor/ivacaftor (Symdeko®, CFTR-ΔF508), or elexacaftor/tezacaftor/ivacaftor (Trikafta™, CFTR-ΔF508), can be employed for correcting protein function for specified mutations. For mutations in the CASR (calcium-sensing-receptor), calcimimetics are at hand [cinacalcet (Mimpara®) and etelcalcetide (Parsabiv®)]; however, trials on therapeutic efficacy to prevent pancreatitis are not yet evident. In conclusion, therapeutic targeting of acinar and duct cell injury is an understudied area.

6.2 Treating Necroptosis to Prevent and Treat Systemic Inflammation

Premature activation of proteases ultimately leads to cell death, and the "danger theory" of the inflammatory response, proposed by Polly Matzinger 20 years ago, suggested that systemic immune responses are triggered by danger signals released by the body's own dying cells [54]. The systemic inflammatory response system leading to multi-organ failure is evoked by necroptosis (receptor mediated regulated cell death) and necrosis of dying acinar cells as well as pyroptosis of innate inflammatory cells (macrophages). Apoptotic cell death as well as autophagy are silent ways of cell death not evoking a systemic inflammatory response. Necroptotic cell death in pancreatitis is triggered by TNF, TRAIL, FasL, type 1 IFN, and TLRs [55]. Downstream RIP1 and RIP3 form a phosphorylated complex (necrosome) phosphorylating MLKL, resulting in membrane rupture and spillage of DAMPs. Forty percent of cells undergo necroptosis in pancreatitis. RIP3 deletion ameliorates severe pancreatitis, and necrostatin treatment is beneficial in mice [25, 56, 57]. Recently, a number of small-molecule inhibitors of necroptosis have been developed, and early clinical testing is expected, although no trials have yet been registered [58].

6.3 Treating Pyroptosis to Prevent and Treat Systemic Inflammation

Pyroptosis, the predominant cell death of macrophages, induces the NLRP3 inflammasome. The inflammasome is a macroscopic cytosolic protein complex (NLRP3, ASC, caspase-1), which proteolytically cleaves pro-IL1β and pro-IL18 and releases HMGB1, leading to spillage of proinflammatory cytokines. NRLP3 activation requires lysosomal rupture and cathepsin release, Ca^{2+} influx, and mitochondrial-derived ROS production, mechanisms all known to be crucially involved in the pathogenesis of pancreatitis [59]. The NLRP3 inflammasome in inflammatory cells is a major sensor of necroptosis, which helps close the vicious cycle of propagation of the inflammatory response. Moreover, there is a direct link between premature cathepsin-B-dependent activation of zymogens in macrophages. In macrophages, engulfed trypsinogen can be activated in a cathepsin B-dependent way resulting in a classically activated polarization as well as activation of the inflammasome and secretion of pro-inflammatory cytokines [6]. Application of lactate [60], beta-hydroxybutyrate, or aspartate ameliorates pancreatitis by blocking the inflammasome pathway. Inhibition of the inflammasome by MCC950, a small-molecule inhibitor, ameliorates pancreatitis and prevents infection. This highlights that inhibition of the inflammasome is an ideal target for the treatment of pancreatitis [11]. At the time of writing, several companies have acquired a portfolio of NLRP3 inhibitors, the most advanced of which has progressed into the clinic. So far though, no company has decided to target acute pancreatitis as a disease indication use case to prove therapeutic efficacy. Nevertheless, treating pancreatitis in this manner would seem a reasonable and logical future target [61].

In conclusion, to overcome the lack of causal treatment in severe acute pancreatitis, one needs to modulate the systemic inflammatory response to avoid an overwhelming pro-inflammatory response but in a way that prevents immunoparalysis. Pancreatic protease inhibition and targeting store-operated calcium channels are both promising targets for the early phase of acute pancreatitis. Also modulating the inflammatory response by targeting the inflammasome and/or the macrophage might also significantly advance the field.

References

1. Geisz A, Sahin-Tóth M. A preclinical model of chronic pancreatitis driven by trypsinogen autoactivation. Nat Commun. 2018;9(1):5033.
2. Kereszturi É, Szmola R, Kukor Z, Simon P, Ulrich Weiss F, Lerch MM, Sahin-Tóth M. Hereditary pancreatitis caused by mutation-induced misfolding of human cationic trypsinogen: a novel disease mechanism. Hum Mutat. 2009;30(4):575–82.
3. Biczo G, Vegh ET, Shalbueva N, Mareninova OA, Elperin J, Lotshaw E, et al. Mitochondrial dysfunction, through impaired autophagy, leads to endoplasmic reticulum stress, deregulated lipid metabolism, and pancreatitis in animal models. Gastroenterology. 2018;154(3):689–703.
4. Mayerle J, Sendler M, Hegyi E, Beyer G, Lerch MM, Sahin-Tóth M. Genetics, cell biology, and pathophysiology of pancreatitis. Gastroenterology. 2019;156(7):1951–1968.e1.
5. Gukovsky I, Gukovskaya AS, Blinman TA, Zaninovic V, Pandol SJ. Early NF-kappaB activation is associated with hormone-induced pancreatitis. Am J Physiol. 1998;275(6):G1402–14.
6. Sendler M, Weiss FU, Golchert J, Homuth G, van den Brandt C, Mahajan UM, et al. Cathepsin B-mediated activation of trypsinogen in endocytosing macrophages increases severity of pancreatitis in mice. Gastroenterology. 2018;154(3):704–718.e10.
7. Sendler M, Dummer A, Weiss FU, Krüger B, Wartmann T, Scharffetter-Kochanek K, et al. Tumour necrosis factor α secretion induces protease activation and acinar cell necrosis in acute experimental pancreatitis in mice. Gut. 2013;62(3):430–9.
8. Perides G, Weiss ER, Michael ES, Laukkarinen JM, Duffield JS, Steer ML. TNF-alpha-dependent regulation of acute pancreatitis severity by Ly-6C(hi) monocytes in mice. J Biol Chem. 2011;286(15):13327–35.
9. Gukovskaya AS, Vaquero E, Zaninovic V, Gorelick FS, Lusis AJ, Brennan ML, et al. Neutrophils and NADPH oxidase mediate intrapancreatic trypsin activation in murine experimental acute pancreatitis. Gastroenterology. 2002;122(4):974–84.
10. Wilden A, Glaubitz J, Otto O, Biedenweg D, Nauck M, Mack M, et al. Mobilization of CD11b+/Ly6chi monocytes causes multi organ dysfunction syndrome in acute pancreatitis. Front Immunol. 2022;13:991295.
11. Sendler M, van den Brandt C, Glaubitz J, Wilden A, Golchert J, Weiss FU, et al. NLRP3 inflammasome regulates development of systemic inflammatory response and compensatory anti-inflammatory response syndromes in mice with acute pancreatitis. Gastroenterology. 2020;158(1):253–269.e14.
12. Glaubitz J, Wilden A, Golchert J, Homuth G, Völker U, Bröker BM, et al. In mouse chronic pancreatitis CD25+FOXP3+ regulatory T cells control pancreatic fibrosis by suppression of the type 2 immune response. Nat Commun. 2022;13(1):4502.
13. Leppkes M, Maueröder C, Hirth S, Nowecki S, Günther C, Billmeier U, et al. Externalized decondensed neutrophil chromatin occludes pancreatic ducts and drives pancreatitis. Nat Commun. 2016;7:10973.
14. Romac JMJ, Shahid RA, Swain SM, Vigna SR, Liddle RA. Piezo1 is a mechanically activated ion channel and mediates pressure induced pancreatitis. Nat Commun. 2018;9(1):1715.
15. Saeki K, Kanai T, Nakano M, Nakamura Y, Miyata N, Sujino T, et al. CCL2-induced migration and SOCS3-mediated activation of macrophages are involved in cerulein-induced pancreatitis in mice. Gastroenterology. 2012;142(4):1010–1020.e9.
16. Xue J, Sharma V, Hsieh MH, Chawla A, Murali R, Pandol SJ, et al. Alternatively activated macrophages promote pancreatic fibrosis in chronic pancreatitis. Nat Commun. 2015;6:7158.

17. Wu J, Zhang L, Shi J, He R, Yang W, Habtezion A, et al. Macrophage phenotypic switch orchestrates the inflammation and repair/regeneration following acute pancreatitis injury. EBioMedicine. 2020;58:102920.

18. Manohar M, Jones EK, Rubin SJS, Subrahmanyam PB, Swaminathan G, Mikhail D, et al. Novel circulating and tissue monocytes as well as macrophages in pancreatitis and recovery. Gastroenterology. 2021;161(6):2014–2029.e14.

19. Zhang Q, Raoof M, Chen Y, Sumi Y, Sursal T, Junger W, et al. Circulating mitochondrial DAMPs cause inflammatory responses to injury. Nature. 2010;464(7285):104–7.

20. Hurst SM, Wilkinson TS, McLoughlin RM, Jones S, Horiuchi S, Yamamoto N, et al. IL-6 and its soluble receptor orchestrate a temporal switch in the pattern of leukocyte recruitment seen during acute inflammation. Immunity. 2001;14(6):705–14.

21. Scheller J, Chalaris A, Schmidt-Arras D, Rose-John S. The pro- and anti-inflammatory properties of the cytokine interleukin-6. Biochim Biophys Acta (BBA) Mol Cell Res. 2011;1813(5):878–88.

22. Samanta J, Singh S, Arora S, Muktesh G, Aggarwal A, Dhaka N, et al. Cytokine profile in prediction of acute lung injury in patients with acute pancreatitis. Pancreatology. 2018;18(8):878–84.

23. Zhang H, Neuhöfer P, Song L, Rabe B, Lesina M, Kurkowski MU, et al. IL-6 trans-signaling promotes pancreatitis-associated lung injury and lethality. J Clin Invest. 2013;123(3):1019–31.

24. Gukovskaya AS, Gukovsky I, Zaninovic V, Song M, Sandoval D, Gukovsky S, et al. Pancreatic acinar cells produce, release, and respond to tumor necrosis factor-alpha. Role in regulating cell death and pancreatitis. J Clin Invest. 1997;100(7):1853–62.

25. He S, Wang L, Miao L, Wang T, Du F, Zhao L, et al. Receptor interacting protein kinase-3 determines cellular necrotic response to TNF-alpha. Cell. 2009;137(6):1100–11.

26. Garlanda C, Dinarello CA, Mantovani A. The interleukin-1 family: back to the future. Immunity. 2013;39(6):1003–18.

27. Hoque R, Sohail M, Malik A, Sarwar S, Luo Y, Shah A, et al. TLR9 and the NLRP3 inflammasome link acinar cell death with inflammation in acute pancreatitis. Gastroenterology. 2011;141(1):358–69.

28. Zhao Q, Wei Y, Pandol SJ, Li L, Habtezion A. STING signaling promotes inflammation in experimental acute pancreatitis. Gastroenterology. 2018;154(6):1822–1835.e2.

29. Glaubitz J, Wilden A, van den Brandt C, Weiss FU, Bröker BM, Mayerle J, et al. Experimental pancreatitis is characterized by rapid T cell activation, Th2 differentiation that parallels disease severity, and improvement after CD4+ T cell depletion. Pancreatology. 2020;20(8):1637–47.

30. Rongione A, Kusske A, Kwan K, Ashley S, Reber H, McFadden D. Interleukin 10 reduces the sever-

ity of acute pancreatitis in rats. Gastroenterology. 1997;112(3):960–7.

31. Hotchkiss RS, Moldawer LL, Opal SM, Reinhart K, Turnbull IR, Vincent JL. Sepsis and septic shock. Nat Rev Dis Primers. 2016;2:16045.

32. Hotchkiss RS, Monneret G, Payen D. Sepsis-induced immunosuppression: from cellular dysfunctions to immunotherapy. Nat Rev Immunol. 2013;13(12):862–74.

33. Xiao W, Mindrinos MN, Seok J, Cuschieri J, Cuenca AG, Gao H, et al. A genomic storm in critically injured humans. J Exp Med. 2011;208(13):2581–90.

34. Zhang R, Shi J, Zhang R, Ni J, Habtezion A, Wang X, et al. Expanded CD14^{hi}CD16$^-$ immunosuppressive monocytes predict disease severity in patients with acute pancreatitis. J Immunol. 2019;202(9):2578–84.

35. Glaubitz J, Wilden A, Frost F, Ameling S, Homuth G, Mazloum H, et al. Activated regulatory T-cells promote duodenal bacterial translocation into necrotic areas in severe acute pancreatitis. Gut. 2023;72:1355–69.

36. van Dijk SM, Hallensleben NDL, van Santvoort HC, Fockens P, van Goor H, Bruno MJ, et al. Acute pancreatitis: recent advances through randomised trials. Gut. 2017;66(11):2024–32.

37. Garg PK, Singh VP. Organ failure due to systemic injury in acute pancreatitis. Gastroenterology. 2019;156(7):2008–23.

38. Hotchkiss RS, Nicholson DW. Apoptosis and caspases regulate death and inflammation in sepsis. Nat Rev Immunol. 2006;6(11):813–22.

39. Geering B, Simon HU. Peculiarities of cell death mechanisms in neutrophils. Cell Death Differ. 2011;18(9):1457–69.

40. Roth S, Cao J, Singh V, Tiedt S, Hundeshagen G, Li T, et al. Post-injury immunosuppression and secondary infections are caused by an AIM2 inflammasome-driven signaling cascade. Immunity. 2021;54(4):648–659.e8.

41. Endo A, Shiraishi A, Fushimi K, Murata K, Otomo Y. Impact of continuous regional arterial infusion in the treatment of acute necrotizing pancreatitis: analysis of a national administrative database. J Gastroenterol. 2018;53(9):1098–106.

42. Cavallini G, Tittobello A, Frulloni L, Masci E, Mariana A, Di Francesco V. Gabexate for the prevention of pancreatic damage related to endoscopic retrograde cholangiopancreatography. Gabexate in digestive endoscopy—Italian group. N Engl J Med. 1996;335(13):919–23.

43. Lerch MM, Halangk W. Human pancreatitis and the role of cathepsin B. Gut. 2006;55(9):1228–30.

44. Kukor Z, Mayerle J, Krüger B, Tóth M, Steed PM, Halangk W, et al. Presence of cathepsin B in the human pancreatic secretory pathway and its role in trypsinogen activation during hereditary pancreatitis. J Biol Chem. 2002;277(24):21389–96.

45. Sendler M, Maertin S, John D, Persike M, Weiss FU, Krüger B, et al. Cathepsin B activity initiates apoptosis via digestive protease activation in pancreatic aci-

nar cells and experimental pancreatitis. J Biol Chem. 2016;291(28):14717–31.

46. Weiss FU, Behn CO, Simon P, Ruthenbürger M, Halangk W, Lerch MM. Cathepsin B gene polymorphism Val26 is not associated with idiopathic chronic pancreatitis in European patients. Gut. 2007;56(9):1322–3.

47. Nagel F, Palm GJ, Geist N, McDonnell TCR, Susemihl A, Girbardt B, et al. Structural and biophysical insights into SPINK1 bound to human cationic trypsin. Int J Mol Sci. 2022;23(7):3468.

48. Kulke M, Nagel F, Schulig L, Geist N, Gabor M, Mayerle J, et al. A hypothesized mechanism for chronic pancreatitis caused by the N34S mutation of serine protease inhibitor Kazal-type 1 based on conformational studies. J Inflamm Res. 2021;14:2111–9.

49. Bourgault J, Abner E, Manikpurage HD, Pujol-Gualdo N, Laisk T, Estonian Biobank Research Team. Proteome-wide Mendelian randomization identifies causal links between blood proteins and acute pancreatitis. Gastroenterology. 2023;164(6):953–965.e3.

50. Lukas J, Pospech J, Oppermann C, Hund C, Iwanov K, Pantoom S, et al. Role of endoplasmic reticulum stress and protein misfolding in disorders of the liver and pancreas. Adv Med Sci. 2019;64(2):315–23.

51. Hegyi P, Wilschanski M, Muallem S, Lukacs GL, Sahin-Tóth M, Uc A, et al. CFTR: a new horizon in the pathomechanism and treatment of pancreatitis. Rev Physiol Biochem Pharmacol. 2016;170:37–66.

52. Weiss FU, Simon P, Bogdanova N, Mayerle J, Dworniczak B, Horst J, et al. Complete cystic fibrosis transmembrane conductance regulator gene sequencing in patients with idiopathic chronic pancreatitis and controls. Gut. 2005;54(10):1456–60.

53. Pallagi P, Madácsy T, Varga Á, Maléth J. Intracellular Ca^{2+} signalling in the pathogenesis of acute pancreatitis: recent advances and translational perspectives. Int J Mol Sci. 2020;21(11):4005.

54. Matzinger P. Tolerance, danger, and the extended family. Annu Rev Immunol. 1994;12:991–1045.

55. He R, Wang Z, Dong S, Chen Z, Zhou W. Understanding necroptosis in pancreatic diseases. Biomolecules. 2022;12(6):828.

56. Louhimo J, Steer ML, Perides G. Necroptosis is an important severity determinant and potential therapeutic target in experimental severe pancreatitis. Cell Mol Gastroenterol Hepatol. 2016;2(4):519–35.

57. He S, Huang S, Shen Z. Biomarkers for the detection of necroptosis. Cell Mol Life Sci. 2016;73(11–12):2177–81.

58. Li Y, Qian L, Yuan J. Small molecule probes for cellular death machines. Curr Opin Chem Biol. 2017;39:74–82.

59. Hoque R, Mehal WZ. Inflammasomes in pancreatic physiology and disease. Am J Physiol Gastrointest Liver Physiol. 2015;308(8):G643–51.

60. Wu BU, Hwang JQ, Gardner TH, Repas K, Delee R, Yu S, et al. Lactated Ringer's solution reduces systemic inflammation compared with saline in patients with acute pancreatitis. Clin Gastroenterol Hepatol. 2011;9(8):710–717.e1.

61. Mullard A. NLRP3 inhibitors stoke anti-inflammatory ambitions. Nat Rev Drug Discov. 2019;18(6):405–7.

Mechanisms of Organ Failure

Vijay P. Singh, Anoop Narayana Pillai,
Prasad Rajalingamgari, and Biswajit Khatua

Key Points

1. Severe acute pancreatitis is characterized by systemic inflammation and multiple organ dysfunction/failure.
2. Numerous potential markers, mediators, and treatment targets of organ failure have been identified, including lipids, proteins, cells, and cellular products.
3. Organ failure is currently managed by generic organ support and there are no specific treatments. This reflects an inadequate understanding of the key mechanisms which drive failure.
4. There are mechanisms of organ failure with strong preclinical evidence and which offer new treatment paradigms with the potential for clinical translation.
5. Visceral fat necrosis (VFN) is a feature of severe acute pancreatitis and, when progressive or extensive, can drive organ failure. This is mediated by pancreatic lipases that cleave the adipocyte triglyceride to unsaturated fatty acids (UFAs), which trigger a cytokine storm, systemic inflammation, cell injury in organs, and a worsening pancreatitis severity.
6. Gut injury is a feature of severe acute pancreatitis and results in significant and toxic changes in the composition of lymph draining the gut, including elevated lipase and UFAs. Bypassing the liver, this toxic lymph drains via the thoracic duct into central veins, impacting the cardiac, respiratory, and renal function.

V. P. Singh (✉) · A. N. Pillai · P. Rajalingamgari · B. Khatua
Division of Gastroenterology and Hepatology, Department of Medicine, Mayo Clinic, Phoenix, AZ, USA
e-mail: singh.vijay@mayo.edu

1 Introduction

While most patients with acute pancreatitis (AP) have a mild clinical course, severe AP can develop in about a fifth of the cases [1], which increases the length of hospital stay and critical care requirements and carries a mortality risk of 8–20% [2–4]. Severity in AP is based on the presence of organ failure as per the Revised Atlanta Criteria [5], which recommends that the severity of organ failure is scored by the modified Marshall score [5, 6]. The modified Marshall scoring system has specific metrics for vital organ systems, among which the respiratory, renal and cardiovascular systems are the most important and frequently involved systems. These metrics include creatinine for the renal system, partial pressure of oxygen for respiratory system and systolic blood pressure for the cardiovascular system. It also includes whether treatments such as oxygen, intravenous fluids and pressors are required. Severe AP is defined

© The Author(s), under exclusive license to Springer Nature Singapore Pte Ltd. 2024
J. A. Windsor et al. (eds.), *Acute Pancreatitis*, https://doi.org/10.1007/978-981-97-3132-9_6

by organ failure lasting >48 h, i.e., persistent organ failure. The duration of organ failure likely depends on the risk factors for severity and the patient's response to treatment [7]. Intravenous fluid resuscitation is the current treatment standard for AP. Aggressive fluid resuscitation [8] can worsen organ failure. Severe AP can develop single or multiple organ failure [5], with the latter being associated with higher mortality [9]. Thus, an increased number of organs with dysfunction during AP is associated with increased severity of AP [5]. Recent large studies show that respiratory and cardiovascular failure are more important in determining mortality in severe AP than renal failure [10]. Here we will focus on the mechanisms underlying organ failure.

Understanding the mechanistic basis of organ failure in humans is helped by considering the risk factors associated with severe AP. These include pre-existing risk factors (including obesity, comorbidities, and age) and those associated with AP (including etiology like hypertriglyceridemia, the systemic inflammatory response, and pancreatic/peri-pancreatic necrosis). The Charlson Comorbidity Index (CCI) [11] is a comprehensive measure of risk-based preexisting morbidities (including age, obesity, and baseline cardiac, respiratory, and renal function). The CCI has been shown to predict mortality in AP [12], including interstitial pancreatitis [13], and also the development of sepsis later in the disease [14]. The ubiquitous presence of lipolytic fat necrosis in AP [15] supports obesity being a risk factor for severe AP [16–26] and also for hypertriglyceridemia to be a risk factor for severity since it is associated with severe AP irrespective of the etiology [27–33].

Organ failure can occur within the first week of pancreatitis or later in the disease [34–36] when it is typically associated with infected pancreatic necrosis [37, 38]. In a landmark study, early persistent organ failure (within the first week) with AP was associated with high mortality [39]. There are some smaller studies that show late mortality from infected necrosis to be more common [40]; however, most studies show that at least half the mortality in AP occurs within 2 weeks of onset, which is attributed to early and persistent organ failure [41–46]. Studies that have followed patients with early organ failure also attribute the majority (>75%) of later septic complications and organ failure to the early phase [39, 45, 46] or show a similar mortality rate with persistent organ failure, irrespective of infection [47, 48]. Interestingly, a recent study shows that infections during pancreatitis are associated with the same lipotoxic mechanisms that cause organ failure [49]. This is due to fatty acids injuring the immune cells that normally clear bacteria [49] that commonly translocate [50, 51].

It is important to understand the pathophysiologic mechanisms driving organ failure in AP, since this may help in designing treatment strategies to improve the outcomes of severe AP. This includes understanding the limitations of different proposed mechanisms, some of which have been extensively studied in clinical trials previously [52–61]. In this chapter, the focus will be on two mechanisms proposed to explain the pathogenesis of early organ failure (in contrast to late organ failure which has a different mechanism, being secondary to infection of pancreatic necrosis), with particular reference to renal failure, hypotension/shock, and lung injury for which the mechanistic and clinical lines of evidence are better established.

2 Approach to Defining Key Mechanisms in Development of Organ Failure

Animal models are important in understanding how pancreatitis is initiated and then progresses to develop local or systemic complications. It is important to distinguish mechanisms that initiate pancreatitis but only result in local inflammation and pancreatic injury from those that make it severe by causing systemic injury. For example, cerulein is a common model of mild acute pancreatitis that causes an increase in serum amylase, lipase, edema of the pancreas with some necrosis, and inflammation [62]. This requires giving rodents high doses of the cholecystokinin (CCK) analog cerulein that binds to the Gαq11 receptors on pancreatic acini (Fig. 1). This binding results in an increase in cytosolic calcium, transcription factor activation, such as NF-κB activation, cytokine upregulation inflammatory cell infiltration, and reactive oxygen species formation, but does not result in organ failure. The increase in serum amylase or lipase is due to leakage of these enzymes from injured acinar cells by mechanisms that inhibit normal secretion (i.e., loss of apical microvilli, due to reorganization of actin), and result in blebbing and basolateral exocytosis. Similarly, the impairment of autophagy by high-dose cerulein that results in trypsin generation has been described in detail [63]; however, as we shall see below, the role of trypsin in organ failure or severe AP is not well supported. Mitochondrial injury that results in caspase and apoptotic activation can also be initiated by cerulein (Fig. 1); however, mitochondrial injury resulting in complex I and V inhibition, mitochondrial swelling [64], and large reductions in ATP resulting in necrosis are not caused by cerulein alone [64, 65]. However, necrosis of the pancreas is caused by unsaturated fatty acids that are released by lipases (leaked into adipose during cerulein pancreatitis) that break down triglycerides stored in the adipocytes, especially in obesity [66, 67]. Obese patients are at increased risk for severe AP (discussed below), and obesity increases the number of adipocytes in and around the pancreas [64, 65]. These unsaturated fatty acids released from adipocyte damage or lipolytic fat necrosis have been shown to cause injury to endothelial cells of blood vessels [68], renal

tubular cells [69, 70], and cells in the alveolar lining, including type-2 pneumocytes that make surfactant [68]. Such cell injury induced by unsaturated fatty acids has been associated with creatinine elevation, renal failure, respiratory failure, and hypotension, i.e., organ failure [68]. These findings mean that models of AP that increase adipose or triglyceride amounts in the abdomen can be used to study the progression of AP from a mild local disease caused by an agent like cerulein to a systemic illness causing organ failure [66, 71]. In the following, we discuss mechanisms elucidated from animal models in the context of risk factors, potential markers, and mediators of severe AP noted in clinical association-type studies in human AP.

Clinical studies looking at the pathogenesis of organ failure during AP often measure pre-existing risk factors (such as obesity [16, 18, 23] and comorbidities [12]) associated with developing severe disease or biomarkers that are typically associated with an increase in severity. Identifying pre-existing risk factors provides important clues to the milieu in which severe AP develops. However, while biomarkers (like cytokines, trypsin, fatty acids) are associated with worse outcome and would appear attractive therapeutic targets, they do not confirm causality with respect to organ failure. For example, cytokine or leucocyte elevation during a disease may be protective or may simply be an epiphenomenon rather than being a harmful causative factor in driving disease severity and organ failure.

Some studies [49, 66, 67] have used the Koch's postulates as a framework to investigate the causality of organ failure during AP. The proof that an agent or a biomarker has a role in causing severe disease, which in the case of AP means persistent organ failure, requires three criteria to be met.

1. The agent can be identified and isolated in pure form during the specific disease state. Several classes of potential agents in AP fulfil this criterion, including cytokines [72–79],

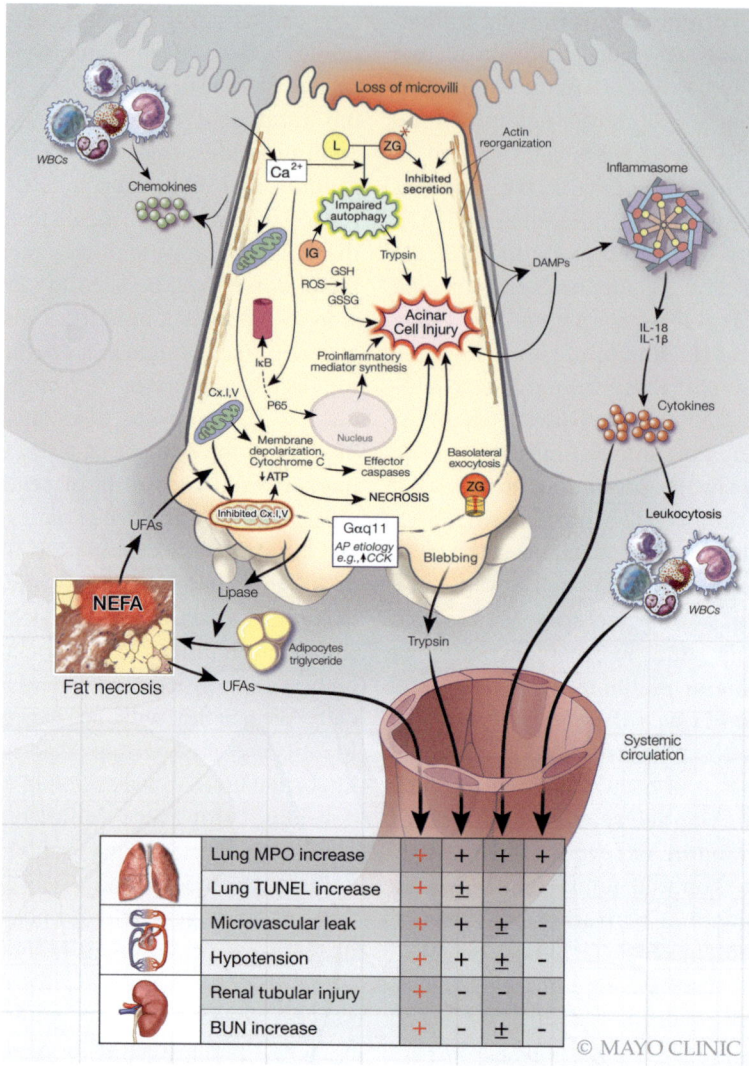

Fig. 1 Schematic describing the transition from mild pancreatitis initiation by cerulein (upper part) to systemic inflammation and organ failure (lower part), along with the evidence for each potential mediator. An injury initiating pancreatitis such as high-dose cerulein or CCK (at the bottom of the yellow cell) initially injures the exocrine acinar cells. This cell injury occurs via receptor (Gαq11) mediated increase in cytosolic calcium (Ca²⁺), actin reorganization, loss of microvilli, and blebbing that results in leakage of their enzymes into the surrounding tissue. There is also an increase in transcription factor activation, such as NF-κB (p65), cytokine increase, trypsin generation via impaired autophagy, reactive oxygen species (ROS) formation, and mitochondrial injury as detailed in the text. This also increases inflammatory mediator synthesis, which include cytokines and chemokines, and thus leads to neutrophil infiltration into the pancreas, along with the release of damage-induced molecular patterns (DAMPs) that can activate the inflammasome and further increase cytokines and leukocytosis. However, cerulein pancreatitis does not result in organ failure. Visceral adipose tissue is present in and around the pancreas as white adipocytes (yellow ovals below the acinar cell), which contain triglycerides containing unsaturated fatty acids. The leaked pancreatic enzymes and lipase from the acinar cell can damage the adipocytes and hydrolyze these triglycerides into nonesterified fatty acids, which are predominantly unsaturated, thus generating excess unsaturated NEFA (UFA). The UFAs so liberated can injure healthy mitochondria (green) and worsen necrosis by inhibiting mitochondrial complexes I and V (Cx. I, V) and reducing ATP levels. When excessive, the UFAs can also enter the systemic circulating and cause systemic mitochondrial injury. The lower part of the figure compares the published evidence of injury to the respiratory, circulatory, and renal systems induced by UFAs, trypsin, cytokines, and inflammatory cells. A red + indicates ≥2 reports citing the outcome induced by an agent, a red + indicates 1 report, and unclear or lack of evidence are shown as ± and −, respectively. The mechanisms and evidence of UFA-induced increases in DAMPs, cytokine storms, and injury to cells in distant organs, like the endothelium, lungs, and kidney tubules, are described in the text

proteases [80, 81], reactive oxygen species [82], inflammatory cells [5, 83], and lipids [64, 66, 67, 84].

2. The agent can reproducibly induce the specific disease state if introduced into a subject. The agents that induce organ failure, and the mechanisms by which these are generated are discussed in the following section.

3. The specific neutralization or reduction of the agent should prevent or reduce the harm in the diseased subject. This criterion has both clinical and experimental evidence to determine which among the various agents mentioned above is a potential mediator of organ failure, and whether neutralisation or reduction of them can decrease the severity of organ dysfunction/failure

Determining the causal mechanisms for organ failure in patients with AP using Koch's postulates is challenging, although some progress has been made in recent years. There are a vast number of potential agents that meet the first postulate. The second postulate cannot be tested with human subjects, since it requires induction of AP, which would not be ethically acceptable. The third postulate requires a therapeutic trial, which is not possible in the absence of a confirmed therapeutic target and would be prohibitive in terms of logistics and cost. A reasonable approach is to address the second and initial third postulates in the laboratory before more definite studies might be performed in human subjects. A large amount of clinical and experimental data has accrued over the last several years. This can help make a reasonable judgement about which agent(s) are likely to mediate organ failure, and potential therapeutic targets to treat severe AP.

The remaining discussion will discuss the evidence for various agents in the light of the above points and then expand on why targeting long-chain unsaturated fatty acids may be the most relevant therapeutic strategy to prevent or mitigate organ failure, reduce the severity of AP, and improve the clinical outcome.

3 Potential Mechanisms Driving Organ Failure

3.1 Adipocyte- and Lipid-Derived Mediators and Visceral Fat Necrosis

Visceral fat averages about 3% of body weight, ranging from 1 to 10% [85–87]. The principal cells in visceral fat are white adipocytes. The triglycerides stored in the adipocyte lipid droplet comprise >80% of an adipocyte's mass [88, 89]. As we shall see below, necrosis of this fat (visceral fat necrosis or VFN) is nearly universal in severe AP. Therefore, the products of adipocytes, including lipids, cytokines, and adipokines, are attractive as potential agents in the pathogenesis and progression to severe AP. Here, we shall first examine the evidence and mechanisms of severe AP for lipid mediators, long-chain unsaturated fatty acids (UFAs), which are also the most abundant constituent of adipose triglyceride and have been extensively studied.

Human studies associating VFN with severity during AP date back to the nineteenth century [90]. The most comprehensive documentations of VFN in human AP were reported separately by surgeons and pathologists. The Finnish surgeon Nordback reported on 79 AP patients he operated on within 4 days of onset [91]. After examining their surgical pathology, he clearly stated "the most vulnerable areas seemed to be the peripancreatic adipose tissue, from where the necrosis spread through the septa towards the pancreatic parenchyma." Similarly the German pathologist Kloppel [15], while reviewing 367 AP patients [92], stated "we recognized only one pattern of injury which was dominated by peripancreatic fat necrosis" and went on to conclude that "fat necrosis is most likely the lesion which definitely marks the beginning of acute pancreatitis… fat necrosis was a constant feature of all cases with AP, irrespective of their duration, severity, and aetiology." Experimental studies have demonstrated that VFN starts within 12 h of cerulein-induced AP in obese mice [67] that went on to develop organ failure by 18 h and had progressively reduced survival over the next 4 days. Thus, VFN is common during AP, occurs early, and may play a pathogenic role during the disease.

3.2 Unsaturated Fatty Acids

Long chain unsaturated fatty acids (UFAs) are fatty acids with chains longer than 12 carbons that have double bonds. This class of fatty acid normally comprises 60–80% of the pool of visceral adipocyte triglyceride [93]. This triglyceride pool undergoes VFN during pancreatitis. The proportion of fatty acids in VFN is similar to the parent visceral fat [94]. This means that if the concentration of each fatty acid (e.g., linoleic acid) in VFN is measured as a percentage of total fatty acid concentration, this is similar to the percentage of linoleic acid in the total triglyceride pool in adipose tissue. Isolated pancreatic parenchymal necrosis is rare during pancreatitis, and it is reported that 95% of pancreatic necrosis events are associated with VFN [15, 91, 95–97]. VFN results from the excessive, rapid breakdown of adipose triglyceride by pancreatic lipases released locally during AP. Thus, VFN mostly starts in and around the fat of the pancreas, though it can spread more extensively over time in the retroperitoneum, in particular. During VFN, triglycerides are hydrolyzed to nonesterified fatty acids (NEFA), and the UFAs, so liberated, are known to enrich the pancreatic necrosis collections in patients undergoing debridement [64, 66]. The excessive and rapid generation of UFAs during VFN can result in organ failure, as we shall see below.

Several studies have analyzed the chemical composition of human VFN and noted this to be enriched in long-chain UFAs [64, 66, 67, 94], with the UFA proportions ranging from 60 to 80% of the total NEFA pool. While these proportions are similar to the fatty acids in the parent visceral triglyceride in human studies [94] and mechanistic rodent studies [67], there is clear evidence that during pancreatitis the adipose triglyceride is degraded to the NEFA found to be present in VFN [67]. NEFA concentrations in the VFN are extremely high, reaching 10 mM [64, 66], perhaps because the starting pure triglyceride in adipocyte lipid droplets (the breakdown of which is the source of NEFA) has a 1 M concentration. This VFN is therefore the likely source of elevated UFAs, such as oleic, linoleic, and arachidonic, noted in the sera of patients with worsening AP [98, 99].

Normally polarized cells of the exocrine pancreas (i.e., acinar cells) secrete their enzymes from the apical portion into the pancreatic ducts that eventually drain into the duodenum. During AP, the acinar cells by various mechanisms [100–106] leak enzymes baslaterally [15, 107–109], into the surrounding visceral fat [15, 108–110]. These enzymes include pancreatic triglyceride lipase (PNLIP), which is the principal lipase in the exocrine pancreas [111]. Genetic deletion studies [67] and molecular techniques [69] show PNLIP is the main enzyme that causes fat necrosis. Moreover, these studies show that PNLIP mediates fat necrosis independent of adipocyte triglyceride lipase [67] (ATGL), which is the principal lipase in adipocytes. To gain access to the adipocyte lipid droplet PNLIP depends on phospholipases of the pancreas that can damage the adipocyte cell membrane [67] and allow PNLIP to hydrolyze the triglyceride within. The resulting NEFAs generated by PNLIP can further worsen fat necrosis and pancreatic necrosis [67], resulting the progression of AP to necrotizing AP or severe AP associated with organ failure [64, 65] (Fig. 1).

Long-chain UFAs in a triglyceride facilitate its interaction with the catalytic pocket of lipases that hydrolyze them [112, 113]. This is because the double bonds in a UFA bring the fatty acid-glycerol ester bond (that needs to be cleaved to generate NEFA) into closer proximity to the catalytic serine in the active site of PNLIP [112]. In contrast, long-chain saturated chain fatty acids (SFA, i.e., those lacking double bonds) interfere with this interaction and thereby decrease the breakdown of the triglyceride [112]. Moreover, when there is excess VFN (e.g., when the several hundred grams of visceral fat breakdown) beyond the binding capacity of albumin (each molecule of which normally carries 6–8 fatty acids [114]), then the remaining albumin unbound UFAs are more aqueous stable than unbound SFAs [112]. Thus, unbound UFAs achieve higher monomeric concentrations than unbound long-chain SFAs [112] in aqueous tissue environments.

Long-chain unbound UFAs are more potent in inducing the lipotoxic signaling relevant to organ failure than long-chain unbound SFAs [68, 112, 113]. Such UFAs inhibit mitochondrial complexes I and V [64], cause mitochondrial depolarization [69, 113] and cytosolic calcium increase [69, 113], and, on electron microscopy, have been shown to cause mitochondrial swelling and inclusions [64]. This results in apoptotic cell death that progresses to necrosis [69]. During severe AP and consequent lipotoxic organ failure in animals, this is seen as an increase in apoptotic cells in the lungs [64, 66, 71, 115] (as in humans with acute respiratory distress syndrome [116–118]), renal tubular injury [64, 66, 115] (supported by direct injury to HEK293 cells [69, 70]), and elevated serum blood urea nitrogen [64, 115, 119, 120] or creatinine [68], endothelial injury [68, 112], and shock [67, 68, 121] that overall reduces survival. Moreover, intravenous infusion of long-chain UFAs is commonly used as a model of acute lung injury [122, 123]. These examples show that while damage to one organ system, such as the vascular system, causing hypotension and vascular leak from endothelial cell injury may contribute to renal failure and worsen lung injury, UFAs can directly injure renal cells (such as HEK293) and induce lung injury. Thus, excess UFA generation can induce multisystem organ failure, which is the hallmark of severe pancreatitis. Interestingly, UFAs can also drastically elevate serum levels of TNF-α, IL-1β, MCP-1, and IL-18 [64, 66–68, 71, 112, 121] by 50–1000-fold over baseline. Moreover, UFAs release damage-associated molecular patterns (DAMPs) that are proinflammatory. For example, lipolysis of visceral triglyceride during pancreatitis increased the serum ds-DNA and fragmented histone-DNA complexes [112, 121], similar to the administration of the long-chain UFA, linoleic acid (C18:2) [68]. Therefore, excess UFAs release can fulfil the second Koch's

postulate by inducing organ failure. Importantly, inhibition of this excessive lipolysis or neutralization of the UFAs can prevent systemic injury, DAMPs release hypercytokinemia, organ failure, and mortality [64, 67, 68, 71, 112, 113, 115, 120], thereby fulfilling the third postulate. Fulfilment of all three Koch's postulates make UFAs highly probable mediators of organ failure and severity during AP. Recently, a novel lipase inhibitor RABI-767 has entered clinical trials (ClinicalTrials.gov ID NCT06080789). It remains to be seen whether lipase inhibition can mitigate or prevent organ failure during human AP.

3.3   Platelet-Activating Factor

Platelet-activating factor (PAF) is a phospholipid (acetyl-glyceryl-ether-phosphorylcholine) produced by platelets, myeloid cells, and endothelial cells. PAF production is catalyzed by phospholipase A2. PAF acts via a G-protein receptor [124] and is degraded by PAF acetylhydrolase [125]. PAF has been extensively targeted in human AP, and its antagonism as a therapy was tested in the largest clinical trial in AP so far [126]. Evidence supporting PAF's role in pancreatitis includes:

1. Intra-arterial delivery of PAFs into the pancreas causes AP [127].
2. PAF increases vascular permeability, worsens inflammation, and causes cell death [128].
3. PAF increases during severe biliary pancreatitis [84] and associated shock and acute lung injury [129].
4. PAF antagonism was protective in biliary pancreatitis, the choline-deficient ethionine-supplemented diet (CDE diet) [130] model in mice, the cerulein model in rats, and severe biliary pancreatitis in opossums [131]; however, the endpoints were focused more on local injury and inflammation than organ failure.

While initial clinical trials using the PAF antagonist lexipafant showed promise [132], the large definitive clinical trial did not reduce organ failure or mortality, despite a reduction in local complications and sepsis [126]. The failure was largely attributed to the presence of early organ failure in the patient cohort in whom lexipafant was tested, but this could also be an inherent limitation of targeting PAF. A critical appraisal of the trial showed that lexipafant was effective in a subgroup of patients who received it within the first 48 h [133].

4 Humoral Mediators Derived From Adipose and Non-Adipose Tissues

4.1 Adipokines and Cytokines

Numerous cytokines, including IL-6 [73–76], IL-1β [72], IL-8 [73, 76, 134], MCP-1 [79], and TNF-α [74] and adipokines, including resistin and visfatin [135, 136], are elevated in the serum of patients during severe AP. These have been used to predict severe pancreatitis [72–79]. Resistin is the adipokine mostly shown to be associated with pancreatitis severity early in the disease [135, 137–139]. Interestingly, IL-6, IL-8, MCP-1, and resistin serum levels peak early in severe AP and then come down within a few days after admission [138, 140]. IL-6 is the most extensively [75] studied cytokine to predict organ failure and AP severity. Consistent with its declining trends over the course of an admission, separate studies have shown IL-6 values [137] >473.4 pg/mL at admission to have an area under the curve (AUC) of 0.78 and day 3 levels >122 pg/mL to have an AUC of 0.82, respectively, for predicting organ failure [141].

The early peak for both adipokines and cytokines and common declining trends over time suggest adipose involvement as a unifying underlying mechanism. Mechanistically this is consistent with adipocytes releasing resistin and fatty acids when they undergo fat necrosis [65]. Moreover, unsaturated fatty acids (but not SFAs) upregulate the mRNA of cytokines, including TNF-α, and the neutrophil chemoattractants CXCL1 and CXCL2 [64] in pancreatic acini. Separately, fat necrosis of UFA-fed mice developing organ failure during severe pancreatitis

showed a 10–1000-fold higher upregulation in the mRNAs of IL-6, TNF-α, MCP-1, and a similar trend in serum levels compared to SFA-fed mice [112]. The administration of linoleic acid (unlike the saturated palmitic acid) to mice also causes the cytokine storm by increasing IL-1β, IL-6, MCP-1, and TNF-α [68] several fold over control values. Similarly, inhibiting lipolysis during experimental severe pancreatitis reduces the increase in serum IL-6, MCP-1, TNF-α [64, 67, 71], IL-β and IL-8 [66, 115] and associated organ failure in mechanistically dissimilar models of pancreatitis. Moreover, DAMPs such as those released during fat necrosis and by linoleic acid [67, 68, 112] can cause the cytokine storm [142–144] and lead to death [145]. Therefore, the parallels noted in adipokines and cytokines during clinically severe AP may have a unifying mechanism in fat necrosis and the consequent UFA-induced cytokine storm.

The benefits of neutralizing or removing cytokines in severe AP are being studied. An important clue about their role is whether these fulfil the second Koch's postulate, by causing harm. In the case of IL-6 infusion, this actually prevented endotoxin-induced TNF-α increase [146] in humans. Over longer periods, it reduced serum iron and caused anemia [147, 148] but did not cause organ failure. IL-6 [149] and TNF-α [150] may protect in experimental AP and do not induce organ failure [151–155]. IL-6 knockout mice were not protected from obesity-induced severe pancreatitis [156]. Therefore, evidence of harm induced by IL-6 during AP is weak. The success of IL-6 neutralization with tocilizumab in another acute illness associated with organ failure, i.e., COVID-19, should be interpreted cautiously. This is because the trials showing a benefit of tocilizumab [125, 157] were done with the majority of patients also receiving corticosteroids as standard of care [158]. Of note, the earlier studies on tocilizumab, when there were fewer patients on steroids, showed weak or no benefits [159, 160]. Therefore, evidence of IL-6 neutralization alone being protective is lacking.

There is also a lack of supportive clinical evidence for targeting TNF-α in acute inflammation.

For example, TNF-α antagonism with etanercept worsened outcomes in alcoholic hepatitis [161]. This was noted despite etanercept showing a benefit in cerulein pancreatitis without fat necrosis [162], though previous studies showed that anti-TNF-α antibodies increased edema in cerulein pancreatitis [150].

In the case of other cytokine targets, IL-1β administration to rats did not induce organ failure [120] despite causing fever and increasing neutrophils in the lungs. Moreover, IL-8 and CXCL1 both reduced the risk of lung infections [163–165] and therefore may have a protective role. Broader approaches have been used to remove cytokines in AP. For example, the removal of cytokines by hemadsorption reduces IL-6 levels, which is associated with improvement of SOFA scores and renal parameters during severe pancreatitis [166]. Similar improvements were also noted during sepsis [167]. However, more definitive studies are needed to gauge improvement in survival or prevention of organ failure. Therefore, while the large increase in cytokines and adipokines early during severe AP makes them potential biomarkers of disease, we need stronger evidence to accept them as mediators, let alone treatment targets, for the organ failure of severe AP.

4.2 Trypsin

The auto-digestive role of trypsin in pancreatitis was proposed over a hundred years ago by Hans Chiari [168]. Trypsinogen is the inactive proenzyme precursor of trypsin normally present in the pancreas [169], and the activation of trypsinogen to trypsin within the pancreas has been shown to occur in experimental models of AP [80, 81, 170, 171] and in humans [80, 81]. Most studies support the role of trypsin in the initiation of pancreatitis [172]. Intravenous infusion of trypsin reduces blood pressure and causes shock [173, 174] and clotting and lung injury independent of neutrophils [175]. Trypsin's role in thrombosis is supported by studies showing elevated D-dimer to predict organ failure with a sensitivity and specificity in the 90% range [176]. Moreover,

thrombosis in the splenic or splanchnic veins is noted in 15–50% of patients with pancreatic necrosis [177, 178]. Mechanistically, the protease activated receptor-2 (PAR-2) [179], which is cleaved and activated by trypsin, may contribute to the deleterious effects of trypsin. For example, an IV infusion of PAR-2 agonists reduces blood pressure [180].

Trypsin is thus an attractive target to reduce acute pancreatitis severity. Interestingly, however, small-molecule trypsin inhibitors have not shown conclusive improvement [52–61] in AP-associated organ failure. Moreover, patients with hereditary pancreatitis due to cationic trypsinogen gene mutations (e.g., PRSS1) rarely develop organ failure in comparison to other cause of AP [181]. Recent studies using dabigatran (a dual trypsin, thrombin inhibitor) has shown it to reduce local injury and the progression of chronic pancreatitis [182, 183]. Circulating anti-proteases such as alpha-2 macroglobulin [184, 185] can inactivate trypsin. Moreover, trypsin is rapidly cleaved itself or by other proteases, resulting in its inactivation [186]. The short-lived nature of trypsin, its presence in AP irrespective of severity, and the natural protective mechanisms to counteract trypsin may explain why trypsin inhibition has not been effective in reducing the severity of acute pancreatitis.

4.3 Damage-Associated Molecular Patterns (DAMPs)

An elevation in the serum DAMPs is associated with severe AP in humans [187–190]. DAMPs are released from cells dying from necrosis and are potential mediators of severity based on animal studies [191, 192]. DAMPs are a heterogeneous class of molecules, which include ATP (a small molecule), proteins including nuclear histones, high-mobility group box 1 (HMGB1), cytoplasmic proteins like S-100, the soluble receptor for advanced glycation end products (sRAGE), other nuclear components (e.g., DNA, nucleosomes), and extracellular matrix molecules including hyaluronic acid. Release of DAMPs such as ds-DNA, histone complexed DNA [112, 121, 193], and HMGB1 [192, 194, 195] has been noted during organ failure in experimental severe AP and also in UFA-induced organ failure [68, 112].

DAMPs can worsen inflammation by causing activation of the inflammasome [191, 196], as shown for ATP (via P2X7), sRAGE, and HMGB1, and also directly by inducing a sterile inflammatory response [197], disrupting the plasmalemma [198], and further increasing HMGB1 release [192]. As mentioned below, histone-DNA complexes in neutrophils may lead to neutrophil extracellular traps (NETs) and therefore worsen pancreatitis by more than one mechanism. HMGB1 is a well-studied DAMP in pancreatitis [194, 195]. HMGB1 has been shown to worsen pancreatic injury via Toll-like receptor-4 (TLR4)-mediated activation of the transcription factor nuclear factor-kB [199]. HMGB1 can also activate NF-kB by acting on RAGE [200]. In experimental pancreatitis, HMGB1 was reduced by N-acetyl cysteine [192] and dexamethasone [201], and in humans, HMGB1 (along with TNF-α) was shown to be reduced in patients given indomethacin to prevent post-ERCP pancreatitis [202]. Serum HMGB1 significantly correlated with AP severity in humans in a meta-analysis [203]. Interestingly, however, neither N-acetyl cysteine [204, 205] nor indomethacin [206] reduced progression of AP, and pancreatitis is listed as an adverse effect of glucocorticoids including dexamethasone [207]. Localized pancreatic hypothermia has also been shown to reduce the release of histone-DNA complexes and ds-DNA [121, 193], along with improving survival during severe pancreatitis. While DAMPs are an attractive target in AP, it remains to be determined if these are one of the dominant mechanisms that worsens AP or if these are part of multiple parallel deleterious pathways, which may not reduce pancreatitis severity if targeted in isolation. This knowledge is important in understanding if modalities targeting DAMPs would

be a reasonable target to reduce the severity of human AP.

5 Inflammatory Cells and Their Mediators

5.1 Neutrophils

Neutrophils from the largest proportion of leukocytes in our circulation [208]. Leukocytosis (>12,000/mm [3]) is part of the systemic inflammatory response syndrome (SIRS) [83], which is often used as an early predictor of severe AP [5]. Neutrophil infiltration into the pancreas [209, 210], intestine [211], and lungs [212, 213], along with an increase in neutrophil products such as myeloperoxidase in the blood, are features of experimental AP [214]. Neutrophil infiltration into the pancreas has been proposed to worsen local injury by converting apoptotic cell death to necrosis [215]. Neutrophil infiltration into the lungs can cause lung injury via vascular leak [164, 165, 213] and reactive oxygen species (ROS) [216] generated by NADPH oxidase [209]. Matrix metalloproteinase-9 (MMP-9) has been suggested as a major neutrophil product that causes lung injury [217]. Additionally, neutrophils can also contribute to neutrophil extracellular traps, which may worsen AP, as described below.

To infiltrate an organ, neutrophils have to first interact with the endothelium [208] via P- and E-selectin on the surface of endothelial cells. These endothelial selectins bind adhesion molecules like L-selectins and β2-integrins on the surface of neutrophils, resulting in neutrophil rolling on the endothelium. Furthermore, neutrophil chemoattractant chemokines (e.g., C-X-C ELR chemokines) released from the tissue increase the affinity state of these integrins, which further bind intercellular adhesion molecule-1 (ICAM-1) or ICAM-2. Agents such as cerulein [218], which cause AP, increase the expression of CXC ELR chemokines in pancreatic acini. Blood levels of P- and E-selectin [219] and ICAM-1 [220] are elevated in experimental AP and also during human AP [221, 222], and these were associated with AP severity and lung injury. Interestingly, UFA administration, which causes organ failure, also increases serum E-selectin and ICAM-1 [68] in rodents.

Infiltrating neutrophils may have multiple roles in worsening AP. This is supported by neutralization of the neutrophil chemoattractant CXC chemokines CXCL2 and CXCL4 reducing lung inflammation [223] during AP. Interestingly, trypsin generation in the late phase of experimental AP has been shown to be neutrophil dependent [175]. This has been proposed to be via NADPH oxidase [209]. Trypsin can also stimulate neutrophils to secrete matrix metalloproteinase-9 [217]. ROS scavengers, inhibitors, and antioxidants have shown promise in reducing the severity of experimental AP [192, 224–226], and neutrophil depletion has been shown to improve microvascular permeability [175, 213, 217, 227], associated with a reduced pulmonary neutrophil infiltration.

However, there are other studies highlighting the physiologic roles of neutrophils and that neutrophil infiltration may not always be deleterious. For example, increasing KC/CXCL1 [163, 164, 228] expression in the lungs increases neutrophil accumulation and does not cause lung injury. Neutrophils have a phagocytic role [208], and loss of neutrophil function results in increased susceptibility to fungal and bacterial infections [163, 164, 228]. Similarly, very low neutrophil counts or neutropenia increases the risk of infections [229–231]. Interestingly, leukopenia (WBC counts <4000/mm [3]) is also a part of SIRS [83], which can be associated with severe AP. Despite the benefits of ROS scavengers, inhibitors, and antioxidants in experimental AP [224–226], these agents have not shown a benefit in human AP [204, 205]. Lastly, the loss of the protective functions of neutrophils may increase this risk of septic complications and infected necrosis in moderate or severe AP

[39, 45, 46]. Therefore, whether neutrophil depletion or reducing neutrophil recruitment will reduce systemic injury in human AP remains to be seen.

5.2   Neutrophil Extracellular Traps

Neutrophil extracellular traps (NETs) are extruded from dying neutrophils and have a web-like structure [208, 232]. NETs were originally shown to be rapidly formed in gram-positive bacterial infections and prevent bacterial dissemination [232]. The contents of NETs include neutrophil granule proteins including myeloperoxidase, elastase, histone-DNA complexes, and chromatin [208]. These are increased in the sera of patients with severe AP [233] and have been recently proposed to worsen the course of AP [234]. In addition, NETs occlude pancreatic ducts in human AP and may perpetuate AP [235]. NETs formation in AP is catalyzed by the enzyme protein arginine deiminase 4 (PAD4) [236], which causes histone modification of arginine residues to citrulline [237]. This modification weakens DNA-histone interactions and allows the neutrophils to expel the de-condensed chromatin. NETs formation has been shown to increase trypsin generation in acini, along with causing activation of the signal transducer and activator of transcription-3 (STAT-3) [233]. NETs formation may also have a protective role during pancreatic necrosis by facilitating its walling off as a barrier between viable and nonviable tissue [238].

Elevated citrullinated histone-3, PAD2, and PAD4 levels were noted in the sera of patients with AP who had developed sepsis compared to AP patients within 72 h of diagnosis who had no infection [239]. Targeting NETs is therapeutically relevant, since reduced NETs formation was noted in humans [240] and rodents after PAD4 inhibition. NETs formation in neutrophils from mice with AP was reduced by the autophagy inhibitor chloroquine [241], which also improved survival in the L-arginine and choline deficient ethionine supplemented (CDE) diet-induced pancreatitis models. Interestingly, previous studies using chloroquine in CDE diet induced AP have shown mixed results [242, 243]. It should be noted that chloroquine also increases lysosomal pH and reduces trypsinogen activation [242, 243]. Whether targeting NETs with chloroquine or other drugs is a possible approach to reduce AP-induced organ failure in humans remains to be studied.

5.3 Inflammasome

The inflammasome family generates the innate immune inflammatory response. These multiprotein oligomers of different proteins from a family of inflammasomes are activated by different stimuli, including DAMPs, extracellular ATP and ROS, and cytosolic ds-DNA. Activation of the inflammasome in macrophages or myeloid cells [244] results in IL-1β [72] and IL-18 [245–247] production and also increases HMGB1 [192, 248].

The inflammasome family may be involved in AP-associated systemic injury [191, 249, 250]. A recent detailed study showed involvement of NOD-, LRR-, and pyrin domain-containing protein 3 (NLRP3) inflammasome and IL-18 in mediating lung myeloperoxidase increase, which was used as a measure of systemic inflammation during duct ligation and L-arginine-induced pancreatitis in mice [250]. Genetic deletion of these reduced T cell activation and Th2 cell-mediated responses. Lysates of cerulein-treated acini activated caspase-1 in macrophages and increased IL-1β levels, which were prevented in NLRP3 knockout macrophages, which are ASC (apoptosis-associated speck-like protein containing a caspase recruitment domain) dependent. IL-18 and ASC levels were also increased in patients with severe AP [250].

Acute pancreatitis can also activate the AIM2 (absent in melanoma 2) inflammasome. This can be via nucleosomes (i.e., DNA-histone complexes) and RAGE [249, 251], which can increase severity and lung inflammation during L-arginine and cerulein pancreatitis [192, 251], or extracellular ATP or NAD released from injured acini activating the P2X7 receptor [191]. TLR 4 and TLR9 can also be activated by DAMPs [191], and antagonism of the latter reduced lung inflammation, but not edema [191].

Interestingly, while IL-1β increases body temperature and lung inflammation, it does not induce lung injury or vascular leak [120]. Similarly, IL-18 (and IL-12) induces AP in lean mice but without the fat necrosis and organ failure that is noted in obese mice [252, 253], which is due to fatty acids [64]. As mentioned above, UFAs can release DAMPs [68, 112], which in turn can trigger inflammasome activation. The role of the inflammasome therefore seems more likely to be downstream of DAMP-mediated IL-1β and IL-18-mediated responses, including fever, inflammatory cell infiltration, and perhaps pancreatic necrosis. The inflammasome's ubiquitous nature (in the absence of known genetic polymorphisms) should otherwise result in a more homogeneous and delayed systemic inflammatory response (because pancreatic necrosis often occurs after the first few days) than what is clinically noted during pancreatitis (i.e., earlier). Future studies are therefore needed to clarify the role and timing of the inflammasome in systemic injury during AP.

In summary, there are various inflammatory arms activated in severe AP. The most potent and upstream one of these appears to be lipolysis of visceral fat, resulting in visceral fat necrosis and generation of UFAs. Once generated, these UFAs cause mitochondrial injury and can exacerbate necrosis, cause DAMPs release, and trigger the cytokine storm, associated with shock, renal failure, and lung injury. Whether these findings can be translated to clinical benefit in clinical trials (NCT 06080789) by decreasing impact of UFAs on the risk of organ failure remains to be seen.

6   Capillary Permeability as a Possible Link Between Systemic Inflammation and Organ Failure

The mechanisms responsible for the transition from transient to persistent systemic inflammation (SIRS) and multiorgan failure (MOF) in AP are beginning to be explored. A fluid compartment model [254] proposes vascular, interstitial, and "third-space" compartments with variable permeability to plasma proteins at the level of the endothelial cell-lined capillaries. Recent studies have shown UFAs, such as oleic and linoleic acid, that are increased in the sera of patients with AP [49, 67, 99, 255] cause endothelial injury [68, 112, 113]. This endothelial injury is evidenced by increased permeability of endothelial monolayers to high-molecular-weight dextran [112, 113], along with a loss of trans-endothelial cell electrical resistance. The findings are relevant to the rapid development of hypoalbuminemia which is a feature of severe AP [256]. This is further supported by evidence that administration of UFAs to mice causes hypoalbuminemia and increased serum levels of E-selectin and ICAM-1, which are endothelial injury markers [112]. This mechanistic data links visceral fat necrosis, which releases fatty acids during AP, to the vascular leak and third spacing of macromolecules and the hypotension and hypoperfusion that develop during progression to MOF.

The compartment model [254] seeks to explain the characteristics of organ systems that typically fail during the transition from SIRS to MOF by using the unregulated loss of large plasma proteins as biomarkers for MOF. In this manner, the exudation of albumin and non-albumin plasma proteins from the vascular compartment during the initial phases of AP was associated with the progression of SIRS to MOF. The resulting intravascular hypovolemia leads to systemic hypotension in visceral organs which suffer disproportional effects. This is possibly aggravated by reflex vasoconstriction of the mesenteric and/or renal arterioles or other mechanisms. Data for the compartment model [254] was obtained from a cohort study of patients at the University of Pittsburgh Medical Center with severe AP ($n = 57$), 18 of whom developed MOF and 5 of whom died. A trajectory analysis compared patients before and after they developed MOF while considering unregulated loss of large plasma proteins by capillary leak. It was hypothesized that this leak led to loss of oncotic pressure and reduced vascular volume, resulting in hypotension with prerenal azotemia and acute renal dysfunction, pancreas necrosis, and pulmonary edema due to increased capillary permeability in the lung with acute respiratory distress syndrome. However, the contribution of oncotic pressure to hypotension and third spacing would appear unlikely because albumin (molecular weight of 60,000 Da) forms about half the mass of plasma proteins, has normal plasma concentrations of 35–55 g/L (0.6–1.0 mM), and contributes minimally to the osmolarity of plasma in the pure form, i.e., 0.6–1.0 milliosmole. Moreover, a large corporation of plasma protein, (globulins with molecular weights >90 kDa) contributes even less to oncotic pressure. It is noteworthy that the albumin molecule binds 6–8 fatty acids [114] that are otherwise toxic in the unbound form [49, 112]. This suggests that fatty acids and other toxic cargo molecules carried by albumin contribute to the osmolarity of albumin in plasma [257] and that pure albumin's contribution to plasma osmotic pressure is relatively minor. A more plausible explanation is that third spacing of plasma proteins and hypoalbuminemia during AP resulting from the endothelial injury is induced by excess albumin unbound fatty acids [49, 68, 112].

These findings are consistent with an increasing hematocrit in patients with MOF and loss of plasma proteins known to be associated with hypoperfusion of the kidneys (increased risk of prerenal azotemia) and pancreas (increased risk of pancreatic necrosis). This model combined with the upstream injury to endothelial cells by fatty acids causing vascular leak [68, 112, 113] and loss of proteins like albumin [68] (i.e., pathological capillary leak syndrome) appear to be important causal mechanisms of organ failure, as well as providing additional relevant biomarkers. Thus, these data clarify a major pathological mechanism of MOF in AP and possibly other disorders in which elevated fatty acids are associated with SIRS and MOF, such as COVID-19 [68, 258], trauma [259], severe burns [260, 261], and sepsis [49, 55, 262].

Trajectory analysis of individual patients using changes in their own biomarker levels while attractive needs to be interpreted with some caution, since the large volume of fluids used during AP treatment can unpredictably perturb vascular volume and also contribute to tissue edema [263]. During a vascular leak, the resuscitation fluid itself can result in fluid overload, third-spacing, and worsening tissue edema. This is important in abdominal compartment syndrome [264, 265] and, recently, in the pulmonary complications of aggressive fluid resuscitation observed in the Waterfall and other studies [8]. Moreover, as shown above, excess UFAs that cause endothelial injury and hypotension can also cause the cytokine storm [49, 67, 68]. These data are consistent with a mechanistic model in which UFA induced leakage of large and small proteins and fluids into the lungs contributing to pulmonary edema and respiratory failure [68]. Further evaluation of modalities to reduce the UFA induced endothelial injury in AP and other diseases with SIRS, capillary leak syndrome, and therapeutic interventions to prevent MOF is needed.

7 Gut Injury and Toxic Gut-Lymph Have a Potential Role in Promoting Systemic Inflammation and Organ Failure

The stereotyped pattern of organ dysfunction and failure is irrespective of etiology, occurring across the range of acute and critical illness (including AP). This suggests the presence of a common mechanism. A feature of severe AP (and other acute and critical illnesses), especially those associated with organ failure, is gut injury [211]. The initial insult is ischemic secondary to reflex splanchnic vasoconstriction, where gut perfusion is sacrificed for perfusion of vital organs. This gut injury can be compounded by

luminal pancreatic enzymes [266] and gut microbiota [267]. Clinical evidence of gut injury includes paralytic ileus and elevated markers of gut injury [268]. However, several examples show gut injury and microbial translocation do not always result in organ failure, including a recent multicenter study in nonocclusive mesenteric ischemia showing survival to be unrelated to intestinal mural enhancement, pneumatosis, wall thickness, or serum lactate on multivariate analysis [269]. Additionally, organ failure in colonic diverticulitis is much less frequent than in pancreatitis [67, 270]. In diverticulitis, there is microperforation of the colon with spillage of fecal contents into the abdomen, but despite the entry of bacteria into the abdomen, i.e., translocation, antibiotics are not recommended in uncomplicated cases [271, 272]. Similarly, sepsis is rare in ulcerative colitis and Crohn's disease [273] despite the presence of extensive ulcerations in the colon that are in contact with fecal material. Moreover, bacteremia has not been noted at the time of surgery for uncontrolled ulcerative colitis that necessitated surgery [274]. The role of bacterial translocation in causing organ failure is further weakened by bacterial translocation being common but transient due to rapid bacterial clearance by competent immune cells. For example, transient bacteriemia is common after tooth brushing, dental extractions [50], and endoscopic procedures [51], for which antibiotics are normally not recommended [275]. Therefore, as recently described [49], lipotoxic immune cell injury during AP, which impairs bacterial clearance by immune cells, links the development of infections during AP to severe AP and the consequent clinical appearance of sepsis. While various conceptual models have been proposed for the role of gut injury in increasing the severity of AP and driving organ failure (including the gut as the "motor" of the septic state, bacterial translocation, and neutrophil activation in the gut wall ('second hit hypothesis') [276]. These models do not provide definitive proof that gut injury causes organ failure.

Most recently, the gut lymph model [211] has been advanced through preclinical and early clinical studies [277]. Lymph transports the interstitial fluid during pancreatitis. The HDL fraction of lymph is rich in triglycerides compared to blood [278], suggesting that the lymphatic system may transport lipid mediators of organ failure generated during visceral fat necrosis. However, lymph also has numerous types of cells and molecules. Agents inducing organ failure have not been isolated in pure form in lymph, which is a requirement of Koch's postulates, and thus gut lymph does not fulfil all these criteria. The evidence supporting the lymphatic route of entry of toxins into the circulation includes:

1. AP induces significant changes in gut lymph composition which are toxic to cells and organs [279]. These include significant increases in pancreatic enzymes including lipase [279]. However, the mediators of toxicity have not all been identified in pure form.
2. AP conditioned gut lymph increases pancreatic edema index and histologic injury [280] and impairs cardiac function [281].
3. External drainage of thoracic duct lymph (the majority of which is gut-lymph) reduces clinical respiratory failure [282] and prevents experimental cardiac failure [281]. Anti-lipase treatment targeting gut-lymph in experimental AP restores blood pressure and decreases biomarkers of end organ injury (in press, personal communication from Professor John Windsor).

The gut lymph model offers two broad treatment paradigms. The first is diversion of thoracic duct lymph by external drainage, which has been offered with an open thoracic duct cannulation approach [277] and now with a minimally invasive radiology approach [283]. The second is pharmacological, targeting drugs to toxic elements of gut-lymph [284].

8 Conclusion

This chapter has summarized current thinking on mechanisms that drive organ failure in AP. These include lipase-induced visceral fat necrosis with release of unsaturated fatty acids and the gut-lymph model in which lymph may be a route for

entry of gut derived toxic and inflammatory factors into the circulation. In the preclinical setting, both of these mechanisms appear to drive organ failure and offer novel strategies for the treatment of organ failure. Clinical trials on whether the novel lipase inhibitor RABI-767, thoracic duct lymphatic diversion or gut-lymph targeted treatments reduce the risk and severity of end-organ dysfunction and failure will shed more light on the relevance of these mechanisms.

References

1. Mederos MA, Reber HA, Girgis MD. Acute pancreatitis: a review. Jama. 2021;325:382–90.
2. Gullo L, Migliori M, Olah A, Farkas G, Levy P, Arvanitakis C, Lankisch P, Beger H. Acute pancreatitis in five European countries: etiology and mortality. Pancreas. 2002;24:223–7.
3. Yasuda H, Horibe M, Sanui M, Sasaki M, Suzuki N, Sawano H, Goto T, Ikeura T, Takeda T, Oda T, Ogura Y, Miyazaki D, Kitamura K, Chiba N, Ozaki T, Yamashita T, Koinuma T, Oshima T, Yamamoto T, Hirota M, Sato M, Miyamoto K, Mine T, Misumi T, Takeda Y, Iwasaki E, Kanai T, Mayumi T. Etiology and mortality in severe acute pancreatitis: a multicenter study in Japan. Pancreatology. 2020;20:307–17.
4. Zhu Y, Pan X, Zeng H, He W, Xia L, Liu P, Zhu Y, Chen Y, Lv N. A study on the etiology, severity, and mortality of 3260 patients with acute pancreatitis according to the revised Atlanta classification in Jiangxi, China over an 8-year period. Pancreas. 2017;46:504–9.
5. Banks PA, Bollen TL, Dervenis C, Gooszen HG, Johnson CD, Sarr MG, Tsiotos GG, Vege SS, Acute Pancreatitis Classification Working Group. Classification of acute pancreatitis—2012: revision of the Atlanta classification and definitions by international consensus. Gut. 2013;62:102–11.
6. Marshall JC, Cook DJ, Christou NV, Bernard GR, Sprung CL, Sibbald WJ. Multiple organ dysfunction score: a reliable descriptor of a complex clinical outcome. Crit Care Med. 1995;23:1638–52.
7. Flint R, Windsor JA. Early physiological response to intensive care as a clinically relevant approach to predicting the outcome in severe acute pancreatitis. Arch Surg. 2004;139:438–43.
8. de-Madaria E, Buxbaum JL, Maisonneuve P, García García de Paredes A, Zapater P, Guilabert L, Vaillo-Rocamora A, Rodríguez-Gandía M, Donate-Ortega J, Lozada-Hernández EE, Collazo Moreno AJR, Lira-Aguilar A, Llovet LP, Mehta R, Tandel R, Navarro P, Sánchez-Pardo AM, Sánchez-Marin C, Cobreros M, Fernández-Cabrera I, Casals-

Seoane F, Casas Deza D, Lauret-Braña E, Martí-Marqués E, Camacho-Montaño LM, Ubieto V, Ganuza M, Bolado F. Aggressive or moderate fluid resuscitation in acute pancreatitis. N Engl J Med. 2022;387:989–1000.

9. Wig JD, Bharathy KG, Kochhar R, Yadav TD, Kudari AK, Doley RP, Gupta V, Babu YR. Correlates of organ failure in severe acute pancreatitis. JOP. 2009;10:271–5.

10. Machicado JD, Gougol A, Tan X, Gao X, Paragomi P, Pothoulakis I, Talukdar R, Kochhar R, Goenka MK, Gulla A, Gonzalez JA, Singh VK, Ferreira M, Stevens T, Barbu ST, Nawaz H, Gutierrez SC, Zarnescu NO, Capurso G, Easler JJ, Triantafyllou K, Pelaez-Luna M, Thakkar S, Ocampo C, de-Madaria E, Cote GA, Wu BU, Conwell DL, Hart PA, Tang G, Papachristou GI. Mortality in acute pancreatitis with persistent organ failure is determined by the number, type, and sequence of organ systems affected. United Eur Gastroenterol J. 2021;9:139–49.

11. Charlson ME, Pompei P, Ales KL, MacKenzie CR. A new method of classifying prognostic comorbidity in longitudinal studies: development and validation. J Chronic Dis. 1987;40:373–83.

12. Szakacs Z, Gede N, Pecsi D, Izbeki F, Papp M, Kovacs G, Feher E, Dobszai D, Kui B, Marta K, Konya K, Szabo I, Torok I, Gajdan L, Takacs T, Sarlos P, Godi S, Varga M, Hamvas J, Vincze A, Szentesi A, Parniczky A, Hegyi P. Aging and comorbidities in acute pancreatitis II.: a cohort-analysis of 1203 prospectively collected cases. Front Physiol. 2018;9:1776.

13. Singh VK, Bollen TL, Wu BU, Repas K, Maurer R, Yu S, Mortele KJ, Conwell DL, Banks PA. An assessment of the severity of interstitial pancreatitis. Clin Gastroenterol Hepatol. 2011;9:1098–103.

14. Feng A, Ao X, Zhou N, Huang T, Li L, Zeng M, Lyu J. A novel risk-prediction scoring system for sepsis among patients with acute pancreatitis: a retrospective analysis of a large clinical database. Int J Clin Pract. 2022;2022:5435656.

15. Kloppel G, Dreyer T, Willemer S, Kern HF, Adler G. Human acute pancreatitis: its pathogenesis in the light of immunocytochemical and ultrastructural findings in acinar cells. Virchows Arch A Pathol Anat Histopathol. 1986;409:791–803.

16. Abu Hilal M, Armstrong T. The impact of obesity on the course and outcome of acute pancreatitis. Obes Surg. 2008;18:326–8.

17. Papachristou GI, Papachristou DJ, Avula H, Slivka A, Whitcomb DC. Obesity increases the severity of acute pancreatitis: performance of APACHE-O score and correlation with the inflammatory response. Pancreatology. 2006;6:279–85.

18. Porter KA, Banks PA. Obesity as a predictor of severity in acute pancreatitis. Int J Pancreatol. 1991;10:247–52.

19. Shin KY, Lee WS, Chung DW, Heo J, Jung MK, Tak WY, Kweon YO, Cho CM. Influence of obesity on the severity and clinical outcome of acute pancreatitis. Gut Liver. 2011;5:335–9.

20. O'Leary DP, O'Neill D, McLaughlin P, O'Neill S, Myers E, Maher MM, Redmond HP. Effects of abdominal fat distribution parameters on severity of acute pancreatitis. World J Surg. 2012;36:1679–85.

21. Sempere L, Martinez J, de Madaria E, Lozano B, Sanchez-Paya J, Jover R, Perez-Mateo M. Obesity and fat distribution imply a greater systemic inflammatory response and a worse prognosis in acute pancreatitis. Pancreatology. 2008;8:257–64.

22. Evans AC, Papachristou GI, Whitcomb DC. Obesity and the risk of severe acute pancreatitis. Minerva Gastroenterol Dietol. 2010;56:169–79.

23. Chen SM, Xiong GS, Wu SM. Is obesity an indicator of complications and mortality in acute pancreatitis? An updated meta-analysis. J Dig Dis. 2012;13:244–51.

24. Sadr-Azodi O, Orsini N, Andren-Sandberg A, Wolk A. Abdominal and total adiposity and the risk of acute pancreatitis: a population-based prospective cohort study. Am J Gastroenterol. 2013;108:133–9.

25. Yashima Y, Isayama H, Tsujino T, Nagano R, Yamamoto K, Mizuno S, Yagioka H, Kawakubo K, Sasaki T, Kogure H, Nakai Y, Hirano K, Sasahira N, Tada M, Kawabe T, Koike K, Omata M. A large volume of visceral adipose tissue leads to severe acute pancreatitis. J Gastroenterol. 2011;46:1213–8.

26. Funnell IC, Bornman PC, Weakley SP, Terblanche J, Marks IN. Obesity: an important prognostic factor in acute pancreatitis. Br J Surg. 1993;80:484–6.

27. Nawaz H, Koutroumpakis E, Easler J, Slivka A, Whitcomb DC, Singh VP, Yadav D, Papachristou GI. Elevated serum triglycerides are independently associated with persistent organ failure in acute pancreatitis. Am J Gastroenterol. 2015;110:1497–503.

28. Pascual I, Sanahuja A, Garcia N, Vazquez P, Moreno O, Tosca J, Pena A, Garayoa A, Lluch P, Mora F. Association of elevated serum triglyceride levels with a more severe course of acute pancreatitis: cohort analysis of 1457 patients. Pancreatology. 2019;19:623–9.

29. Wan J, He W, Zhu Y, Zhu Y, Zeng H, Liu P, Xia L, Lu N. Stratified analysis and clinical significance of elevated serum triglyceride levels in early acute pancreatitis: a retrospective study. Lipids Health Dis. 2017;16:124.

30. Zhang R, Deng L, Jin T, Zhu P, Shi N, Jiang K, Li L, Yang X, Guo J, Yang X, Liu T, Mukherjee R, Singh VK, Windsor JA, Sutton R, Huang W, Xia Q. Hypertriglyceridaemia-associated acute pancreatitis: diagnosis and impact on severity. HPB (Oxford). 2019;21:1240–9.

31. Zhang Q, Qin M, Liang Z, Huang H, Tang Y, Qin L, Wei Z, Xu M, Tang G. The relationship between serum triglyceride levels and acute pancreatitis in an animal model and a 14-year retrospective clinical study. Lipids Health Dis. 2019;18:183.

32. Bálint ER, Fűr G, Kiss L, Németh DI, Soós A, Hegyi P, Szakács Z, Tinusz B, Varjú P, Vincze Á, Erőss B, Czimmer J, Szepes Z, Varga G, Rakonczay Z Jr. Assessment of the course of acute pancreatitis in the light of aetiology: a systematic review and meta-analysis. Sci Rep. 2020;10:17936.

33. Kiss L, Fűr G, Pisipati S, Rajalingamgari P, Ewald N, Singh V, Rakonczay Z Jr. Mechanisms linking hypertriglyceridemia to acute pancreatitis. Acta Physiol (Oxf). 2023;237:e13916.

34. Isenmann R, Rau B, Beger HG. Early severe acute pancreatitis: characteristics of a new subgroup. Pancreas. 2001;22:274–8.

35. Sharma M, Banerjee D, Garg PK. Characterization of newer subgroups of fulminant and subfulminant pancreatitis associated with a high early mortality. Am J Gastroenterol. 2007;102:2688–95.

36. Mofidi R, Duff MD, Wigmore SJ, Madhavan KK, Garden OJ, Parks RW. Association between early systemic inflammatory response, severity of multiorgan dysfunction and death in acute pancreatitis. Br J Surg. 2006;93:738–44.

37. Lu JD, Cao F, Ding YX, Wu YD, Guo YL, Li F. Timing, distribution, and microbiology of infectious complications after necrotizing pancreatitis. World J Gastroenterol. 2019;25:5162–73.

38. Ni T, Wen Y, Zhao B, Ning N, Chen E, Mao E, Zhou W. Characteristics and risk factors for extrapancreatic infection in patients with moderate or severe acute pancreatitis. Heliyon. 2023;9:e13131.

39. Johnson CD, Abu-Hilal M. Persistent organ failure during the first week as a marker of fatal outcome in acute pancreatitis. Gut. 2004;53:1340–4.

40. Gloor B, Muller CA, Worni M, Martignoni ME, Uhl W, Buchler MW. Late mortality in patients with severe acute pancreatitis. Br J Surg. 2001;88:975–9.

41. Fu CY, Yeh CN, Hsu JT, Jan YY, Hwang TL. Timing of mortality in severe acute pancreatitis: experience from 643 patients. World J Gastroenterol. 2007;13:1966–9.

42. Carnovale A, Rabitti PG, Manes G, Esposito P, Pacelli L, Uomo G. Mortality in acute pancreatitis: is it an early or a late event? JOP. 2005;6:438–44.

43. Mutinga M, Rosenbluth A, Tenner SM, Odze RR, Sica GT, Banks PA. Does mortality occur early or late in acute pancreatitis? Int J Pancreatol. 2000;28:91–5.

44. McKay CJ, Evans S, Sinclair M, Carter CR, Imrie CW. High early mortality rate from acute pancreatitis in Scotland, 1984–1995. Br J Surg. 1999;86:1302–5.

45. Lytras D, Manes K, Triantopoulou C, Paraskeva C, Delis S, Avgerinos C, Dervenis C. Persistent early organ failure: defining the high-risk group of patients with severe acute pancreatitis? Pancreas. 2008;36:249–54.

46. Padhan RK, Jain S, Agarwal S, Harikrishnan S, Vadiraja P, Behera S, Jain SK, Dhingra R, Dash NR, Sahni P, Garg PK. Primary and secondary organ failures cause mortality differentially in acute pancreatitis and should be distinguished. Pancreas. 2018;47:302–7.

47. Schepers NJ, Bakker OJ, Besselink MG, Ahmed Ali U, Bollen TL, Gooszen HG, van Santvoort HC, Bruno MJ. Impact of characteristics of organ failure and infected necrosis on mortality in necrotising pancreatitis. Gut. 2019;68:1044–51.

48. Sternby H, Bolado F, Canaval-Zuleta HJ, Marra-López C, Hernando-Alonso AI, del-Val-Antoñana A, García-Rayado G, Rivera-Irigoin R, Grau-García FJ, Oms L, Millastre-Bocos J, Pascual-Moreno I, Martínez-Ares D, Rodríguez-Oballe JA, López-Serrano A, Ruiz-Rebollo ML, Viejo-Almanzor A, González-de-la-Higuera B, Orive-Calzada A, Gómez-Anta I, Pamies-Guilabert J, Fernández-Gutiérrez-del-Álamo F, Iranzo-González-Cruz I, Pérez-Muñante ME, Esteba MD, Pardillos-Tomé A, Zapater P, de-Madaria E. Determinants of severity in acute pancreatitis: a nation-wide multicenter prospective cohort study. Ann Surg. 2019;270:348–55.

49. Kostenko S, Khatua B, Trivedi S, Pillai AN, McFayden B, Morsy M, Rajalingamgari P, Sharma V, Noel P, Patel K, El-Kurdi B, Borges da Silva H, Chen X, Chandan V, Navina S, Vela S, Cartin-Ceba R, Snozek C, Singh VP. Amphipathic liponecrosis impairs bacterial clearance and causes infection during sterile inflammation. Gastroenterology. 2023;165:999.

50. Lockhart PB, Brennan MT, Sasser HC, Fox PC, Paster BJ, Bahrani-Mougeot FK. Bacteremia associated with toothbrushing and dental extraction. Circulation. 2008;117:3118–25.

51. Shorvon PJ, Eykyn SJ, Cotton PB. Gastrointestinal instrumentation, bacteraemia, and endocarditis. Gut. 1983;24:1078–93.

52. Andriulli A, Caruso N, Quitadamo M, Forlano R, Leandro G, Spirito F, De Maio G. Antisecretory vs. antiproteasic drugs in the prevention of post-ERCP pancreatitis: the evidence-based medicine derived from a meta-analysis study. JOP. 2003;4:41–8.

53. Andriulli A, Leandro G, Clemente R, Festa V, Caruso N, Annese V, Lezzi G, Lichino E, Bruno F, Perri F. Meta-analysis of somatostatin, octreotide and gabexate mesilate in the therapy of acute pancreatitis. Aliment Pharmacol Ther. 1998;12:237–45.

54. Asang E. Changes in the therapy of inflammatory diseases of the pancreas. A report on 1 year of therapy and prophylaxis with the kallikrein- and trypsin inactivator trasylol (Bayer). Langenbecks Arch Klin Chir Ver Dtsch Z Chir. 1960;293:645–70.

55. Buchler M, Malfertheiner P, Uhl W, Scholmerich J, Stockmann F, Adler G, Gaus W, Rolle K, Beger HG. Gabexate mesilate in human acute pancreatitis. German Pancreatitis Study Group. Gastroenterology. 1993;104:1165–70.

56. Chen HM, Chen JC, Hwang TL, Jan YY, Chen MF. Prospective and randomized study of gabexate mesilate for the treatment of severe acute pancreatitis with organ dysfunction. Hepato-Gastroenterology. 2000;47:1147–50.

57. Park KT, Kang DH, Choi CW, Cho M, Park SB, Kim HW, Kim DU, Chung CW, Yoon KT. Is high-dose nafamostat mesilate effective for the prevention of post-ERCP pancreatitis, especially in high-risk patients? Pancreas. 2011;40:1215–9.

58. Seta T, Noguchi Y, Shimada T, Shikata S, Fukui T. Treatment of acute pancreatitis with protease inhibitors: a meta-analysis. Eur J Gastroenterol Hepatol. 2004;16:1287–93.

59. Trapnell JE, Rigby CC, Talbot CH, Duncan EH. Proceedings: Aprotinin in the treatment of acute pancreatitis. Gut. 1973;14:828.

60. Trapnell JE, Rigby CC, Talbot CH, Duncan EH. A controlled trial of trasylol in the treatment of acute pancreatitis. Br J Surg. 1974;61:177–82.

61. Trapnell JE, Talbot CH, Capper WM. Trasylol in acute pancreatitis. Am J Dig Dis. 1967;12:409–12.

62. Lerch MM, Gorelick FS. Models of acute and chronic pancreatitis. Gastroenterology. 2013;144:1180–93.

63. Mareninova OA, Hermann K, French SW, O'Konski MS, Pandol SJ, Webster P, Erickson AH, Katunuma N, Gorelick FS, Gukovsky I, Gukovskaya AS. Impaired autophagic flux mediates acinar cell vacuole formation and trypsinogen activation in rodent models of acute pancreatitis. J Clin Invest. 2009;119:3340–55.

64. Navina S, Acharya C, DeLany JP, Orlichenko LS, Baty CJ, Shiva SS, Durgampudi C, Karlsson JM, Lee K, Bae KT, Furlan A, Behari J, Liu S, McHale T, Nichols L, Papachristou GI, Yadav D, Singh VP. Lipotoxicity causes multisystem organ failure and exacerbates acute pancreatitis in obesity. Sci Transl Med. 2011;3:107ra10.

65. Acharya C, Cline RA, Jaligama D, Noel P, Delany JP, Bae K, Furlan A, Baty CJ, Karlsson JM, Rosario BL, Patel K, Mishra V, Dugampudi C, Yadav D, Navina S, Singh VP. Fibrosis reduces severity of acute-on-chronic pancreatitis in humans. Gastroenterology. 2013;145:466–75.

66. Noel P, Patel K, Durgampudi C, Trivedi RN, de Oliveira C, Crowell MD, Pannala R, Lee K, Brand R, Chennat J, Slivka A, Papachristou GI, Khalid A, Whitcomb DC, DeLany JP, Cline RA, Acharya C, Jaligama D, Murad FM, Yadav D, Navina S, Singh VP. Peripancreatic fat necrosis worsens acute pancreatitis independent of pancreatic necrosis via unsaturated fatty acids increased in human pancreatic necrosis collections. Gut. 2016;65:100–11.

67. de Oliveira C, Khatua B, Noel P, Kostenko S, Bag A, Balakrishnan B, Patel KS, Guerra AA, Martinez MN, Trivedi S, McCullough A, Lam-Himlin DM, Navina S, Faigel DO, Fukami N, Pannala R, Phillips AE, Papachristou GI, Kershaw EE, Lowe ME, Singh VP. Pancreatic triglyceride lipase mediates lipotoxic systemic inflammation. J Clin Invest. 2020;130:1931–47.

68. Cartin-Ceba R, Khatua B, El-Kurdi B, Trivedi S, Kostenko S, Imam Z, Smith R, Snozek C, Navina S, Sharma V, McFayden B, Ionescu F, Stolow E, Keiser S, Tejani A, Harrington A, Acosta P, Kuwelker S, Echavarria J, Nair GB, Bataineh A, Singh VP. Evidence showing lipotoxicity worsens outcomes in Covid-19 patients and insights about the underlying mechanisms. iScience. 2022;25:104322.

69. Khatua B, Trivedi RN, Noel P, Patel K, Singh R, de Oliveira C, Trivedi S, Mishra V, Lowe M, Singh VP. Carboxyl ester lipase may not mediate lipotoxic injury during severe acute pancreatitis. Am J Pathol. 2019;189:1226–40.

70. Khatua B, Yaron JR, El-Kurdi B, Kostenko S, Papachristou GI, Singh VP. Ringer's lactate prevents early organ failure by providing extracellular calcium. J Clin Med. 2020;9:9.

71. Patel K, Trivedi RN, Durgampudi C, Noel P, Cline RA, DeLany JP, Navina S, Singh VP. Lipolysis of visceral adipocyte triglyceride by pancreatic lipases converts mild acute pancreatitis to severe pancreatitis independent of necrosis and inflammation. Am J Pathol. 2015;185:808–19.

72. Hirota M, Nozawa F, Okabe A, Shibata M, Beppu T, Shimada S, Egami H, Yamaguchi Y, Ikei S, Okajima T, Okamoto K, Ogawa M. Relationship between plasma cytokine concentration and multiple organ failure in patients with acute pancreatitis. Pancreas. 2000;21:141–6.

73. Messmann H, Vogt W, Falk W, Vogl D, Zirngibl H, Leser HG, Scholmerich J. Interleukins and their antagonists but not TNF and its receptors are released in post-ERP pancreatitis. Eur J Gastroenterol Hepatol. 1998;10:611–7.

74. Brivet FG, Emilie D, Galanaud P. Pro- and anti-inflammatory cytokines during acute severe pancreatitis: an early and sustained response, although unpredictable of death. Parisian Study Group on Acute Pancreatitis. Crit Care Med. 1999;27:749–55.

75. Dambrauskas Z, Giese N, Gulbinas A, Giese T, Berberat PO, Pundzius J, Barauskas G, Friess H. Different profiles of cytokine expression during mild and severe acute pancreatitis. World J Gastroenterol. 2010;16:1845–53.

76. Aoun E, Chen J, Reighard D, Gleeson FC, Whitcomb DC, Papachristou GI. Diagnostic accuracy of interleukin-6 and interleukin-8 in predicting severe acute pancreatitis: a meta-analysis. Pancreatology. 2009;9:777–85.

77. Daniel P, Lesniowski B, Mokrowiecka A, Jasinska A, Pietruczuk M, Malecka-Panas E. Circulating levels of visfatin, resistin and pro-inflammatory cytokine interleukin-8 in acute pancreatitis. Pancreatology. 2010;10:477–82.

78. Ueda T, Takeyama Y, Yasuda T, Matsumura N, Sawa H, Nakajima T, Ajiki T, Fujino Y, Suzuki Y, Kuroda Y. Significant elevation of serum interleukin-18 levels in patients with acute pancreatitis. J Gastroenterol. 2006;41:158–65.

79. Regner S, Appelros S, Hjalmarsson C, Manjer J, Sadic J, Borgstrom A. Monocyte chemoattractant protein 1, active carboxypeptidase B and CAPAP at hospital admission are predictive markers for severe acute pancreatitis. Pancreatology. 2008;8:42–9.

80. Geokas MC, Rinderknecht H, Brodrick JW, Largman C. Studies on the ascites fluid of acute pancreatitis in man. Am J Dig Dis. 1978;23:182–8.

81. Renner IG, Rinderknecht H, Douglas AP. Profiles of pure pancreatic secretions in patients with acute pancreatitis: the possible role of proteolytic enzymes in pathogenesis. Gastroenterology. 1978;75:1090–8.

82. Wozniak B, Wisniewska-Jarosinska M, Drzewoski J. Evaluation of selected parameters of the inflammatory response to endoscopic retrograde cholangiopancreatography. Pancreas. 2001;23:349–55.

83. Bone RC, Balk RA, Cerra FB, Dellinger RP, Fein AM, Knaus WA, Schein RM, Sibbald WJ. Definitions for sepsis and organ failure and guidelines for the use of innovative therapies in sepsis. The ACCP/SCCM Consensus Conference Committee. American College of Chest Physicians/Society of Critical Care Medicine. Chest. 1992;101:1644–55.

84. Ais G, Lopez-Farre A, Gomez-Garre DN, Novo C, Romeo JM, Braquet P, Lopez-Novoa JM. Role of platelet-activating factor in hemodynamic derangements in an acute rodent pancreatic model. Gastroenterology. 1992;102:181–7.

85. Demerath EW, Reed D, Choh AC, Soloway L, Lee M, Czerwinski SA, Chumlea WC, Siervogel RM, Towne B. Rapid postnatal weight gain and visceral adiposity in adulthood: the Fels longitudinal study. Obesity (Silver Spring). 2009;17:2060–6.

86. Choh AC, Demerath EW, Lee M, Williams KD, Towne B, Siervogel RM, Cole SA, Czerwinski SA. Genetic analysis of self-reported physical activity and adiposity: the Southwest Ohio family study. Public Health Nutr. 2009;12:1052–60.

87. Camhi SM, Bray GA, Bouchard C, Greenway FL, Johnson WD, Newton RL, Ravussin E, Ryan DH, Smith SR, Katzmarzyk PT. The relationship of waist circumference and BMI to visceral, subcutaneous, and total body fat: sex and race differences. Obesity (Silver Spring). 2011;19:402–8.

88. Thomas LW. The chemical composition of adipose tissue of man and mice. Q J Exp Physiol Cogn Med Sci. 1962;47:179–88.

89. Ren J, Dimitrov I, Sherry AD, Malloy CR. Composition of adipose tissue and marrow fat in humans by 1H NMR at 7 tesla. J Lipid Res. 2008;49:2055–62.

90. Fitz RH. Acute pancreatitis: a consideration of pancreatic hemorrhage, hemorrhagic, suppurative, and gangrenous pancreatitis, and of disseminated fat-necrosis. Boston Med Surg J. 1889;120:181.

91. Nordback I, Lauslahti K. Clinical pathology of acute necrotising pancreatitis. J Clin Pathol. 1986;39:68–74.

92. Kloppel G, Von Gerkan R, Dreyer T. Pathomorphology of acute pancreatitis. Analysis of 367 autopsy cases and 3 surgical specimens. Oxford; 1984.

93. Pinnick KE, Collins SC, Londos C, Gauguier D, Clark A, Fielding BA. Pancreatic ectopic fat is characterized by adipocyte infiltration and altered lipid composition. Obesity (Silver Spring). 2008;16:522–30.

94. Panek J, Sztefko K, Drozdz W. Composition of free fatty acid and triglyceride fractions in human necrotic pancreatic tissue. Med Sci Monit. 2001;7:894–8.

95. Bakker OJ, van Santvoort H, Besselink MG, Boermeester MA, van Eijck C, Dejong K, van Goor H, Hofker S, Ahmed Ali U, Gooszen HG, Bollen TL. Extrapancreatic necrosis without pancreatic parenchymal necrosis: a separate entity in necrotising pancreatitis? Gut. 2013;62:1475–80.

96. Kloppel G, Maillet B. Pseudocysts in chronic pancreatitis: a morphological analysis of 57 resection specimens and 9 autopsy pancreata. Pancreas. 1991;6:266–74.

97. Schmitz-Moormann P. Comparative radiological and morphological study of the human pancreas. IV. Acute necrotizing pancreatitis in man. Pathol Res Pract. 1981;171:325–35.

98. Domschke S, Malfertheiner P, Uhl W, Buchler M, Domschke W. Free fatty acids in serum of patients with acute necrotizing or edematous pancreatitis. Int J Pancreatol. 1993;13:105–10.

99. Sztefko K, Panek J. Serum free fatty acid concentration in patients with acute pancreatitis. Pancreatology. 2001;1:230–6.

100. Torgerson RR, McNiven MA. Agonist-induced changes in cell shape during regulated secretion in rat pancreatic acini. J Cell Physiol. 2000;182:438–47.

101. Torgerson RR, McNiven MA. The actin–myosin cytoskeleton mediates reversible agonist-induced membrane blebbing. J Cell Sci. 1998;111(Pt 19):2911–22.

102. Singh VP, McNiven MA. Src-mediated cortactin phosphorylation regulates actin localization and injurious blebbing in acinar cells. Mol Biol Cell. 2008;19:2339–47.

103. Lam PP, Cosen Binker LI, Lugea A, Pandol SJ, Gaisano HY. Alcohol redirects CCK-mediated apical exocytosis to the acinar basolateral membrane in alcoholic pancreatitis. Traffic. 2007;8:605–17.

104. Gaisano HY, Lutz MP, Leser J, Sheu L, Lynch G, Tang L, Tamori Y, Trimble WS, Salapatek AM. Supramaximal cholecystokinin displaces Munc18c from the pancreatic acinar basal surface, redirecting apical exocytosis to the basal membrane. J Clin Invest. 2001;108:1597–611.

105. Cosen-Binker LI, Lam PP, Binker MG, Reeve J, Pandol S, Gaisano HY. Alcohol/cholecystokinin-evoked pancreatic acinar basolateral exocytosis is mediated by protein kinase C alpha phosphorylation of Munc18c. J Biol Chem. 2007;282:13047–58.

106. Cosen-Binker LI, Binker MG, Wang CC, Hong W, Gaisano HY. VAMP8 is the v-SNARE that mediates basolateral exocytosis in a mouse model of alcoholic pancreatitis. J Clin Invest. 2008;118:2535–51.

107. Watanabe O, Baccino FM, Steer ML, Meldolesi J. Supramaximal caerulein stimulation and ultrastructure of rat pancreatic acinar cell: early morpho-

logical changes during development of experimental pancreatitis. Am J Phys. 1984;246:G457–67.

108. Aho HJ, Sternby B, Kallajoki M, Nevalainen TJ. Carboxyl ester lipase in human tissues and in acute pancreatitis. Int J Pancreatol. 1989;5:123–34.

109. Aho HJ, Sternby B, Nevalainen TJ. Fat necrosis in human acute pancreatitis; an immunohistological study. Acta Pathol Microbiol Immunol Scand Ser A Pathol. 1986;94:101–5.

110. Willemer S, Elsasser HP, Kern HF, Adler G. Tubular complexes in cerulein- and oleic acid-induced pancreatitis in rats: glycoconjugate pattern, immunocytochemical, and ultrastructural findings. Pancreas. 1987;2:669–75.

111. Lowe ME. The triglyceride lipases of the pancreas. J Lipid Res. 2002;43:2007–16.

112. Khatua B, El-Kurdi B, Patel K, Rood C, Noel P, Crowell M, Yaron JR, Kostenko S, Guerra A, Faigel DO, Lowe M, Singh VP. Adipose saturation reduces lipotoxic systemic inflammation and explains the obesity paradox. Sci Adv. 2021;7:7.

113. El-Kurdi B, Khatua B, Rood C, Snozek C, Cartin-Ceba R, Singh VP. Lipotoxicity in C-SG: mortality from coronavirus disease 2019 increases with unsaturated fat and may be reduced by early calcium and albumin supplementation. Gastroenterology. 2020;159:1015–8.

114. Ashbrook JD, Spector AA, Santos EC, Fletcher JE. Long chain fatty acid binding to human plasma albumin. J Biol Chem. 1975;250:2333–8.

115. Durgampudi C, Noel P, Patel K, Cline R, Trivedi RN, DeLany JP, Yadav D, Papachristou GI, Lee K, Acharya C, Jaligama D, Navina S, Murad F, Singh VP. Acute lipotoxicity regulates severity of biliary acute pancreatitis without affecting its initiation. Am J Pathol. 2014;184:1773–84.

116. Goncalves-de-Albuquerque CF, Burth P, Silva AR, de Moraes IM, de Jesus Oliveira FM, Santelli RE, Freire AS, Bozza PT, Younes-Ibrahim M, de Castro-Faria-Neto HC, de Castro-Faria MV. Oleic acid inhibits lung Na/K-ATPase in mice and induces injury with lipid body formation in leukocytes and eicosanoid production. J Inflamm (Lond). 2013;10:34.

117. Hussain N, Wu F, Zhu L, Thrall RS, Kresch MJ. Neutrophil apoptosis during the development and resolution of oleic acid-induced acute lung injury in the rat. Am J Respir Cell Mol Biol. 1998;19:867–74.

118. Matthay MA, Zemans RL. The acute respiratory distress syndrome: pathogenesis and treatment. Annu Rev Pathol. 2011;6:147–63.

119. Patel K, Durgampudi C, Noel P, Trivedi RN, de Oliveira C, Singh VP. Fatty acid ethyl esters are less toxic than their parent fatty acids generated during acute pancreatitis. Am J Pathol. 2016;186:874–84.

120. Noel P, Patel K, Durgampudi C, Trivedi RN, de Oliveira C, Crowell MD, Pannala R, Lee K, Brand R, Chennat J, Slivka A, Papachristou GI, Khalid A, Whitcomb DC, DeLany JP, Cline RA, Acharya C, Jaligama D, Murad FM, Yadav D, Navina S, Singh VP. Peripancreatic fat necrosis worsens acute pancreatitis independent of pancreatic necrosis via unsaturated fatty acids increased in human pancreatic necrosis collections. Gut. 2014;65:100.

121. de Oliveira C, Khatua B, Bag A, El-Kurdi B, Patel K, Mishra V, Navina S, Singh VP. Multimodal transgastric local pancreatic hypothermia reduces severity of acute pancreatitis in rats and increases survival. Gastroenterology. 2019;156:735–47.

122. Kamuf J, Garcia-Bardon A, Ziebart A, Thomas R, Rümmler R, Möllmann C, Hartmann EK. Oleic acid-injection in pigs as a model for acute respiratory distress syndrome. J Vis Exp. 2018;140:e57783.

123. Moriuchi H, Zaha M, Fukumoto T, Yuizono T. Activation of polymorphonuclear leukocytes in oleic acid-induced lung injury. Intensive Care Med. 1998;24:709–15.

124. Seyfried CE, Schweickart VL, Godiska R, Gray PW. The human platelet-activating factor receptor gene (PTAFR) contains no introns and maps to chromosome 1. Genomics. 1992;13:832–4.

125. Prescott SM, Zimmerman GA, Stafforini DM, McIntyre TM. Platelet-activating factor and related lipid mediators. Annu Rev Biochem. 2000;69:419–45.

126. Johnson CD, Kingsnorth AN, Imrie CW, McMahon MJ, Neoptolemos JP, McKay C, Toh SK, Skaife P, Leeder PC, Wilson P, Larvin M, Curtis LD. Double blind, randomised, placebo controlled study of a platelet activating factor antagonist, lexipafant, in the treatment and prevention of organ failure in predicted severe acute pancreatitis. Gut. 2001;48:62–9.

127. Emanuelli G, Montrucchio G, Gaia E, Dughera L, Corvetti G, Gubetta L. Experimental acute pancreatitis induced by platelet activating factor in rabbits. Am J Pathol. 1989;134:315–26.

128. Liu LR, Xia SH. Role of platelet-activating factor in the pathogenesis of acute pancreatitis. World J Gastroenterol. 2006;12:539–45.

129. Zhou W, McCollum MO, Levine BA, Olson MS. Role of platelet-activating factor in pancreatitis-associated acute lung injury in the rat. Am J Pathol. 1992;140:971–9.

130. Leonhardt U, Fayyazzi A, Seidensticker F, Stockmann F, Soling HD, Creutzfeldt W. Influence of a platelet-activating factor antagonist on severe pancreatitis in two experimental models. Int J Pancreatol. 1992;12:161–6.

131. Hofbauer B, Saluja AK, Bhatia M, Frossard JL, Lee HS, Bhagat L, Steer ML. Effect of recombinant platelet-activating factor acetylhydrolase on two models of experimental acute pancreatitis. Gastroenterology. 1998;115:1238–47.

132. McKay CJ, Curran F, Sharples C, Baxter JN, Imrie CW. Prospective placebo-controlled randomized trial of lexipafant in predicted severe acute pancreatitis. Br J Surg. 1997;84:1239–43.

133. Abu-Zidan FM, Windsor JA. Lexipafant and acute pancreatitis: a critical appraisal of the clinical trials. Eur J Surg. 2002;168:215–9.

134. Amin M, Simerman A, Cho M, Singh P, Briton-Jones C, Hill D, Grogan T, Elashoff D, Clarke NJ, Chazenbalk GD, Dumesic DA. 21-Hydroxylase-derived steroids in follicles of nonobese women undergoing ovarian stimulation for in vitro fertilization (IVF) positively correlate with lipid content of luteinized granulosa cells (LGCs) as a source of cholesterol for steroid synthesis. J Clin Endocrinol Metab. 2014;99:1299–306.

135. Schaffler A, Hamer O, Dickopf J, Goetz A, Landfried K, Voelk M, Herfarth H, Kopp A, Buchler C, Scholmerich J, Brunnler T. Admission resistin levels predict peripancreatic necrosis and clinical severity in acute pancreatitis. Am J Gastroenterol. 2010;105:2474–84.

136. Schaffler A, Hamer OW, Dickopf J, Goetz A, Landfried K, Voelk M, Herfarth H, Kopp A, Buechler C, Scholmerich J, Brunnler T. Admission visfatin levels predict pancreatic and peripancreatic necrosis in acute pancreatitis and correlate with clinical severity. Am J Gastroenterol. 2011;106:957–67.

137. Karpavicius A, Dambrauskas Z, Gradauskas A, Samuilis A, Zviniene K, Kupcinskas J, Brimas G, Meckovski A, Sileikis A, Strupas K. The clinical value of adipokines in predicting the severity and outcome of acute pancreatitis. BMC Gastroenterol. 2016;16:99.

138. Greer PJ, Lee PJ, Paragomi P, Stello KM, Phillips A, Hart P, Speake C, Lacy-Hulbert A, Whitcomb DC, Papachristou GI. Severe acute pancreatitis exhibits distinct cytokine signatures and trajectories in humans: a prospective observational study. Am J Physiol Gastrointest Liver Physiol. 2022;323:G428.

139. Schaffler A, Landfried K, Volk M, Furst A, Buchler C, Scholmerich J, Herfarth H. Potential of adipocytokines in predicting peripancreatic necrosis and severity in acute pancreatitis: pilot study. J Gastroenterol Hepatol. 2007;22:326–34.

140. Zhong Y, Yu Z, Wang L, Yang X. Combined detection of procalcitonin, heparin-binding protein, and interleukin-6 is a promising assay to diagnose and predict acute pancreatitis. J Clin Lab Anal. 2021;35:e23869.

141. Sathyanarayan G, Garg PK, Prasad H, Tandon RK. Elevated level of interleukin-6 predicts organ failure and severe disease in patients with acute pancreatitis. J Gastroenterol Hepatol. 2007;22:550–4.

142. Andersson U, Ottestad W, Tracey KJ. Extracellular HMGB1: a therapeutic target in severe pulmonary inflammation including COVID-19? Mol Med. 2020;26:42.

143. Yang H, Wang H, Andersson U. Targeting inflammation driven by HMGB1. Front Immunol. 2020;11:484.

144. Hegyi P, Szakacs Z, Sahin-Toth M. Lipotoxicity and cytokine storm in severe acute pancreatitis and COVID-19. Gastroenterology. 2020;159:824.

145. Xu J, Zhang X, Pelayo R, Monestier M, Ammollo CT, Semeraro F, Taylor FB, Esmon NL, Lupu F, Esmon CT. Extracellular histones are major mediators of death in sepsis. Nat Med. 2009;15:1318–21.

146. Starkie R, Ostrowski SR, Jauffred S, Febbraio M, Pedersen BK. Exercise and IL-6 infusion inhibit endotoxin-induced TNF-alpha production in humans. FASEB J. 2003;17:884–6.

147. Nieken J, Mulder NH, Buter J, Vellenga E, Limburg PC, Piers DA, de Vries EG. Recombinant human interleukin-6 induces a rapid and reversible anemia in cancer patients. Blood. 1995;86:900–5.

148. Nemeth E, Rivera S, Gabayan V, Keller C, Taudorf S, Pedersen BK, Ganz T. IL-6 mediates hypoferremia of inflammation by inducing the synthesis of the iron regulatory hormone hepcidin. J Clin Invest. 2004;113:1271–6.

149. Cuzzocrea S, Mazzon E, Dugo L, Centorrino T, Ciccolo A, McDonald MC, de Sarro A, Caputi AP, Thiemermann C. Absence of endogenous interleukin-6 enhances the inflammatory response during acute pancreatitis induced by cerulein in mice. Cytokine. 2002;18:274–85.

150. Guice KS, Oldham KT, Remick DG, Kunkel SL, Ward PA. Anti-tumor necrosis factor antibody augments edema formation in caerulein-induced acute pancreatitis. J Surg Res. 1991;51:495–9.

151. Wang LZ, Su JY, Lu CY, Zhou BH, Ma DL. Effects of recombinant human endothelial-derived interleukin-8 on hemorrhagic shock in rats. Zhongguo Yao Li Xue Bao. 1997;18:434–6.

152. Morimoto K, Morimoto A, Nakamori T, Tan N, Minagawa T, Murakami N. Cardiovascular responses induced in free-moving rats by immune cytokines. J Physiol. 1992;448:307–20.

153. Wogensen L, Jensen M, Svensson P, Worsaae H, Welinder B, Nerup J. Pancreatic beta-cell function and interleukin-1 beta in plasma during the acute phase response in patients with major burn injuries. Eur J Clin Investig. 1993;23:311–9.

154. Li S, Ballou LR, Morham SG, Blatteis CM. Cyclooxygenase-2 mediates the febrile response of mice to interleukin-1beta. Brain Res. 2001;910:163–73.

155. Bhargava R, Janssen W, Altmann C, Andres-Hernando A, Okamura K, Vandivier RW, Ahuja N, Faubel S. Intratracheal IL-6 protects against lung inflammation in direct, but not indirect, causes of acute lung injury in mice. PLoS One. 2013;8:e61405.

156. Pini M, Rhodes DH, Castellanos KJ, Hall AR, Cabay RJ, Chennuri R, Grady EF, Fantuzzi G. Role of IL-6 in the resolution of pancreatitis in obese mice. J Leukoc Biol. 2012;91:957–66.

157. Investigators R-C, Gordon AC, Mouncey PR, Al-Beidh F, Rowan KM, Nichol AD, Arabi YM, Annane D, Beane A, van Bentum-Puijk W, Berry LR, Bhimani Z, Bonten MJM, Bradbury CA, Brunkhorst FM, Buzgau A, Cheng AC, Detry MA, Duffy EJ, Estcourt LJ, Fitzgerald M, Goossens

H, Haniffa R, Higgins AM, Hills TE, Horvat CM, Lamontagne F, Lawler PR, Leavis HL, Linstrum KM, Litton E, Lorenzi E, Marshall JC, Mayr FB, McAuley DF, McGlothlin A, McGuinness SP, McVerry BJ, Montgomery SK, Morpeth SC, Murthy S, Orr K, Parke RL, Parker JC, Patanwala AE, Pettila V, Rademaker E, Santos MS, Saunders CT, Seymour CW, Shankar-Hari M, Sligl WI, Turgeon AF, Turner AM, van de Veerdonk FL, Zarychanski R, Green C, Lewis RJ, Angus DC, McArthur CJ, Berry S, Webb SA, Derde LPG. Interleukin-6 receptor antagonists in critically ill patients with Covid-19. N Engl J Med. 2021;384:1491–502.

158. WHO Rapid Evidence Appraisal for COVID-19 Therapies (REACT) Working Group. Association between administration of IL-6 antagonists and mortality among patients hospitalized for COVID-19: a meta-analysis. JAMA. 2021;326:499–518.

159. Stone JH, Frigault MJ, Serling-Boyd NJ, Fernandes AD, Harvey L, Foulkes AS, Horick NK, Healy BC, Shah R, Bensaci AM, Woolley AE, Nikiforow S, Lin N, Sagar M, Schrager H, Huckins DS, Axelrod M, Pincus MD, Fleisher J, Sacks CA, Dougan M, North CM, Halvorsen Y-D, Thurber TK, Dagher Z, Scherer A, Wallwork RS, Kim AY, Schoenfeld S, Sen P, Neilan TG, Perugino CA, Unizony SH, Collier DS, Matza MA, Yinh JM, Bowman KA, Meyerowitz E, Zafar A, Drobni ZD, Bolster MB, Kohler M, D'Silva KM, Dau J, Lockwood MM, Cubbison C, Weber BN, Mansour MK. Efficacy of tocilizumab in patients hospitalized with Covid-19. N Engl J Med. 2020;383:2333–44.

160. Rosas IO, Diaz G, Gottlieb RL, Lobo SM, Robinson P, Hunter BD, Cavalcante AW, Overcash JS, Hanania NA, Skarbnik A, Garcia-Diaz J, Gordeev I, Carratalà J, Gordon O, Graham E, Lewin-Koh N, Tsai L, Tuckwell K, Cao H, Brainard D, Olsson JK. Tocilizumab and remdesivir in hospitalized patients with severe COVID-19 pneumonia: a randomized clinical trial. Intensive Care Med. 2021;47:1258–70.

161. Boetticher NC, Peine CJ, Kwo P, Abrams GA, Patel T, Aqel B, Boardman L, Gores GJ, Harmsen WS, McClain CJ, Kamath PS, Shah VH. A randomized, double-blinded, placebo-controlled multicenter trial of etanercept in the treatment of alcoholic hepatitis. Gastroenterology. 2008;135:1953–60.

162. Malleo G, Mazzon E, Genovese T, Di Paola R, Muia C, Centorrino T, Siriwardena AK, Cuzzocrea S. Etanercept attenuates the development of cerulein-induced acute pancreatitis in mice: a comparison with TNF-alpha genetic deletion. Shock. 2007;27:542–51.

163. Tsai WC, Strieter RM, Wilkowski JM, Bucknell KA, Burdick MD, Lira SA, Standiford TJ. Lung-specific transgenic expression of KC enhances resistance to Klebsiella pneumoniae in mice. J Immunol. 1998;161:2435–40.

164. Mehrad B, Wiekowski M, Morrison BE, Chen SC, Coronel EC, Manfra DJ, Lira SA. Transient lung-specific expression of the chemokine KC improves outcome in invasive aspergillosis. Am J Respir Crit Care Med. 2002;166:1263–8.

165. Batra S, Cai S, Balamayooran G, Jeyaseelan S. Intrapulmonary administration of leukotriene B(4) augments neutrophil accumulation and responses in the lung to Klebsiella infection in CXCL1 knockout mice. J Immunol. 2012;188:3458–68.

166. Rasch S, Sancak S, Erber J, Wiessner J, Schulz D, Huberle C, Algul H, Schmid RM, Lahmer T. Influence of extracorporeal cytokine adsorption on hemodynamics in severe acute pancreatitis: results of the matched cohort pancreatitis cytosorbents inflammatory cytokine removal (PACIFIC) study. Artif Organs. 2022;46:1019–26.

167. Paul R, Sathe P, Kumar S, Prasad S, Aleem M, Sakhalvalkar P. Multicentered prospective investigator initiated study to evaluate the clinical outcomes with extracorporeal cytokine adsorption device (CytoSorb((R))) in patients with sepsis and septic shock. World J Crit Care Med. 2021;10:22–34.

168. Chiari H. Ueber Selbstverdauung des menschlichen Pankreas. Zeitschrift für Heilkunde. 1896;17:69–96.

169. Saluja A, Dudeja V, Dawra R, Sah RP. Early intra-acinar events in pathogenesis of pancreatitis. Gastroenterology. 2019;156:1979–93.

170. Buchler M, Malfertheiner P, Uhl W, Wolf HR, Schwab G, Beger HG. Gabexate mesilate in the therapy of acute pancreatitis. Multicenter study of tolerance of a high intravenous dose (4 g/day). Med Klin (Munich). 1988;83:320–4.

171. Berling R, Borgstrom A, Ohlsson K. Peritoneal lavage with aprotinin in patients with severe acute pancreatitis. Effects on plasma and peritoneal levels of trypsin and leukocyte proteases and their major inhibitors. Int J Pancreatol. 1998;24:9–17.

172. Hegyi E, Sahin-Toth M. Genetic risk in chronic pancreatitis: the trypsin-dependent pathway. Dig Dis Sci. 2017;62:1692–701.

173. Jobling JW, Petersen W, Eggstein AA. Serum ferments and antiferment during trypsin shock : studies on ferment action. J Exp Med. 1915;22:141–53.

174. Tagnon HJ. The nature of the mechanism of the shock produced by the injection of trypsin and thrombin. J Clin Invest. 1945;24:1–10.

175. Hartwig W, Werner J, Jimenez RE, Z'Graggen K, Weimann J, Lewandrowski KB, Warshaw AL, Fernandez-del Castillo C. Trypsin and activation of circulating trypsinogen contribute to pancreatitis-associated lung injury. Am J Phys. 1999;277:G1008–16.

176. Radenkovic D, Bajec D, Ivancevic N, Milic N, Bumbasirevic V, Jeremic V, Djukic V, Stefanovic B, Stefanovic B, Milosevic-Zbutega G, Gregoric P. D-dimer in acute pancreatitis: a new approach for an early assessment of organ failure. Pancreas. 2009;38:655–60.

177. Easler J, Muddana V, Furlan A, Dasyam A, Vipperla K, Slivka A, Whitcomb DC, Papachristou GI, Yadav D. Portosplenomesenteric venous

thrombosis in patients with acute pancreatitis is associated with pancreatic necrosis and usually has a benign course. Clin Gastroenterol Hepatol. 2014;12:854–62.

178. Ding L, Deng F, Yu C, He WH, Xia L, Zhou M, Huang X, Lei YP, Zhou XJ, Zhu Y, Lu NH. Portosplenomesenteric vein thrombosis in patients with early-stage severe acute pancreatitis. World J Gastroenterol. 2018;24:4054–60.

179. Singh VP, Bhagat L, Navina S, Sharif R, Dawra RK, Saluja AK. Protease-activated receptor-2 protects against pancreatitis by stimulating exocrine secretion. Gut. 2007;56:958–64.

180. Namkung W, Han W, Luo X, Muallem S, Cho KH, Kim KH, Lee MG. Protease-activated receptor 2 exerts local protection and mediates some systemic complications in acute pancreatitis. Gastroenterology. 2004;126:1844–59.

181. Rebours V, Boutron-Ruault MC, Jooste V, Bouvier AM, Hammel P, Ruszniewski P, Levy P. Mortality rate and risk factors in patients with hereditary pancreatitis: uni- and multidimensional analyses. Am J Gastroenterol. 2009;104:2312–7.

182. Gui F, Zhang Y, Wan J, Zhan X, Yao Y, Li Y, Haddock AN, Shi J, Guo J, Chen J, Zhu X, Edenfield BH, Zhuang L, Hu C, Wang Y, Mukhopadhyay D, Radisky ES, Zhang L, Lugea A, Pandol SJ, Bi Y, Ji B. Trypsin activity governs increased susceptibility to pancreatitis in mice expressing human PRSS1R122H. J Clin Invest. 2020;130:189–202.

183. Pesei ZG, Jancso Z, Demcsak A, Nemeth BC, Vajda S, Sahin-Toth M. Preclinical testing of dabigatran in trypsin-dependent pancreatitis. JCI Insight. 2022;7(21):e161145.

184. Nakae Y, Hayakawa T, Kondo T, Shibata T, Kitagawa M, Sakai Y, Sobajima H, Ishiguro H, Tanikawa M. Serum alpha 2-macroglobulin-trypsin complex and early recognition of severe acute pancreatitis after endoscopic retrograde pancreatography. J Gastroenterol Hepatol. 1994;9:272–6.

185. McMahon MJ, Bowen M, Mayer AD, Cooper EH. Relation of alpha 2-macroglobulin and other antiproteases to the clinical features of acute pancreatitis. Am J Surg. 1984;147:164–70.

186. Szmola R, Sahin-Toth M. Chymotrypsin C (caldecrin) promotes degradation of human cationic trypsin: identity with Rinderknecht's enzyme Y. Proc Natl Acad Sci USA. 2007;104:11227–32.

187. Penttila AK, Rouhiainen A, Kylanpaa L, Mustonen H, Puolakkainen P, Rauvala H, Repo H. Circulating nucleosomes as predictive markers of severe acute pancreatitis. J Intensive Care. 2016;4:14.

188. Yasuda T, Ueda T, Takeyama Y, Shinzeki M, Sawa H, Nakajima T, Ajiki T, Fujino Y, Suzuki Y, Kuroda Y. Significant increase of serum high-mobility group box chromosomal protein 1 levels in patients with severe acute pancreatitis. Pancreas. 2006;33:359–63.

189. Lindstrom O, Tukiainen E, Kylanpaa L, Mentula P, Rouhiainen A, Puolakkainen P, Rauvala H, Repo H. Circulating levels of a soluble form of receptor for advanced glycation end products and high-mobility group box chromosomal protein 1 in patients with acute pancreatitis. Pancreas. 2009;38:e215–20.

190. Liu T, Huang W, Szatmary P, Abrams ST, Alhamdi Y, Lin Z, Greenhalf W, Wang G, Sutton R, Toh CH. Accuracy of circulating histones in predicting persistent organ failure and mortality in patients with acute pancreatitis. Br J Surg. 2017;104:1215.

191. Hoque R, Sohail M, Malik A, Sarwar S, Luo Y, Shah A, Barrat F, Flavell R, Gorelick F, Husain S, Mehal W. TLR9 and the NLRP3 inflammasome link acinar cell death with inflammation in acute pancreatitis. Gastroenterology. 2011;141:358–69.

192. Kang R, Zhang Q, Hou W, Yan Z, Chen R, Bonaroti J, Bansal P, Billiar TR, Tsung A, Wang Q, Bartlett DL, Whitcomb DC, Chang EB, Zhu X, Wang H, Lu B, Tracey KJ, Cao L, Fan XG, Lotze MT, Zeh HJ 3rd, Tang D. Intracellular Hmgb1 inhibits inflammatory nucleosome release and limits acute pancreatitis in mice. Gastroenterology. 2014;146:1097–107.

193. de Oliveira C, Khatua B, El-Kurdi B, Patel K, Mishra V, Navina S, Grim BJ, Gupta S, Belohlavek M, Cherry B, Yarger J, Green MD, Singh VP. Thermodynamic interference with bile acid demicelleization reduces systemic entry and injury during cholestasis. Sci Rep. 2020;10:8462.

194. Linders J, Madhi R, Rahman M, Mörgelin M, Regner S, Brenner M, Wang P, Thorlacius H. Extracellular cold-inducible RNA-binding protein regulates neutrophil extracellular trap formation and tissue damage in acute pancreatitis. Lab Investig. 2020;100:1618–30.

195. Cheng BQ, Liu CT, Li WJ, Fan W, Zhong N, Zhang Y, Jia XQ, Zhang SZ. Ethyl pyruvate improves survival and ameliorates distant organ injury in rats with severe acute pancreatitis. Pancreas. 2007;35:256–61.

196. Hoque R, Mehal WZ. Inflammasomes in pancreatic physiology and disease. Am J Physiol Gastrointest Liver Physiol. 2015;308:G643–51.

197. Hoque R, Malik AF, Gorelick F, Mehal WZ. Sterile inflammatory response in acute pancreatitis. Pancreas. 2012;41:353–7.

198. Szatmary P, Liu T, Abrams ST, Voronina S, Wen L, Chvanov M, Huang W, Wang G, Criddle DN, Tepikin AV, Toh CH, Sutton R. Systemic histone release disrupts plasmalemma and contributes to necrosis in acute pancreatitis. Pancreatology. 2017;17:884–92.

199. Li G, Wu X, Yang L, He Y, Liu Y, Jin X, Yuan H. TLR4-mediated NF-kappaB signaling pathway mediates HMGB1-induced pancreatic injury in mice with severe acute pancreatitis. Int J Mol Med. 2016;37:99–107.

200. Kierdorf K, Fritz G. RAGE regulation and signaling in inflammation and beyond. J Leukoc Biol. 2013;94:55.

201. Zhao S, Yang J, Liu T, Zeng J, Mi L, Xiang K. Dexamethasone inhibits NF-κBp65 and HMGB1 expression in the pancreas of rats with severe acute pancreatitis. Mol Med Rep. 2018;18:5345–52.

202. Li L, Liu M, Zhang T, Jia Y, Zhang Y, Yuan H, Zhang G, He C. Indomethacin down-regulating HMGB1 and TNF-α to prevent pancreatitis after endoscopic retrograde cholangiopancreatography. Scand J Gastroenterol. 2019;54:793–9.

203. Lin Y, Lin LJ, Jin Y, Cao Y, Zhang Y, Zheng CQ, Liu JL, Yang SL. Correlation between serum levels of high mobility group box-1 protein and pancreatitis: a meta-analysis. Biomed Res Int. 2015;2015:430185.

204. Siriwardena AK, Mason JM, Balachandra S, Bagul A, Galloway S, Formela L, Hardman JG, Jamdar S. Randomised, double blind, placebo controlled trial of intravenous antioxidant (n-acetylcysteine, selenium, vitamin C) therapy in severe acute pancreatitis. Gut. 2007;56:1439–44.

205. Sharer NM, Scott PD, Deardon DJ, Lee SH, Taylor PM, Braganza JM. Clinical trial of 24 h treatment with glutathione precursors in acute pancreatitis. Clin Drug Investig. 1995;10:147–57.

206. Machicado JD, Mounzer R, Paragomi P, Pothoulakis I, Hart PA, Conwell DL, de-Madaria E, Greer P, Yadav D, Whitcomb DC, Lee PJ, Hinton A, Papachristou GI. Rectal indomethacin does not mitigate the systemic inflammatory response syndrome in acute pancreatitis: a randomized trial. Clin Transl Gastroenterol. 2021;12:e00415.

207. Nango D, Hirose Y, Goto M, Echizen H. Analysis of the Association of Administration of various glucocorticoids with development of acute pancreatitis using US Food and Drug Administration adverse event reporting system (FAERS). J Pharm Health Care Sci. 2019;5:5.

208. Rosales C. Neutrophil: a cell with many roles in inflammation or several cell types? Front Physiol. 2018;9:113.

209. Gukovskaya AS, Vaquero E, Zaninovic V, Gorelick FS, Lusis AJ, Brennan ML, Holland S, Pandol SJ. Neutrophils and NADPH oxidase mediate intrapancreatic trypsin activation in murine experimental acute pancreatitis. Gastroenterology. 2002;122:974–84.

210. Rakonczay Z Jr, Hegyi P, Dósa S, Iványi B, Jármay K, Biczó G, Hracskó Z, Varga IS, Karg E, Kaszaki J, Varró A, Lonovics J, Boros I, Gukovsky I, Gukovskaya AS, Pandol SJ, Takács T. A new severe acute necrotizing pancreatitis model induced by L-ornithine in rats. Crit Care Med. 2008;36:2117–27.

211. Windsor JA, Trevaskis NL, Phillips AJ. The gut-lymph model gives new treatment strategies for organ failure. JAMA Surg. 2022;157:540–1.

212. Zhang H, Neuhofer P, Song L, Rabe B, Lesina M, Kurkowski MU, Treiber M, Wartmann T, Regner S, Thorlacius H, Saur D, Weirich G, Yoshimura A, Halangk W, Mizgerd JP, Schmid RM, Rose-John S, Algul H. IL-6 trans-signaling promotes pancreatitis-associated lung injury and lethality. J Clin Invest. 2013;123:1019–31.

213. Bhatia M, Saluja AK, Hofbauer B, Lee HS, Frossard JL, Steer ML. The effects of neutrophil depletion on a completely noninvasive model of acute pancreatitis-associated lung injury. Int J Pancreatol. 1998;24:77–83.

214. Tokoro T, Makino I, Harada S, Okamoto K, Nakanuma S, Sakai S, Kinoshita J, Nakamura K, Miyashita T, Tajima H, Ninomiya I, Fushida S, Ohta T. Interactions between neutrophils and platelets in the progression of acute pancreatitis. Pancreas. 2020;49:830–6.

215. Sandoval D, Gukovskaya A, Reavey P, Gukovsky S, Sisk A, Braquet P, Pandol SJ, Poucell-Hatton S. The role of neutrophils and platelet-activating factor in mediating experimental pancreatitis. Gastroenterology. 1996;111:1081–91.

216. Liu D, Wen L, Wang Z, Hai Y, Yang D, Zhang Y, Bai M, Song B, Wang Y. The mechanism of lung and intestinal injury in acute pancreatitis: a review. Front Med (Lausanne). 2022;9:904078.

217. Keck T, Balcom JH 4th, Fernández-del Castillo C, Antoniu BA, Warshaw AL. Matrix metalloproteinase-9 promotes neutrophil migration and alveolar capillary leakage in pancreatitis-associated lung injury in the rat. Gastroenterology. 2002;122:188–201.

218. Orlichenko LS, Behari J, Yeh TH, Liu S, Stolz DB, Saluja AK, Singh VP. Transcriptional regulation of CXC-ELR chemokines KC and MIP-2 in mouse pancreatic acini. Am J Physiol Gastrointest Liver Physiol. 2010;299:G867–76.

219. Telek G, Ducroc R, Scoazec JY, Pasquier C, Feldmann G, Roze C. Differential upregulation of cellular adhesion molecules at the sites of oxidative stress in experimental acute pancreatitis. J Surg Res. 2001;96:56–67.

220. Frossard JL, Saluja A, Bhagat L, Lee HS, Bhatia M, Hofbauer B, Steer ML. The role of intercellular adhesion molecule 1 and neutrophils in acute pancreatitis and pancreatitis-associated lung injury. Gastroenterology. 1999;116:694–701.

221. Powell JJ, Siriwardena AK, Fearon KC, Ross JA. Endothelial-derived selectins in the development of organ dysfunction in acute pancreatitis. Crit Care Med. 2001;29:567–72.

222. Perejaslov A, Chooklin S, Bihalskyy I. Implication of interleukin 18 and intercellular adhesion molecule (ICAM)-1 in acute pancreatitis. Hepato-Gastroenterology. 2008;55:1806–13.

223. Wetterholm E, Linders J, Merza M, Regner S, Thorlacius H. Platelet-derived CXCL4 regulates neutrophil infiltration and tissue damage in severe acute pancreatitis. Transl Res. 2016;176:105–18.

224. Du BQ, Yang YM, Chen YH, Liu XB, Mai G. N-Acetylcysteine improves pancreatic microcirculation and alleviates the severity of acute necrotizing pancreatitis. Gut Liver. 2013;7:357–62.

225. Manso MA, Ramudo L, De Dios I. Extrapancreatic organ impairment during acute pancreatitis induced by bile-pancreatic duct obstruction. Effect of N-acetylcysteine. Int J Exp Pathol. 2007;88:343–9.

226. Shi C, Zhao X, Wang X, Andersson R. Role of nuclear factor-kappaB, reactive oxygen species and

cellular signaling in the early phase of acute pancreatitis. Scand J Gastroenterol. 2005;40:103–8.

227. Inoue S, Nakao A, Kishimoto W, Murakami H, Itoh K, Itoh T, Harada A, Nonami T, Takagi H. Antineutrophil antibody attenuates the severity of acute lung injury in rats with experimental acute pancreatitis. Arch Surg. 1995;130:93–8.

228. Lira SA. Genetic approaches to study chemokine function. J Leukoc Biol. 1996;59:45–52.

229. Cryz SJ Jr, Furer E, Germanier R. Simple model for the study of *Pseudomonas aeruginosa* infections in leukopenic mice. Infect Immun. 1983;39:1067–71.

230. Uchida K, Yamamoto Y, Klein TW, Friedman H, Yamaguchi H. Granulocyte-colony stimulating factor facilitates the restoration of resistance to opportunistic fungi in leukopenic mice. J Med Vet Mycol. 1992;30:293–300.

231. Wang E, Simard M, Ouellet N, Bergeron Y, Beauchamp D, Bergeron MG. Pathogenesis of pneumococcal pneumonia in cyclophosphamide-induced leukopenia in mice. Infect Immun. 2002;70:4226–38.

232. Yipp BG, Petri B, Salina D, Jenne CN, Scott BN, Zbytnuik LD, Pittman K, Asaduzzaman M, Wu K, Meijndert HC, Malawista SE, de Boisfleury CA, Zhang K, Conly J, Kubes P. Infection-induced NETosis is a dynamic process involving neutrophil multitasking in vivo. Nat Med. 2012;18:1386–93.

233. Merza M, Hartman H, Rahman M, Hwaiz R, Zhang E, Renström E, Luo L, Mörgelin M, Regner S, Thorlacius H. Neutrophil extracellular traps induce trypsin activation, inflammation, and tissue damage in mice with severe acute pancreatitis. Gastroenterology. 2015;149:1920–31.e8.

234. Li H, Zhao L, Wang Y, Zhang MC, Qiao C. Roles, detection, and visualization of neutrophil extracellular traps in acute pancreatitis. Front Immunol. 2022;13:974821.

235. Leppkes M, Maueroder C, Hirth S, Nowecki S, Gunther C, Billmeier U, Paulus S, Biermann M, Munoz LE, Hoffmann M, Wildner D, Croxford AL, Waisman A, Mowen K, Jenne DE, Krenn V, Mayerle J, Lerch MM, Schett G, Wirtz S, Neurath MF, Herrmann M, Becker C. Externalized decondensed neutrophil chromatin occludes pancreatic ducts and drives pancreatitis. Nat Commun. 2016;7:10973.

236. Bicker KL, Thompson PR. The protein arginine deiminases: structure, function, inhibition, and disease. Biopolymers. 2013;99:155–63.

237. Wang Y, Li M, Stadler S, Correll S, Li P, Wang D, Hayama R, Leonelli L, Han H, Grigoryev SA, Allis CD, Coonrod SA. Histone hypercitrullination mediates chromatin decondensation and neutrophil extracellular trap formation. J Cell Biol. 2009;184:205–13.

238. Bilyy R, Fedorov V, Vovk V, Leppkes M, Dumych T, Chopyak V, Schett G, Herrmann M. Neutrophil extracellular traps form a barrier between necrotic and viable areas in acute abdominal inflammation. Front Immunol. 2016;7:424.

239. Pan B, Li Y, Liu Y, Wang W, Huang G, Ouyang Y. Circulating CitH3 is a reliable diagnostic and prognostic biomarker of septic patients in acute pancreatitis. Front Immunol. 2021;12:766391.

240. Lewis HD, Liddle J, Coote JE, Atkinson SJ, Barker MD, Bax BD, Bicker KL, Bingham RP, Campbell M, Chen YH, Chung CW, Craggs PD, Davis RP, Eberhard D, Joberty G, Lind KE, Locke K, Maller C, Martinod K, Patten C, Polyakova O, Rise CE, Rudiger M, Sheppard RJ, Slade DJ, Thomas P, Thorpe J, Yao G, Drewes G, Wagner DD, Thompson PR, Prinjha RK, Wilson DM. Inhibition of PAD4 activity is sufficient to disrupt mouse and human NET formation. Nat Chem Biol. 2015;11:189–91.

241. Murthy P, Singhi AD, Ross MA, Loughran P, Paragomi P, Papachristou GI, Whitcomb DC, Zureikat AH, Lotze MT, Zeh Iii HJ, Boone BA. Enhanced neutrophil extracellular trap formation in acute pancreatitis contributes to disease severity and is reduced by chloroquine. Front Immunol. 2019;10:28.

242. Lerch MM, Saluja AK, Dawra R, Saluja M, Steer ML. The effect of chloroquine administration on two experimental models of acute pancreatitis. Gastroenterology. 1993;104:1768–79.

243. Guillaumes S, Blanco I, Villanueva A, Sans MD, Clavé P, Chabás A, Farré A, Lluís F. Chloroquine stabilizes pancreatic lysosomes and improves survival of mice with diet-induced acute pancreatitis. Pancreas. 1997;14:262–6.

244. Martinon F, Burns K, Tschopp J. The inflammasome: a molecular platform triggering activation of inflammatory caspases and processing of proIL-beta. Mol Cell. 2002;10:417–26.

245. Martin MA, Saracibar E, Santamaria A, Arranz E, Garrote JA, Almaraz A, del Olmo ML, Garcia-Pajares F, Fernandez-Orcajo P, Velicia R, Blanco-Quiros A, Caro-Paton A. Interleukin 18 (IL-18) and other immunological parameters as markers of severity in acute pancreatitis. Rev Esp Enferm Dig. 2008;100:768–73.

246. Zhang XH, Li ML, Wang B, Guo MX, Zhu RM. Caspase-1 inhibition alleviates acute renal injury in rats with severe acute pancreatitis. World J Gastroenterol. 2014;20:10457–63.

247. Janiak A, Lesniowski B, Jasinska A, Pietruczuk M, Malecka-Panas E. Interleukin 18 as an early marker or prognostic factor in acute pancreatitis. Prz Gastroenterol. 2015;10:203–7.

248. Yuan H, Jin X, Sun J, Li F, Feng Q, Zhang C, Cao Y, Wang Y. Protective effect of HMGB1 a box on organ injury of acute pancreatitis in mice. Pancreas. 2009;38:143–8.

249. Algaba-Chueca F, de-Madaria E, Lozano-Ruiz B, Martinez-Cardona C, Quesada-Vazquez N, Bachiller V, Tarin F, Such J, Frances R, Zapater P, Gonzalez-Navajas JM. The expression and activation of the AIM2 inflammasome correlates with inflammation and disease severity in patients with acute pancreatitis. Pancreatology. 2017;17:364–71.

250. Sendler M, van den Brandt C, Glaubitz J, Wilden A, Golchert J, Weiss FU, Homuth G, De Freitas Chama LL, Mishra N, Mahajan UM, Bossaller L, Völker U, Bröker BM, Mayerle J, Lerch MM. NLRP3 inflammasome regulates development of systemic inflammatory response and compensatory anti-inflammatory response syndromes in mice with acute pancreatitis. Gastroenterology. 2020;158:253–69. e14.

251. Kang R, Chen R, Xie M, Cao L, Lotze MT, Tang D, Zeh HJ 3rd. The receptor for advanced glycation end products activates the AIM2 inflammasome in acute pancreatitis. J Immunol. 2016;196:4331–7.

252. Sennello JA, Fayad R, Pini M, Gove ME, Ponemone V, Cabay RJ, Siegmund B, Dinarello CA, Fantuzzi G. Interleukin-18, together with interleukin-12, induces severe acute pancreatitis in obese but not in nonobese leptin-deficient mice. Proc Natl Acad Sci USA. 2008;105:8085–90.

253. Pini M, Sennello JA, Cabay RJ, Fantuzzi G. Effect of diet-induced obesity on acute pancreatitis induced by administration of interleukin-12 plus interleukin-18 in mice. Obesity (Silver Spring). 2010;18:476–81.

254. Komara NL, Paragomi P, Greer PJ, Wilson AS, Breze C, Papachristou GI, Whitcomb DC. Severe acute pancreatitis: capillary permeability model linking systemic inflammation to multiorgan failure. Am J Physiol Gastrointest Liver Physiol. 2020;319:G573–G83.

255. Phillips AE, Wilson AS, Greer PJ, Hinton A, Culp S, Paragomi P, Pothoulakis I, Singh V, Lee PJ, Lahooti I, Whitcomb DC, Papachristou GI. Relationship of circulating levels of long-chain fatty acids to persistent organ failure in acute pancreatitis. Am J Physiol Gastrointest Liver Physiol. 2023;325:G279–G85.

256. Blamey SL, Imrie CW, O'Neill J, Gilmour WH, Carter DC. Prognostic factors in acute pancreatitis. Gut. 1984;25:1340–6.

257. Michelis R, Sela S, Zeitun T, Geron R, Kristal B. Unexpected normal colloid osmotic pressure in clinical states with low serum albumin. PLoS One. 2016;11:e0159839.

258. Thomas T, Stefanoni D, Reisz JA, Nemkov T, Bertolone L, Francis RO, Hudson KE, Zimring JC, Hansen KC, Hod EA, Spitalnik SL, D'Alessandro A. COVID-19 infection alters kynurenine and fatty acid metabolism, correlating with IL-6 levels and renal status. JCI Insight. 2020;5:5.

259. Fiandaca MS, Mapstone M, Mahmoodi A, Gross T, Macciardi F, Cheema AK, Merchant-Borna K, Bazarian J, Federoff HJ. Plasma metabolomic biomarkers accurately classify acute mild traumatic brain injury from controls. PLoS One. 2018;13:e0195318.

260. Rieu M, Rautu L, Wassermann D, Schlotterer M. Evolution of blood fatty acid levels in severe burns. Anesth Analg (Paris). 1977;34:1323–9.

261. Wolfe RR, Herndon DN, Jahoor F, Miyoshi H, Wolfe M. Effect of severe burn injury on substrate cycling by glucose and fatty acids. N Engl J Med. 1987;317:403–8.

262. Kamisoglu K, Haimovich B, Calvano SE, Coyle SM, Corbett SA, Langley RJ, Kingsmore SF, Androulakis IP. Human metabolic response to systemic inflammation: assessment of the concordance between experimental endotoxemia and clinical cases of sepsis/SIRS. Crit Care. 2015;19:71.

263. Lee PJ, Papachristou GI. Management of severe acute pancreatitis. Curr Treat Options Gastroenterol. 2020;18:670–81.

264. Gad MM, Simons-Linares CR. Is aggressive intravenous fluid resuscitation beneficial in acute pancreatitis? A meta-analysis of randomized control trials and cohort studies. World J Gastroenterol. 2020;26:1098–106.

265. Kuwabara K, Matsuda S, Fushimi K, Ishikawa KB, Horiguchi H, Fujimori K. Early crystalloid fluid volume management in acute pancreatitis: association with mortality and organ failure. Pancreatology. 2011;11:351–61.

266. Schmid-Schonbein GW, Chang M. The autodigestion hypothesis for shock and multi-organ failure. Ann Biomed Eng. 2014;42:405–14.

267. Zhu Y, He C, Li X, Cai Y, Hu J, Liao Y, Zhao J, Xia L, He W, Liu L, Luo C, Shu X, Cai Q, Chen Y, Lu N. Gut microbiota dysbiosis worsens the severity of acute pancreatitis in patients and mice. J Gastroenterol. 2019;54:347–58.

268. Evennett NJ, Petrov MS, Mittal A, Windsor JA. Systematic review and pooled estimates for the diagnostic accuracy of serological markers for intestinal ischemia. World J Surg. 2009;33:1374–83.

269. Murata T, Yamaguchi N, Shimomoto Y, Mikajiri Y, Sasaki Y, Konagaya K, Igarashi Y, Sawamura N, Yamamoto K, Kume N, Suno Y, Kurata S, Kasetani T, Kato I, Nishida T, Hirata H, Miyake K, Oonishi T, Isogai N, Fukai R, Kanomata H, Shimoyama R, Kashiwagi H, Takenoue T, Terashima T, Murayama H, Kohriki S, Morita T, Takaki M, Ogino H, Kanemaru T, Sano K, Kurogi N, Watanabe K, Hirata M, Kawachi J. Preoperative prognostic predictors and treatment strategies for surgical procedure focused on the sequential organ failure assessment score in nonocclusive mesenteric ischemia: a multicenter retrospective cohort study. Int J Surg. 2023;109:4119–25.

270. Floch MH, Bina I. The natural history of diverticulitis: fact and theory. J Clin Gastroenterol. 2004;38:S2–7.

271. Hall J, Hardiman K, Lee S, Lightner A, Stocchi L, Paquette IM, Steele SR, Feingold DL. The American Society of Colon and Rectal Surgeons clinical practice guidelines for the treatment of left-sided colonic diverticulitis. Dis Colon Rectum. 2020;63:728–47.

272. Cirocchi R, Randolph JJ, Binda GA, Gioia S, Henry BM, Tomaszewski KA, Allegritti M, Arezzo A,

Marzaioli R, Ruscelli P. Is the outpatient management of acute diverticulitis safe and effective? A systematic review and meta-analysis. Tech Coloproctol. 2019;23:87–100.

273. Colombel JF, Sands BE, Rutgeerts P, Sandborn W, Danese S, D'Haens G, Panaccione R, Loftus EV Jr, Sankoh S, Fox I, Parikh A, Milch C, Abhyankar B, Feagan BG. The safety of vedolizumab for ulcerative colitis and Crohn's disease. Gut. 2017;66:839–51.

274. Palmer KR, Duerden BI, Holdsworth CD. Bacteriological and endotoxin studies in cases of ulcerative colitis submitted to surgery. Gut. 1980;21:851–4.

275. Rey JR, Axon A, Budzynska A, Kruse A, Nowak A. Guidelines of the European Society of Gastrointestinal Endoscopy (E.S.G.E.) antibiotic prophylaxis for gastrointestinal endoscopy. European Society of Gastrointestinal Endoscopy. Endoscopy. 1998;30:318–24.

276. Mittal R, Coopersmith CM. Redefining the gut as the motor of critical illness. Trends Mol Med. 2014;20:214–23.

277. Wang HW, Escott AB, Phang KL, Petrov MS, Phillips AR, Windsor JA. Indications, techniques, and clinical outcomes of thoracic duct interventions in patients: a forgotten literature? J Surg Res. 2016;204:213–27.

278. Sloop CH, Dory L, Roheim PS. Interstitial fluid lipoproteins. J Lipid Res. 1987;28:225–37.

279. Mittal A, Phillips AR, Middleditch M, Ruggiero K, Loveday B, Delahunt B, Cooper GJ, Windsor JA. The proteome of mesenteric lymph during acute pancreatitis and implications for treatment. JOP. 2009;10:130–42.

280. Flint RS, Phillips AR, Power SE, Dunbar PR, Brown C, Delahunt B, Cooper GJ, Windsor JA. Acute pancreatitis severity is exacerbated by intestinal ischemia-reperfusion conditioned mesenteric lymph. Surgery. 2008;143:404–13.

281. Shanbhag ST, Choong B, Petrov M, Delahunt B, Windsor JA, Phillips ARJ. Acute pancreatitis conditioned mesenteric lymph causes cardiac dysfunction in rats independent of hypotension. Surgery. 2018;163:1097–105.

282. Dugernier T, Reynaert MS, Deby-Dupont G, Roeseler JJ, Carlier M, Squifflet JP, Deby C, Pincemail J, Lamy M, De Maeght S, et al. Prospective evaluation of thoracic-duct drainage in the treatment of respiratory failure complicating severe acute pancreatitis. Intensive Care Med. 1989;15:372–8.

283. Itkin M, Nadolski GJ. Modern techniques of lymphangiography and interventions: current status and future development. Cardiovasc Intervent Radiol. 2018;41:366–76.

284. Trevaskis NL, Kaminskas LM, Porter CJ. From sewer to saviour—targeting the lymphatic system to promote drug exposure and activity. Nat Rev Drug Discov. 2015;14:781–803.

Part II

Clinical Management

Post-ERCP Pancreatitis and Prevention

Venkata S. Akshintala and Vikesh K. Singh

1 Introduction

Pancreatitis following endoscopic retrograde cholangiopancreatography (PEP) represents the most common adverse outcome of the procedure, affecting 2–15% of individuals, leading to significant morbidity, occasional fatalities, and a rise in healthcare costs [1, 2]. Annually, PEP contributes more than $200 million to healthcare expenses in the United States [3, 4]. From 2011 to 2017, there was a 15.3% surge in hospital admissions due to PEP, primarily because ERCP is increasingly utilized for complex therapeutic purposes rather than diagnostic ones [5]. Progress in understanding PEP's pathophysiology, better selection of patients, enhancements in the techniques used during the procedure, and the introduction of more effective measures for PEP prevention have been achieved. This chapter is dedicated to presenting a strategy grounded in scientific evidence for preventing PEP, along with a discussion on the continuous efforts to decrease its incidence.

2 Pathophysiology of PEP

Understanding the pathophysiology of post-ERCP pancreatitis (PEP) is challenging, yet various potential causes have been suggested, including (a) damage to the duodenal papillae, the pancreatic sphincter, and the pancreatic duct; (b) injury to the ductal system caused by the pressure of contrast injections; (c) harm from the contrast material itself; (d) infections due to gut bacteria; (e) burns or shocks from the use of electrosurgical devices; and (f) neuronal damage [6–9]. These hypothesized mechanisms underlie the procedural risk factors for PEP and inform the preventive strategies currently in practice. Furthermore, research using mouse models has shed light on the inflammatory processes associated with PEP, particularly pointing to the activation of calcineurin as a significant factor [10].

PEP's onset is influenced by multiple factors, yet the key process involves the early activation of zymogens within the pancreas, leading to the initiation of the inflammatory response. The blockage of pancreatic duct (PD) outflow and the ensuing activation of trypsinogen within the ducts, often due to swelling of the papilla, are a recognized cause of PEP [11]. Studies using electron microscopy on the duodenal papilla and the ampulla of Vater have revealed a distinctive pattern resembling layers of onion skin made up of mucosal folds that appear as tongue-like flaps oriented toward the papillary opening (Fig. 1a) [12, 13]. These flaps form cul-de-sacs which,

V. S. Akshintala · V. K. Singh (✉)
Division of Gastroenterology, Johns Hopkins University School of Medicine, Baltimore, MD, USA
e-mail: vakshin1@jhmi.edu; vsingh1@jhmi.edu

© The Author(s), under exclusive license to Springer Nature Singapore Pte Ltd. 2024
J. A. Windsor et al. (eds.), *Acute Pancreatitis*, https://doi.org/10.1007/978-981-97-3132-9_7

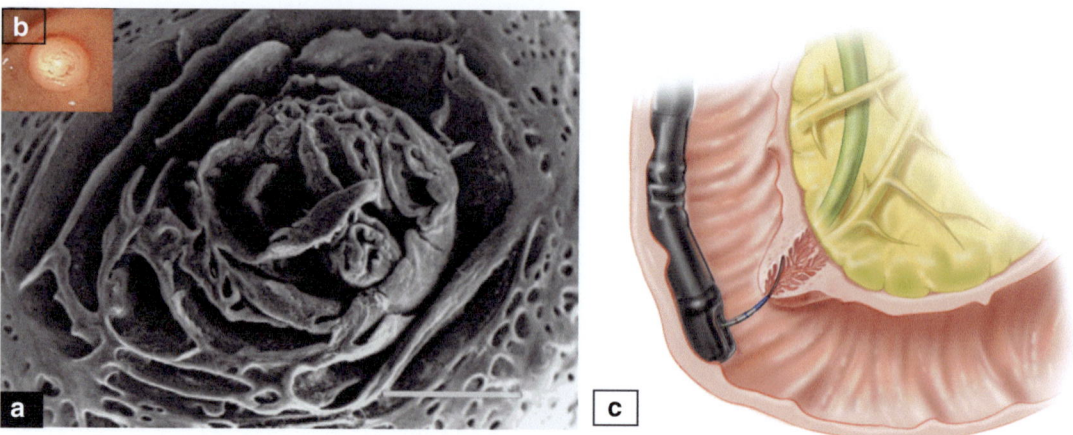

Fig. 1 (**a**) Electron microscopy view of the major duodenal papilla demonstrating mucosal duplications. (**b**) Endoscopy view of the major papilla. * (**c**) Guidewire and sphincterotome trapped within the cul-de-sacs under the tongue-shaped mucosal flaps within the duodenal papilla or ampulla #. (*Adapted with permission from Paulson FP et al. # From Johns Hopkins University)

along with the filamentous terminal septum, may cause difficulty in cannulation due to entrapment of the cannula or guidewire (Fig. 1c). Moreover, these mucosal folds are richly supplied with blood and contain numerous sero-mucinous glands. Any edema in the mucosa significantly increases the outflow pressure of the PD and contributes to pancreatic enzyme activation within the PD [12]. Recognized procedural risk factors for PEP, such as difficult cannulation, as well as procedures like pancreatic sphincterotomy and pre-cut sphincterotomy, may induce PEP by causing papillary edema [14, 15]. Type 3, or bulky protruding, duodenal papillae are known to be associated with difficult cannulation as these are densely filled by these mucosal flaps and increase the risk of PEP [16, 17].

The better understanding of these mechanistic characteristics has guided PEP prevention methods toward enhanced cannulation techniques [18, 19], as well as the use of pharmacological interventions to lessen papillary edema [20, 21]. Interventions such as pancreatic stent placement, protease inhibitors that target zymogen activation, non-steroidal anti-inflammatory (NSAIDs) to decrease inflammation and intravenous fluids have also been used for PEP prophylaxis.

3 Diagnostic Criteria for PEP

The diagnosis and severity grading of PEP use either the consensus criteria or the Revised Atlanta Classification (RAC). According to the consensus criteria established in 1991, PEP is defined as new onset or increased upper abdominal pain and pancreatic amylase (or lipase) elevation of three times greater than the upper limit of normal at least 24 h after ERCP and resulting in hospitalization or prolongation of ongoing hospitalization of 2 or more nights [22]. The RAC revised in 2012, defines PEP as the presence of two of the following three criteria: (1) abdominal pain consistent with AP (acute onset of a persistent, severe, epigastric pain often radiating to the back); (2) serum lipase (or amylase) level at least three times greater than the upper limit of normal; and (3) characteristic findings of AP on contrast-enhanced computed tomography (CECT), magnetic resonance imaging (MRI), or transabdominal ultrasonography [23].

The definitions of PEP used in clinical trials have been inconsistent, but the consensus criteria has increasingly been used as the standard over the last three decades [1]. Smeets et al. compared the consensus criteria and RAC definitions for

PEP. They found the RAC to be more sensitive (100 vs. 55%) and specific (98 vs. 72%) and to have a higher positive predictive value (58 vs. 5%) [24]. The RAC is superior in grading the severity of PEP since the consensus criteria rely primarily on hospital length of stay, which may be influenced by factors unrelated to PEP, such as comorbidity.

Both PEP definitions are, however, limited by the subjective nature of abdominal pain, the timing of lipase or amylase measurement, and routine hospital admission for observation following ERCP which all affect the accuracy of PEP diagnosis. This also introduces heterogeneity among clinical studies of PEP and caution must be advised when interpreting these results. In addition, ERCP can cause abdominal pain without AP, and lipase elevation may occur following ERCP due to pancreatic duct instrumentation without activation of the inflammatory cascade [25–27]. In uncertain clinical situations, a CT scan provides a more accurate diagnosis of PEP and will also help assess for other ERCP-related complications such as duodenal perforation.

4 Patient Selection

The best strategy to prevent PEP is prudent patient selection for ERCP which is recommended by several professional society guidelines [3, 28]. There has been an increase in the utilization of ERCPs in the past decade, but the downside has been a 15.3% increase in the incidence of PEP from 2011 to 2017 [5, 29, 30]. Diagnostic ERCPs have been largely abandoned since the advent of magnetic resonance cholangiopancreatography (MRCP) and endoscopic ultrasound (EUS) [31–33]. ERCP is now only performed for therapeutic purposes. Therapeutic ERCP has become increasingly complex which likely explains the recent increase in PEP. Interventional EUS provides an alternative to ERCP for biliary drainage in difficult-to-access anatomy and with obstructive pathologies, potentially reducing the risk of PEP [34, 35]. Improvements in EUS accessories, such as steerable needles that facilitate

and simplify biliary access, will likely further reduce the risk of PEP [36].

However, ERCPs continue to be performed on an empirical basis for some indications. For example, sphincterotomy is often performed for sphincter of Oddi dysfunction (SOD), particularly for type 1 and 2 SOD. The sham-controlled EPISOD trial conclusively demonstrated the lack of benefit of sphincterotomy for patients with type 3 SOD, who are at increased risk of developing PEP [37]. The results of the EPISOD trial have led to a significant decrease in the number of ERCPs performed for SOD since 2013 [38]. This is also reflected in the fact that RCTs evaluating PEP prophylaxis in high-risk patients are enrolling fewer with suspected SOD with 82% in the landmark trial showing the efficacy of rectal indomethacin over placebo in 2012 but only 26% in the recent SVI trial. ERCP with sphincterotomy for type 2 SOD and idiopathic recurrent AP due to type 1 pancreatic sphincter of Oddi dysfunction or pancreas divisum are being prospectively evaluated in the ReSPOND study and the SHARP trial, respectively [39, 40]. The results of these studies will likely further steer endoscopists away from pursuing ERCP in patients with these conditions, and this should correspondingly reduce rates of PEP.

5 PEP Risk Stratification

5.1 Risk Factors

The patient- and procedure-related risk factors for PEP have been well defined (Table 1). Recognition of these risk factors can assist with ERCP procedural planning and selection of PEP prophylaxis. ERCP procedures involving difficult or failed cannulation, pancreatic sphincterotomy, pre-cut sphincterotomy, brush cytology, pneumatic biliary dilation without biliary sphincterotomy, more than two PD guidewire passes, more than two PD contrast injections, pancreatic acinarization, and trainee involvement in the procedure have all been associated with an increased risk of PEP [14, 41–49]. Patient-related risk factors have been identified that increase the risk of

Table 1 Patient- and procedure-related risk factors for the development of post-ERCP pancreatitis

Patient-related risk factors	Procedure-related risk factors
History of recurrent acute pancreatitis	Difficult cannulation
History of post-ERCP pancreatitis	Pancreatic or pre-cut sphincterotomy
Suspected sphincter of Oddi dysfunction	Multiple pancreatic duct injections
Young age and female gender	Multiple pancreatic duct guidewire passes
Chronic pancreatitis (protective)	Pancreatic acinarization
Pancreas head mass (protective)	Short-duration balloon dilation of an intact biliary sphincter
Prior sphincterotomy (protective)	

PEP including female sex, age <50 years, SOD, history of AP, and prior history of PEP [50, 51]. Primary sclerosing cholangitis (PSC) was previously suspected to be an independent risk factor for PEP, but this was not confirmed in larger studies [52]. Patients with chronic calcific pancreatitis and pancreatic head neoplasms have a reduced risk for the development of PEP [48]. Similarly, patients with prior biliary sphincterotomy are at a reduced risk of accidental PD cannulation and are at a decreased risk of PEP. These patient and procedural risk factors have consistently been shown to be significant and have been incorporated into ERCP quality reporting metrics to improve the performance and safety of ERCP procedures [53].

5.2   Risk Stratification Methods

Endoscopists face difficulties in accurately determining the risk of post-ERCP pancreatitis (PEP) in individual patients due to the large number, differential weight, and synergistic effect of the risk factors for PEP. Although a few prognostic scoring systems have been developed to stratify patients based on their risk of developing PEP by using multivariable regression models, none of them are in widespread clinical use or endorsed by professional society guidelines [54–59]. Retrospective and non-randomized data incorporating a small number of risk factors and limited ability to account for the interaction between risk factors have limited the PEP scoring systems [55–57]. These models were not adjusted for PEP prophylaxis strategies such as rectal NSAIDs, aggressive hydration, or prophylactic PD stenting [60]. Data from randomized controlled trials (RCTs) and the application of

novel machine learning techniques have been used to develop improved risk stratification models [61]. Web-based applications that can be integrated into the electronic medical records systems are currently being developed that will provide real-time prediction of the PEP risk and may also help in appropriate PEP prophylaxis selection [57].

A priori quantification of the patient's PEP risk profile will help with the discussion with the patient of potential procedural risks and alternatives to ERCP. Prophylactic PD stent placement can be reserved for high-risk patients due to technical challenges and costs associated with stent placement and removal. NSAIDs may be used selectively for those at moderate-to-high risk of PEP, while avoiding those at low risk, especially due to the increase in the cost of rectal NSAIDs in countries like the United States (see below) [62]. Post-procedure hospital admission for observation is highly variable between centers, with some admitting every patient, even after an uneventful elective ERCP procedure. However, this is cost-prohibitive in most settings. Patients at the highest risk of developing PEP or those with early signs of PEP during the post-procedure period should be considered for hospital admission. An elevation in serum lipase levels more than three times the upper limit of normal within 2–4 h of the ERCP procedure may be a useful biomarker to identify patients who may eventually develop PEP and would more likely benefit from an inpatient admission. However, this strategy requires prospective validation in a larger cohort [63]. Other inflammatory biomarkers such as interleukins (IL-6, IL-10) and tumor necrosis factor alpha (TNFα) do not assist in the early detection of PEP [64]. To determine biomarkers that can aid in the identification of patients with high-risk PEP, as well as early detection of PEP, further research is necessary. This research should utilize the biorepositories of large-scale PEP-related studies that are currently ongoing. The identification of such biomarkers would allow for improved selection of patients for prophylaxis and admission for observation following an ERCP procedure.

6 ERCP Procedure

Having a thorough understanding of the pathophysiology and risk factors associated with PEP is crucial in refining the procedural technique of ERCP to minimize the risk of PEP. In this regard, there are several technical considerations that need to be taken into account when selecting the appropriate methods and technologies during the ERCP procedure.

Adverse events that are associated with ERCP, such as PEP, can be indicative of the quality of the procedure. This quality can be dependent on several factors such as the patient selection process, the use of appropriate procedural techniques, the identification of factors that may lead to adverse events, and the implementation of strategies to mitigate the risks associated with such events. These factors are crucial in ensuring the safety and efficacy of ERCP procedures. Due to its intricate nature, ERCP has a long learning curve, and adequate training is essential to achieve proficiency in the relevant aspects of the procedure to reduce the risk of adverse events. It is worth noting that there is a strong emphasis on establishing clearly defined and rigorously validated competency thresholds during training evaluations. Such thresholds are particularly critical in the context of ERCP, where the ability to competently perform this complex procedure is essential for ensuring positive patient outcomes [65]. Studies have demonstrated that implementing transparent reporting and auditing of the quality indicators can effectively mitigate the risk of procedural complications [66, 67]. Standardized quality report cards have been developed for the ERCP procedure, and at the authors' institution, wherein an auto-mated system that captures the quality metrics related to ERCP for each endoscopist is in use [68, 69].

Difficult cannulation leading to edema of the duodenal papilla can result in obstruction of the PD outflow and an increased risk of PEP. This is often attributed to an inadequate understanding of the complex anatomy of the papilla, including the intricate papillary projections within (Fig. 1). Using a suitable method such as the compact disc technique, proposed by Takenaka et al. can effectively navigate the ERCP cannula or other catheters while taking into account the papilla's anatomical features. This enables selective biliary cannulation, which reduces the risk of PD trauma (Fig. 2) [18]. Alternate methods such as double-wire cannulation and pre-cut sphincterotomy should be considered in the setting of difficult cannulation [70]. It is now established that the preceding difficult cannulation and papillary edema truly increase the PEP risk rather than such maneuvers, with the odds ratio (OR) increasing by 1.072 for each additional minute spent attempting cannulation [71]. Several studies have confirmed that early use of pre-cut sphincterotomy reduces the risk of PEP when compared to late pre-cut after repeated papillary cannulation attempts which again validate this hypothesis [19]. It is pertinent to receive sufficient training

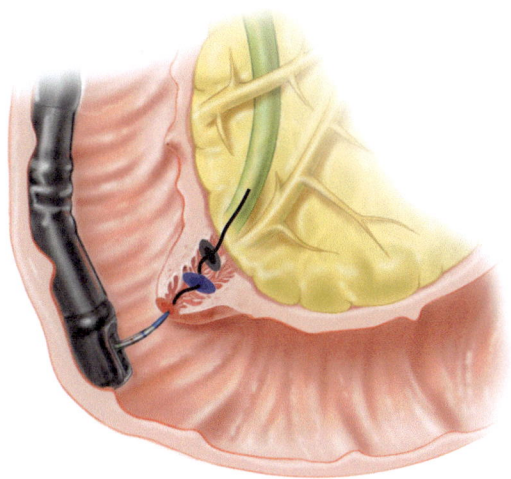

Fig. 2 Cannulation using the disc method, maneuvering around the mucosal projections in the papilla/ampulla

in such alternate cannulation techniques and be able to recognize the appropriate time to switch to these, typically after 5–10 min of standard cannulation, along with the use of combination PEP prophylactic strategies as described below. Blended current is preferred over pure-cut current, while iso-osmolar contrast agents are preferred over hyperosmolar contrast agents. These options have been widely acknowledged to be safer and are now considered the standard of care [72, 73].

In the past, the standard method for cannulation involved using a cannula to engage the papilla and then injecting contrast in the desired duct's direction. In recent years, the use of guidewire-assisted cannulation as a technique for bile duct cannulation has become more popular without the use of contrast. This approach has shown to be effective in increasing the success rates of cannulation while also being a safer option [74]. Freeman et al. observed that the risk of PEP increases significantly with the passage of one or more deep guidewires into the PD. Additionally, if the pancreatic guidewire is manipulated during attempts to place a stent or if stent placement is unsuccessful, this also increases the risk of PEP [75]. An additional RCT demonstrated a higher risk of PEP when there were more than two guidewire passes into the PD, or when pancreatic brush cytology was performed [76]. This indicates that the trauma caused by guidewires or other accessories in the pancreatic duct or its side branches may play a significant role in the development of PEP (Fig. 3). This RCT also showed that 13.7% of patients with >2 guidewire passes into the PD developed PEP despite receiving rectal indomethacin. This suggests that a PD stent should be inserted in these patients as is recommended by the ESGE guidelines [77]. The double guidewire is another technique to achieve biliary cannulation in the setting of repeat unintentional passage of the guidewire into the PD, where the guidewire is left in the PD to straighten the common channel and repeat the biliary cannulation attempts. A PD stent can similarly be used in this context to reduce the risk of PEP while increasing the success of biliary cannulation [78].

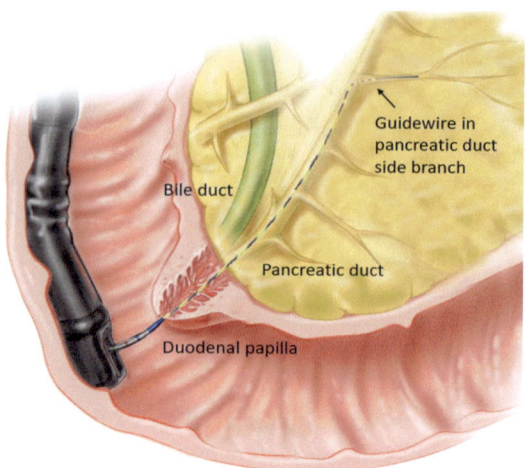

Fig. 3 Trauma to the pancreatic duct side branches from guidewire passage

The risk of PEP is higher in patients with large bile duct stones who undergo mechanical lithotripsy [49]. Endoscopic papillary large balloon dilation (EPLBD) is another technique that involves focal dilation of the biliary sphincter with, or without, preceding sphincterotomy [79]. Performing biliary sphincterotomy in this context results in a "controlled disruption" of the biliary sphincter with papillary edema and is the recommended approach [80]. Societal guidelines from ASGE and ESGE recommend using EPLBD combined with limited sphincterotomy as the initial approach for large bile duct stones [81, 82].

7 PEP Prophylaxis

Since 1977, several prophylactic agents for PEP prophylaxis have been tested in RCTs [83]. The use of rectal NSAIDs [84], high-volume IVF [85, 86], and PD stent placement have the strongest evidence in preventing PEP [87]. Recent studies suggest that combining these strategies leads to a cumulative additive benefit, although there are limited head-to-head RCTs on this topic [60]. According to the ESGE guidelines, rectal NSAIDs should be used routinely for all inpatients, PD stents for those at high risk, and IVF for those unable to receive rectal NSAIDs [77]. The revised ASGE guidelines also recommend the use of rectal NSAIDs for all patients, with aggressive peri- and post-procedural IVF and limiting PD stent use for high-risk patients [28].

7.1 NSAIDs

It is widely accepted that PEP occurs due to uncontrolled activation of the inflammatory cascade after injury caused by the ERCP procedure. However, there is limited understanding about the primary inflammatory mediators that play a role in this process. One of the proinflammatory mediators, cyclooxygenase-2 (COX-2), has been identified as being involved in this process. Pharmacologic inhibition or selective genetic deletion of COX-2 in animal models resulted in a decrease in the severity of pancreatitis [88]. Several clinical trials have been conducted evaluating the efficacy of NSAIDs for PEP prophylaxis, and a recent comprehensive review and network meta-analysis (NMA) have compared at least 11 different NSAID regimens using diclofenac, indomethacin, celecoxib, naproxen, or ketoprofen in various doses and routes of delivery (Fig. 4) [60]. The variation in patient population, along with the type, route, and dose of NSAIDs used, led to heterogenous results. It is possible that the variations in the levels of cytochrome P450 2C9 enzyme, responsible for the metabolism of NSAIDs, contributed to the heterogeneity observed in some cases [89]. In general, the administration of rectal NSAIDs was found to be more effective than the oral route. It is probable that the improved effectiveness of NSAIDs when administered rectally is due to superior bioavailability, as this delivery method bypasses the first-pass metabolism in the liver (that results in only 50–60% of the orally administered drug reaching systemic circulation) [90]. Pharmacokinetic studies have shown that when indomethacin is delivered through the rectum, it remains at its highest concentration in the body for a longer period of time compared to when it is administered through intravenous or intramuscular routes [91].

After a milestone clinical trial was published in 2012, rectal indomethacin became a com-monly used prophylaxis both in the United States and internationally [92, 93]. PEP risk was reduced by around 50% with the use of rectal indomethacin. All prophylactic strategies for PEP prophylaxis, including the use of rectal indomethacin, were deemed cost-effective due to the economic implications of PEP [94]. There has been a marked rise in the cost of the use of rectal indomethacin in the United States (from $2 in 2005 to $340 for 100 mg in 2021) [62]. The increase in price puts pressure on the healthcare system and can cause patients to incur out-of-pocket expenses. Alternative agents or other NSAIDs have been studied as a potential replacement for rectal indomethacin. At least 15 RCTs were conducted to evaluate the effectiveness of rectal indomethacin 100 mg, while 9 RCTs were conducted to evaluate rectal diclofenac 100 mg. It is worth noting that rectal diclofenac 100 mg was found to be more effective than rectal indomethacin 100 mg (OR 0.59; 95% CI, 0.40–0.89) or at least equally effective [60]. Interestingly, another two recent RCTs evaluated an increased dose of rectal indomethacin administered to 200 mg but did not find this to be superior to 100 mg of rectal indomethacin [60].

7.2 Intravenous Fluid

The cornerstone management of AP and PEP prophylaxis is IVF. The use of IVF potentially reduces the inflammation that may occur in the pancreas after the ERCP procedure. Lactuated Ringers solution is more effective than normal saline under specific circumstances. The superiority of LR is likely due to the immunomodulatory mechanisms of lactate, which provides anti-inflammatory effects, and the effect of lactate on acidosis in the context of AP [95]. In a recent NMA, the authors found aggressive hydration with LR or NS to be more effective when compared to placebo or standard volume hydration for PEP prophylaxis [60]. The RCTs investigated different IVF regimens that varred based on whether patients are admitted for observation following ERCP. One randomized controlled trial found that providing aggressive hydration for a

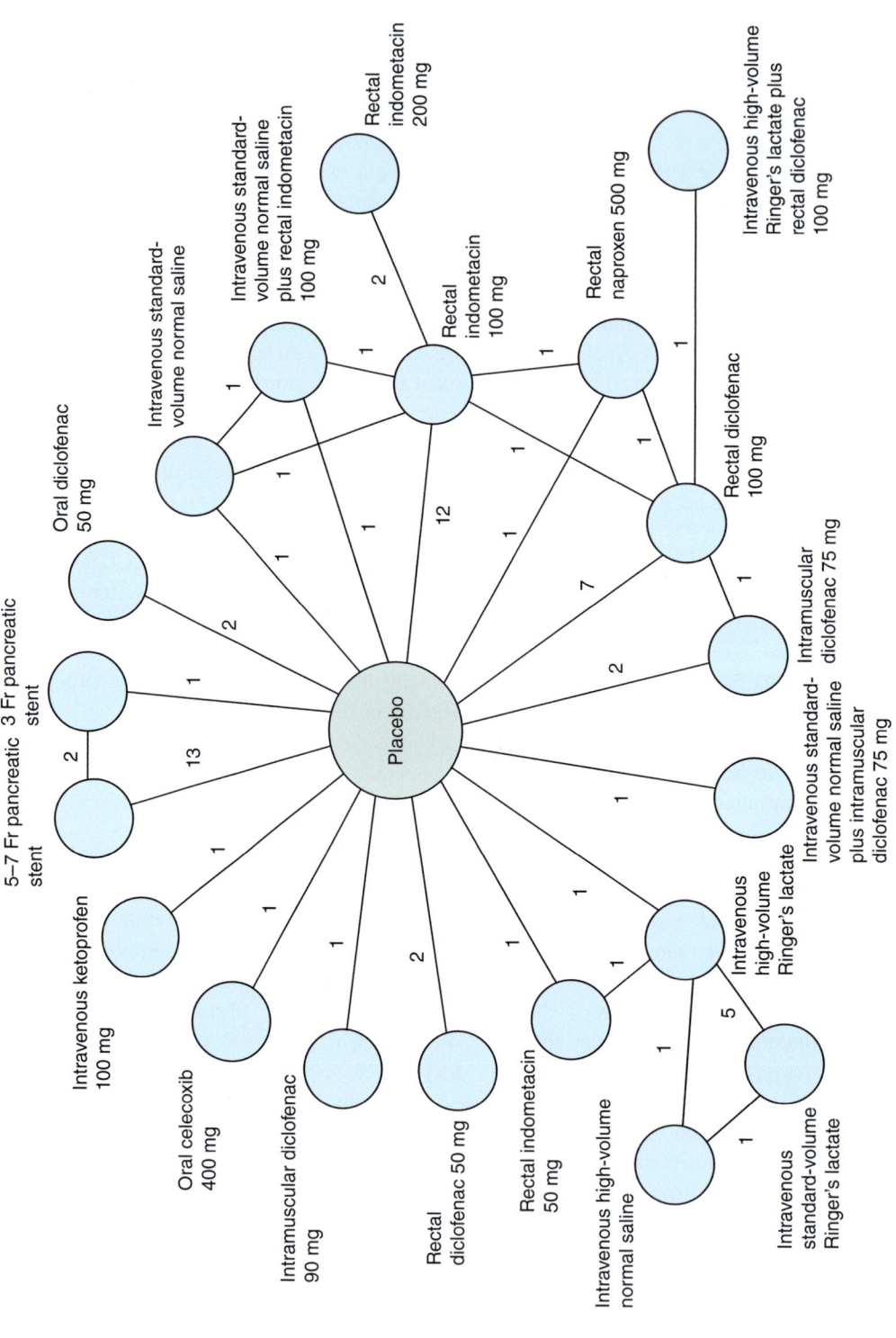

Fig. 4 Network of randomized controlled trials comparing NSAIDs, pancreatic stents, and intravenous fluids, or combinations of these. (Used with permission from Akshintala VS et al. [60])

duration of 8 h after ERCP did not show any significant advantage over moderate hydration [96]. Aggressively hydrating for an extended period of tim increases the fluid overload [97]. It is currently unclear what the best approach is for IVF treatment. However, it may be advisable to administer 2–3 L of LR fluid in the perioperative period for patients undergoing ERCP, with adjustments made for those with renal or cardiopulmonary comorbidities. Patients experiencing pain after undergoing ERCP procedure should be closely monitored for any signs of fluid overload while providing them with extra hydration. There is inconsistent evidence regarding the potential benefits of using a combination of IVF and NSAIDs together. The benefits of this combination are still unclear and requires further investigation [96]. It is plausible that combining IVF and rectal NSAIDs could lead to additional benefits due to their distinct mechanisms of action.

7.3 Pancreatic Duct Stent

The placement of a prophylactic PD stent is thought to enhance the flow from the pancreatic duct, thus preventing ductal hypertension in the presence of papillary edema and other factors associated with the development of PEP, as described earlier. RCTs and meta-analyses have repeatedly demonstrated the effectiveness of PD stents in preventing PEP, and also decreasing the severity of PEP [60, 98]. There are different types of PD stents, including different diameters, lengths, presence of internal flanges, and configuration (straight or single pigtail). Comparisons by NMAs have been of PD stents, and the results indicate that 5-Fr PD stents outperform 3-Fr PD stents [99]. The duration for which the PD stent is required to remain in place for PEP prophylaxis is uncertain, as is the length of the PD stent [99]. Some studies have reported lower PEP rates when the PD stent is placed in the body or tail of the pancreas, while other studies have found no significant difference in PEP rates among different lengths of PD stents used [87, 100]. Although PD stents can be effective, they come with a few downsides. These include the expenses and inconveniences associated with follow-up imaging and repeat endoscopy, which is necessary in 5–10% of the procedures, for stent removal [101, 102]. In addition, the placement of PD stents can be a complex procedure, and multiple attempts to insert the stent after cannulation of the PD can increase the risk of PEP [103]. If a guidewire has already entered the PD, particularly after multiple guidewire passes, placement of a PD stent is likely to be beneficial in preventing PEP. Pharmaco-prophylaxis offers several benefits compared to PD stents, as explained earlier. Additionally, when it comes to combination treatments, the network meta-analysis did not find any significant difference between using a 5–7 Fr PD stent and a combination of IVF and rectal NSAIDs [60]. It is necessary to conduct a prospective RCT to determine whether a combination of NSAIDs and IVF can replace PD stent. A large ongoing RCT is currently exploring this topic, and we are eagerly awaiting its results [104]. It is presently advised by societal guidelines to utilize PD stents for patients who are at a high risk of developing PEP [28, 77].

7.4 Pharmacological Prophylaxis

Numerous preventive measures for PEP have been investigated, and among them, more than 40 pharmacological prophylactic agents have been tested. However, only a few of these agents have consistently shown promising results [83]. Animal models in recent studies have found potential new mediators involved in the development of PEP such as calcium-dependent serine, threonine phosphatase calcineurin (Cn), and Cn inhibitors such as tacrolimus which are being considered for prophylaxis against PEP [10, 105].

7.5 Conclusion

Despite advancements in the understanding of its pathophysiology and the availability of prophylactic strategies, the incidence of PEP remains high. It is important to continue research to improve methods of PEP prophylaxis, particularly through pharmacological options. Additionally, efforts should be made to refine procedural techniques and enhance risk stratification approaches. It is recommended that a personalized prophylactic strategy be developed for each patient, taking into consideration their individual risk factors. The key strategies to prevent PEP is through careful patient selection, use of the appropriate ERCP techniques, and the recommended PEP prophylaxis.

Disclosure Statement The authors have no disclosures relevant to this publication.

References

1. Kochar B, Akshintala VS, Afghani E, et al. Incidence, severity, and mortality of post-ERCP pancreatitis: a systematic review by using randomized, controlled trials. Gastrointest Endosc. 2015;81:143–9.
2. Akshintala VS, Kanthasamy K, Bhullar FA, et al. Incidence, severity and mortality of post ERCP pancreatitis: an updated systematic review and meta-analysis of 145 randomized controlled trials. Gastrointest Endosc. 2023;98:1.
3. Dumonceau JM, Kapral C, Aabakken L, et al. ERCP-related adverse events: European Society of Gastrointestinal Endoscopy (ESGE) guideline. Endoscopy. 2020;52:127–49.
4. Cotton PB. Analysis of 59 ERCP lawsuits; mainly about indications. Gastrointest Endosc. 2006;63:378–82.
5. Mutneja HR, Vohra I, Go A, et al. Temporal trends and mortality of post-ERCP pancreatitis in the United States: a nationwide analysis. Endoscopy. 2020;53(4):357–66.
6. Freeman ML, Guda NM. Prevention of post-ERCP pancreatitis: a comprehensive review. Gastrointest Endosc. 2004;59:845–64.
7. Pezzilli R, Romboli E, Campana D, et al. Mechanisms involved in the onset of post-ERCP pancreatitis. JOP. 2002;3:162–8.
8. Akashi R, Kiyozumi T, Tanaka T, et al. Mechanism of pancreatitis caused by ERCP. Gastrointest Endosc. 2002;55:50–4.
9. Li C, Zhu Y, Shenoy M, et al. Anatomical and functional characterization of a duodeno-pancreatic neural reflex that can induce acute pancreatitis. Am J Physiol Gastrointest Liver Physiol. 2013;304:G490–500.
10. Wen L, Javed TA, Yimlamai D, et al. Transient high pressure in pancreatic ducts promotes inflammation

11. Rinderknecht H. Activation of pancreatic zymogens. Normal activation, premature intrapancreatic activation, protective mechanisms against inappropriate activation. Dig Dis Sci. 1986;31:314–21.
12. Paulsen FP, Bobka T, Tsokos M, et al. Functional anatomy of the papilla vateri: biomechanical aspects and impact of difficult endoscopic intubation. Surg Endosc. 2002;16:296–301.
13. Brown JO, Echenberg RJ. Mucosal reduplications associated with the ampullary portion of the major duodenal papilla in humans. Anat Rec. 1964;150:293–301.
14. Cheng CL, Sherman S, Watkins JL, et al. Risk factors for post-ERCP pancreatitis: a prospective multicenter study. Am J Gastroenterol. 2006;101:139–47.
15. Wang P, Li ZS, Liu F, et al. Risk factors for ERCP-related complications: a prospective multicenter study. Am J Gastroenterol. 2009;104:31–40.
16. Haraldsson E, Kylanpaa L, Gronroos J, et al. Macroscopic appearance of the major duodenal papilla influences bile duct cannulation: a prospective multicenter study by the Scandinavian Association for Digestive Endoscopy Study Group for ERCP. Gastrointest Endosc. 2019;90:957–63.
17. Mohamed R, Lethebe BC, Gonzalez-Moreno E, et al. Morphology of the major papilla predicts ERCP procedural outcomes and adverse events. Surg Endosc. 2021;35:6455–65.
18. Takenaka M, Yoshikawa T, Minaga K, et al. A novel teaching tool for visualizing the invisible bile duct axis in 3 dimensions during biliary cannulation (compact disc method). VideoGIE. 2020;5:389–94.
19. Mariani A, Di Leo M, Giardullo N, et al. Early pre-cut sphincterotomy for difficult biliary access to reduce post-ERCP pancreatitis: a randomized trial. Endoscopy. 2016;48:530–5.
20. Ohno T, Katori M, Nishiyama K, et al. Direct observation of microcirculation of the basal region of rat gastric mucosa. J Gastroenterol. 1995;30:557–64.
21. Igawa M, Miyaoka M, Saitoh T. Influence of topical epinephrine application on microcirculatory disturbance in subjects with ulcerative colitis evaluated by laser Doppler flowmetry and transmission electron microscopy. Dig Endosc. 2000;12:126–30.
22. Cotton PB, Lehman G, Vennes J, et al. Endoscopic sphincterotomy complications and their management: an attempt at consensus. Gastrointest Endosc. 1991;37:383–93.
23. Banks PA, Bollen TL, Dervenis C, et al. Classification of acute pancreatitis—2012: revision of the Atlanta classification and definitions by international consensus. Gut. 2013;62:102–11.
24. Smeets X, Bouhouch N, Buxbaum J, et al. The revised Atlanta criteria more accurately reflect severity of post-ERCP pancreatitis compared to the consensus criteria. United Eur Gastroenterol J. 2019;7:557–64.

25. Hameed AM, Lam VW, Pleass HC. Significant elevations of serum lipase not caused by pancreatitis: a systematic review. HPB (Oxford). 2015;17:99–112.

26. Prat F, Amaris J, Ducot B, et al. Nifedipine for prevention of post-ERCP pancreatitis: a prospective, double-blind randomized study. Gastrointest Endosc. 2002;56:202–8.

27. Shah R, Raphael KL, Mekaroonkamol P, et al. Non-pancreatitis-related abdominal pain following ERCP in patients with pancreas Divisum: 91. Am Coll Gastroenterol. 2017;112(S42):S44.

28. Buxbaum JL, Freeman M, Amateau SK, et al. American Society for Gastrointestinal Endoscopy guideline on post-ERCP pancreatitis prevention strategies: summary and recommendations. Gastrointest Endosc. 2023;97:153–62.

29. Coelho-Prabhu N, Shah ND, Van Houten H, et al. Endoscopic retrograde cholangiopancreatography: utilisation and outcomes in a 10-year population-based cohort. BMJ Open. 2013;3:3.

30. Kroner PT, Bilal M, Samuel R, et al. Use of ERCP in the United States over the past decade. Endosc Int Open. 2020;8:E761–9.

31. Moffatt DC, Yu BN, Yie W, et al. Trends in utilization of diagnostic and therapeutic ERCP and cholecystectomy over the past 25 years: a population-based study. Gastrointest Endosc. 2014;79:615–22.

32. Huang RJ, Thosani NC, Barakat MT, et al. Evolution in the utilization of biliary interventions in the United States: results of a nationwide longitudinal study from 1998 to 2013. Gastrointest Endosc. 2017;86:319–26.

33. Ahmed M, Kanotra R, Savani GT, et al. Utilization trends in inpatient endoscopic retrograde cholangiopancreatography (ERCP): a cross-sectional US experience. Endosc Int Open. 2017;5:E261–71.

34. Kakked G, Salameh H, Cheesman AR, et al. Primary EUS-guided biliary drainage versus ERCP drainage for the management of malignant biliary obstruction: a systematic review and meta-analysis. Endosc Ultrasound. 2020;9:298–307.

35. Logiudice FP, Bernardo WM, Galetti F, et al. Endoscopic ultrasound-guided vs endoscopic retrograde cholangiopancreatography biliary drainage for obstructed distal malignant biliary strictures: a systematic review and meta-analysis. World J Gastrointest Endosc. 2019;11:281–91.

36. Lakhtakia S, Chavan R, Ramchandani M, et al. EUS-guided rendezvous with a steerable access needle in choledocholithiasis. VideoGIE. 2020;5:359–61.

37. Cotton PB, Durkalski V, Romagnuolo J, et al. Effect of endoscopic sphincterotomy for suspected sphincter of Oddi dysfunction on pain-related disability following cholecystectomy: the EPISOD randomized clinical trial. JAMA. 2014;311:2101–9.

38. Smith ZL, Shah R, Elmunzer BJ, et al. The next EPISOD: trends in utilization of endoscopic sphincterotomy for sphincter of Oddi dysfunction from 2010 to 2019. Clin Gastroenterol Hepatol. 2022;20:e600–9.

39. Cote GA, Durkalski-Mauldin VL, Serrano J, et al. SpHincterotomy for acute recurrent pancreatitis randomized trial: rationale, methodology, and potential implications. Pancreas. 2019;48:1061–7.

40. Cote GA, Nitchie H, Elmunzer BJ, et al. Characteristics of patients undergoing endoscopic retrograde cholangiopancreatography for sphincter of Oddi disorders. Clin Gastroenterol Hepatol. 2022;20:e627–34.

41. Vandervoort J, Soetikno RM, Tham TC, et al. Risk factors for complications after performance of ERCP. Gastrointest Endosc. 2002;56:652–6.

42. Rabenstein T, Schneider HT, Bulling D, et al. Analysis of the risk factors associated with endoscopic sphincterotomy techniques: preliminary results of a prospective study, with emphasis on the reduced risk of acute pancreatitis with low-dose anticoagulation treatment. Endoscopy. 2000;32:10–9.

43. Christoforidis E, Goulimaris I, Kanellos I, et al. Post-ERCP pancreatitis and hyperamylasemia: patient-related and operative risk factors. Endoscopy. 2002;34:286–92.

44. Hookey LC, RioTinto R, Delhaye M, et al. Risk factors for pancreatitis after pancreatic sphincterotomy: a review of 572 cases. Endoscopy. 2006;38:670–6.

45. Boender J, Nix GA, de Ridder MA, et al. Endoscopic papillotomy for common bile duct stones: factors influencing the complication rate. Endoscopy. 1994;26:209–16.

46. Christensen M, Matzen P, Schulze S, et al. Complications of ERCP: a prospective study. Gastrointest Endosc. 2004;60:721–31.

47. Masci E, Toti G, Mariani A, et al. Complications of diagnostic and therapeutic ERCP: a prospective multicenter study. Am J Gastroenterol. 2001;96:417–23.

48. Freeman ML, DiSario JA, Nelson DB, et al. Risk factors for post-ERCP pancreatitis: a prospective, multicenter study. Gastrointest Endosc. 2001;54:425–34.

49. Freeman ML. Complications of endoscopic sphincterotomy. Endoscopy. 1998;30:A216–20.

50. Chen JJ, Wang XM, Liu XQ, et al. Risk factors for post-ERCP pancreatitis: a systematic review of clinical trials with a large sample size in the past 10 years. Eur J Med Res. 2014;19:26.

51. Ding X, Zhang F, Wang Y. Risk factors for post-ERCP pancreatitis: a systematic review and meta-analysis. Surgeon. 2015;13:218–29.

52. Natt N, Michael F, Michael H, et al. ERCP-related adverse events in primary sclerosing cholangitis: a systematic review and meta-analysis. Can J Gastroenterol Hepatol. 2022;2022:2372257.

53. Keswani RN, Duloy A, Nieto JM, et al. Interventions to improve the performance of ERCP and EUS quality indicators. Gastrointest Endosc. 2023;97:825.

54. Friedland S, Soetikno RM, Vandervoort J, et al. Bedside scoring system to predict the risk of developing pancreatitis following ERCP. Endoscopy. 2002;34:483–8.

55. Park CH, Park SW, Yang MJ, et al. Pre- and post-procedure risk prediction models for post-

endoscopic retrograde cholangiopancreatography pancreatitis. Surg Endosc. 2021;36(3):2052–61.

56. Chiba M, Kato M, Kinoshita Y, et al. The milestone for preventing post-ERCP pancreatitis using novel simplified predictive scoring system: a propensity score analysis. Surg Endosc. 2020;35(12):6696–707.

57. Rodrigues-Pinto E, Morais R, Sousa-Pinto B, et al. Development of an online app to predict post-endoscopic retrograde cholangiopancreatography adverse events using a single-center retrospective cohort. Dig Dis. 2021;39:283–93.

58. Kamal A, Akshintala VS, Elmunzer BJ, Lehman GA, Andriulli A, Talukdar R, Goenka MK, Kochhar R, Faghih M, Kumbhari V, Ngamruengphong S, Khashab MA, Kalloo AN, Duvvur NR, Singh V. Development and validation of a risk stratification score for post-endoscopic retrograde cholangiopancreatography (ERCP) pancreatitis. Gastrointest Endosc. 2018;87(6):AB573.

59. Rex DK, Schoenfeld PS, Cohen J, et al. Quality indicators for colonoscopy. Gastrointest Endosc. 2015;81:31–53.

60. Akshintala VS, Sperna Weiland CJ, Bhullar FA, et al. Non-steroidal anti-inflammatory drugs, intravenous fluids, pancreatic stents, or their combinations for the prevention of post-endoscopic retrograde cholangiopancreatography pancreatitis: a systematic review and network meta-analysis. Lancet Gastroenterol Hepatol. 2021;6(9):733–42.

61. Akshintala VS, Kuo A, Kamal A, et al. Development, validation of a post-ERCP pancreatitis risk calculator and machine learning based decision making tool for prophylaxis selection. Gastroenterology. 2019;156:S-116.

62. McKee K, Singh VK, Akshintala VS. Rectal nonsteroidal anti-inflammatory drugs for post-endoscopic retrograde cholangiopancreatography pancreatitis prophylaxis: a case study in a price-escalation era. Gastroenterology. 2022;163:543–6.

63. Goyal H, Sachdeva S, Sherazi SAA, et al. Early prediction of post-ERCP pancreatitis by post-procedure amylase and lipase levels: a systematic review and meta-analysis. Endosc Int Open. 2022;10:E952–70.

64. Concepcion-Martin M, Gomez-Oliva C, Juanes A, et al. IL-6, IL-10 and TNFalpha do not improve early detection of post-endoscopic retrograde cholangiopancreatography acute pancreatitis: a prospective cohort study. Sci Rep. 2016;6:33492.

65. Wani S, Hall M, Wang AY, et al. Variation in learning curves and competence for ERCP among advanced endoscopy trainees by using cumulative sum analysis. Gastrointest Endosc. 2016;83:711–9.

66. Adler DG, Lieb JG 2nd, Cohen J, et al. Quality indicators for ERCP. Gastrointest Endosc. 2015;81:54–66.

67. Shao H, Fonseca V, Furman R, et al. Impact of quality improvement (QI) program on 5-year risk of diabetes-related complications: a simulation study. Diabetes Care. 2020;43:2847–52.

68. Cote GA, Elmunzer BJ, Forster E, et al. Development of an automated ERCP quality report Card using structured data fields. Tech Innov Gastrointest Endosc. 2021;23:129–38.

69. Singh A, Brenner TA, Bujnak B, et al. Development of an automated real-time ERCP quality report CARD. Gastrointest Endosc. 2022;95:AB100–1.

70. Elmunzer BJ. Reducing the risk of post-endoscopic retrograde cholangiopancreatography pancreatitis. Dig Endosc. 2017;29:749–57.

71. Canena J, Lopes L, Fernandes J, et al. Efficacy and safety of primary, early and late needle-knife fistulotomy for biliary access. Sci Rep. 2021;11:16658.

72. Verma D, Kapadia A, Adler DG. Pure versus mixed electrosurgical current for endoscopic biliary sphincterotomy: a meta-analysis of adverse outcomes. Gastrointest Endosc. 2007;66:283–90.

73. Ogura T, Imoto A, Okuda A, et al. Can iodixanol prevent post-endoscopic retrograde cholangiopancreatography pancreatitis? A prospective, randomized, controlled trial. Dig Dis. 2019;37:255–61.

74. Tse F, Liu J, Yuan Y, et al. Guidewire-assisted cannulation of the common bile duct for the prevention of post-endoscopic retrograde cholangiopancreatography (ERCP) pancreatitis. Cochrane Database Syst Rev. 2022;2022:CD009662.

75. Freeman ML, Overby C, Qi D. Pancreatic stent insertion: consequences of failure and results of a modified technique to maximize success. Gastrointest Endosc. 2004;59:8–14.

76. Kamal A, Akshintala VS, Talukdar R, et al. A randomized trial of topical epinephrine and rectal indomethacin for preventing post-endoscopic retrograde cholangiopancreatography pancreatitis in high-risk patients. Am J Gastroenterol. 2019;114:339–47.

77. Dumonceau JM, Andriulli A, Elmunzer BJ, et al. Prophylaxis of post-ERCP pancreatitis: European Society of Gastrointestinal Endoscopy (ESGE) guideline—updated June 2014. Endoscopy. 2014;46:799–815.

78. Ito K, Fujita N, Noda Y, et al. Can pancreatic duct stenting prevent post-ERCP pancreatitis in patients who undergo pancreatic duct guidewire placement for achieving selective biliary cannulation? A prospective randomized controlled trial. J Gastroenterol. 2010;45:1183–91.

79. Draganov PV, Evans W, Fazel A, et al. Large size balloon dilation of the ampulla after biliary sphincterotomy can facilitate endoscopic extraction of difficult bile duct stones. J Clin Gastroenterol. 2009;43:782–6.

80. Attasaranya S, Cheon YK, Vittal H, et al. Large-diameter biliary orifice balloon dilation to aid in endoscopic bile duct stone removal: a multicenter series. Gastrointest Endosc. 2008;67:1046–52.

81. ASGE Standards of Practice Committee, Buxbaum JL, Abbas Fehmi SM, et al. ASGE guideline on the role of endoscopy in the evaluation and management of choledocholithiasis. Gastrointest Endosc. 2019;89:1075–105.

82. Manes G, Paspatis G, Aabakken L, et al. Endoscopic management of common bile duct stones: European

Society of Gastrointestinal Endoscopy (ESGE) guideline. Endoscopy. 2019;51:472–91.

83. Akshintala VS, Hutfless SM, Colantuoni E, et al. Systematic review with network meta-analysis: pharmacological prophylaxis against post-ERCP pancreatitis. Aliment Pharmacol Ther. 2013;38:1325–37.

84. Serrano JPR, de Moura DTH, Bernardo WM, et al. Nonsteroidal anti-inflammatory drugs versus placebo for post-endoscopic retrograde cholangiopancreatography pancreatitis: a systematic review and meta-analysis. Endosc Int Open. 2019;7:E477–86.

85. Choi JH, Kim HJ, Lee BU, et al. Vigorous periprocedural hydration with lactated Ringer's solution reduces the risk of pancreatitis after retrograde cholangiopancreatography in hospitalized patients. Clin Gastroenterol Hepatol. 2017;15:86–92.

86. Park CH, Paik WH, Park ET, et al. Aggressive intravenous hydration with lactated Ringer's solution for prevention of post-ERCP pancreatitis: a prospective randomized multicenter clinical trial. Endoscopy. 2018;50:378–85.

87. Phillip V, Pukitis A, Epstein A, et al. Pancreatic stenting to prevent post-ERCP pancreatitis: a randomized multicenter trial. Endosc Int Open. 2019;7:E860–8.

88. Ethridge RT, Chung DH, Slogoff M, et al. Cyclooxygenase-2 gene disruption attenuates the severity of acute pancreatitis and pancreatitis-associated lung injury. Gastroenterology. 2002;123:1311–22.

89. Bruno A, Tacconelli S, Patrignani P. Variability in the response to non-steroidal anti-inflammatory drugs: mechanisms and perspectives. Basic Clin Pharmacol Toxicol. 2014;114:56–63.

90. Willis JV, Kendall MJ, Flinn RM, et al. The pharmacokinetics of diclofenac sodium following intravenous and oral administration. Eur J Clin Pharmacol. 1979;16:405–10.

91. Jensen KM, Grenabo L. Bioavailability of indomethacin after intramuscular injection and rectal administration of solution and suppositories. Acta Pharmacol Toxicol (Copenh). 1985;57:322–7.

92. Elmunzer BJ, Scheiman JM, Lehman GA, et al. A randomized trial of rectal indomethacin to prevent post-ERCP pancreatitis. N Engl J Med. 2012;366:1414–22.

93. Avila P, Holmes I, Kouanda A, et al. Practice patterns of post-ERCP pancreatitis prophylaxis techniques in the United States: a survey of advanced endoscopists. Gastrointest Endosc. 2020;91:568–73.

94. Thiruvengadam NR, Saumoy M, Schneider Y, et al. A cost-effectiveness analysis for post-endoscopic retrograde cholangiopancreatography pancreatitis prophylaxis in the United States. Clin Gastroenterol Hepatol. 2022;20:216–26.

95. de-Madaria E, Herrera-Marante I, Gonzalez-Camacho V, et al. Fluid resuscitation with lactated Ringer's solution vs normal saline in acute pancreatitis: a triple-blind, randomized, controlled trial. United Eur Gastroenterol J. 2018;6:63–72.

96. Sperna Weiland CJ, Smeets X, Kievit W, et al. Aggressive fluid hydration plus non-steroidal anti-inflammatory drugs versus non-steroidal anti-inflammatory drugs alone for post-endoscopic retrograde cholangiopancreatography pancreatitis (FLUYT): a multicentre, open-label, randomised, controlled trial. Lancet Gastroenterol Hepatol. 2021;6:350–8.

97. de-Madaria E, Buxbaum JL, Maisonneuve P, et al. Aggressive or moderate fluid resuscitation in acute pancreatitis. N Engl J Med. 2022;387:989–1000.

98. Mazaki T, Mado K, Masuda H, et al. Prophylactic pancreatic stent placement and post-ERCP pancreatitis: an updated meta-analysis. J Gastroenterol. 2013;49:343.

99. Afghani E, Akshintala VS, Khashab MA, et al. 5-Fr vs. 3-Fr pancreatic stents for the prevention of post-ERCP pancreatitis in high-risk patients: a systematic review and network meta-analysis. Endoscopy. 2014;46:573–80.

100. Sugimoto M, Takagi T, Suzuki R, et al. Pancreatic stents for the prevention of post-endoscopic retrograde cholangiopancreatography pancreatitis should be inserted up to the pancreatic body or tail. World J Gastroenterol. 2018;24:2392–9.

101. Brackbill S, Young S, Schoenfeld P, et al. A survey of physician practices on prophylactic pancreatic stents. Gastrointest Endosc. 2006;64:45–52.

102. Chahal P, Baron TH, Petersen BT, et al. Pancreatic stent prophylaxis of post endoscopic retrograde cholangiopancreatography pancreatitis: spontaneous migration rates and clinical outcomes. Minerva Gastroenterol Dietol. 2007;53:225–30.

103. Choksi NS, Fogel EL, Cote GA, et al. The risk of post-ERCP pancreatitis and the protective effect of rectal indomethacin in cases of attempted but unsuccessful prophylactic pancreatic stent placement. Gastrointest Endosc. 2015;81:150–5.

104. Elmunzer BJ, Serrano J, Chak A, et al. Rectal indomethacin alone versus indomethacin and prophylactic pancreatic stent placement for preventing pancreatitis after ERCP: study protocol for a randomized controlled trial. Trials. 2016;17:120.

105. Akshintala VS, Husain SZ, Brenner TA, et al. Rectal INdomethacin, oral TacROlimus, or their combination for the prevention of post-ERCP pancreatitis (INTRO trial): protocol for a randomized, controlled, double-blinded trial. Pancreatology. 2022;22:887–93.

Diagnosis and Severity of Acute Pancreatitis

Enrique de-Madaria and Gabriele Capurso

Key Points

1. Diagnosis of acute pancreatitis is based on acute-onset upper abdominal pain associated with increased (> 3 × the upper level of normal) serum amylase or lipase activity.
2. Patients with atypical signs or symptoms, delayed presentation, or nondiagnostic enzyme levels require a CT scan for differential diagnosis.
3. Prediction of acute pancreatitis severity helps with clinical decisions relating to triage, transfer, treatment, and trials.
4. Current clinical, radiological, and biochemical factors only have moderate accuracy in predicting severity.
5. The classification of severity is useful for categorizing patient groups with similar outcomes.

E. de-Madaria (✉)
Gastroenterology Department, Dr. Balmis General University Hospital, Alicante Institute for Health and Biomedical Research (ISABIAL), Miguel Hernandez University, Alicante, Spain

G. Capurso
Pancreato-Biliary Endoscopy and Endosonography Division, Pancreas Translational and Clinical Research Center, San Raffaele Scientific Institute IRCCS, Vita-Salute San Raffaele University, Milan, Italy

1 Introduction

The most frequent presentation of acute pancreatitis (AP) is acute-onset upper abdominal pain, so intense that most patients seek urgent medical attention early in the course of the disease. Abdominal pain is almost universal, but it may not be apparent due to special circumstances like sedation (e.g., AP in the postoperative period), dementia, or immunosuppression. An increase in pancreatic enzyme serum activity is very frequent in AP, and a key diagnostic criterion, but it is not a perfect test, since some patients have normal levels (lowering sensitivity) and many diseases can be associated with an elevated serum pancreatic enzyme activity (lowering specificity) [1]. Overall, patients with AP have variable outcomes, with most patients having a mild course of the disease, while others develop complications or fulminant disease. Local and systemic complications develop in one-third of patients with more severe disease, and have an increased risk of death [2].

In considering the severity of acute pancreatitis, it is important to distinguish two concepts: prediction and classification. The *prediction of severity* is about identifying patients with a higher risk of developing severe disease. This amounts to a probability of a future event, as the patient may or may not develop severe disease. This is useful for clinical decisions about triage, transfer, treatment, and trial allocation. The *classification of severity* is about the actual severity of AP

© The Author(s), under exclusive license to Springer Nature Singapore Pte Ltd. 2024
J. A. Windsor et al. (eds.), *Acute Pancreatitis*, https://doi.org/10.1007/978-981-97-3132-9_8

at that time and is not a probability. It is useful in monitoring patients, communicating, and clinical audit. In this chapter, we will review the diagnosis, prediction of severity, and classification of severity of AP.

2　Diagnosis of Acute Pancreatitis

2.1　Clinical Factors

Pain is typically acute onset, severe, and belt-like, across the upper abdomen, and it often radiates to the mid-back. Nausea and vomiting are very frequent at presentation. Patients with choledocholithiasis may have jaundice. A low-grade fever is frequent, but high-grade fever with rigors suggests concomitant acute cholangitis in gallstone-associated acute pancreatitis. Some patients may develop paralytic ileus, often related to retroperitoneal and abdominal inflammation. The most important symptoms of AP can be measured with a validated patient-reported outcome measure, the PAN-PROMISE scale [3] (Table 1).

Skin signs are infrequent, but clinicians must recognize them, as they are associated with more severe disease. The infiltration of subcutaneous fat tissue by necro-hemorrhagic exudate that tracks from the peripancreatic retroperitoneum inducing ecchymoses of the skin at the periumbilical region (Cullen's sign), flanks (Grey Turner's sign), inguinal ligament (Fox's sign), or scrotum (Bryant's sign) (Fig. 1). Some patients can develop painful focal lesions, more like a cellulitis than ecchymoses. Subcutaneous nodules due to lipase digestion of subcutaneous fat are called pancreatic panniculitis (Fig. 2) but are very rare. Some patients with moderately severe to severe disease may experience psychiatric symptoms: the so-called pancreatic encephalopathy. Purtscher retinopathy is a very rare complication of pancreatitis associated with painless diminished visual acuity.

2.2　Laboratory Factors

Most (but not all) patients with AP have an increase in amylase and lipase serum activity, to at least three times the upper limit of normal. The peak of serum amylase activity is at 12–72 h and normalizes approximately on the fifth day. Lipase peaks within 4–8 h and remains high longer, up to 8–14 days, so patients presenting after several days of abdominal pain may have normal amylase activity but increased lipase levels [1]. Besides this, there is no clear advantage in using lipase over amylase in the diagnosis of AP [4]. There are other useful laboratory tests like urinary trypsinogen-2 and urinary amylase, but they are not widely used and, again, do not have advantages over serum amylase and lipase [4]. Patients with hypertriglyceridemia may present with falsely normal serum enzymes due to the interference of the triglycerides with the measurement. In this case, serum can be diluted and the enzymes measured again.

Table 1 PAN-PROMISE symptom scale (patient-reported outcome measurement)

PAN-PROMISE symptom scale	Score (0–10)
Pain, especially in the abdomen, chest, or back	
Abdominal distention (bloating, sensation of excess gas)	
Difficulty eating, sensation of food being stuck in the stomach	
Difficulty with bowel movements (constipation or straining on bowel movements)	
Nausea and/or vomiting	
Thirst	
Weakness, lack of energy, fatigue, difficulty moving	
Total score	

Each item is scored from 0 to 10 (worst score in the last 24 h; 0, none; 10, the highest possible intensity. de-Madaria et al., Gut 2021

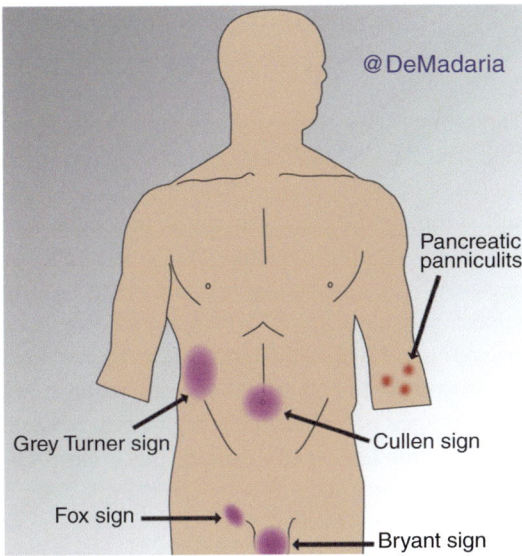

Fig. 1 Classic cutaneous signs in acute pancreatitis. [Courtesy of Dr. Enrique de-Madaria]

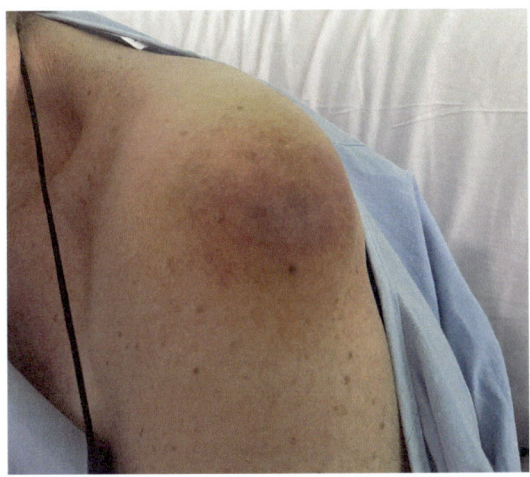

Fig. 2 Pancreatic panniculitis. [Patient with biopsy-confirmed pancreatic panniculitis, courtesy of Dr. Enrique de-Madaria]

2.3 Imaging Factors

CT scanning is a useful imaging technique to confirm AP in patients with atypical signs or symptoms with diagnostic uncertainty, or with delayed presentation and nondiagnostic pancreatic enzyme levels. A CT scan performed in the first 2–3 days may not detect local complications like pancreatic or peripancreatic fat necrosis, so early scans are encouraged only for differential diagnosis, and not to predict severity or to diagnose local complications. Intravenous contrast should be avoided in the presence of azotemia/renal failure, as peripancreatic fat stranding, indicative of AP, is easily detected without contrast, although its absence does not rule out AP. Abdominal ultrasonography can be used to diagnose gallstones, acute cholecystitis or other biliary complication, but its accuracy in diagnosing AP is operator-dependent and hindered by overlying bowel gas. MRI is useful to diagnose pancreatitis, but it is mainly used to investigate the biliary tract, as it is more expensive and a proportion of patients do not tolerate it or have difficulty with breath holding (particularly older patients). An MR and ultrasound scans are useful in determining the extent of solid necrosum within a local collection, which is not possible with a CT scan.

A CT scan is key diagnosing local complications when a patient has predicted severe AP and shows evidence of deterioration by symptoms, signs, or laboratory abnormalities. In general, local complications should be diagnosed by CT scan at least after 3–4 days after disease onset, since necrosis can continue to evolve and demarcate.

2.4 Diagnostic Criteria and Differential Diagnosis

The most widely accepted way to diagnose of AP involves the presence of at least two of these three criteria [5]:

1. Typical abdominal pain
2. Increased blood levels of pancreatic enzymes (at least three times greater than the upper limit of normality)
3. Imaging compatible with AP (CT scan, MRI, or ultrasonography)

In typical cases, the first two criteria are enough to diagnose AP. Importantly, any cause of acute abdomen can be associated with abdominal pain plus an increase in amylase and/or lipase blood level, e.g., acute cholangitis, cholecystitis, gastrointestinal tract perforation, acute mesenteric ischemia, acute gynecologic problems, or inflammation of the small or large bowel. Diabetic ketoacidosis and complicated abdominal aortic aneurysm can also induce pain and increase pancreatic enzymes. These problems are associated with atypical symptoms and signs (peritonism, Murphy's sign, diarrhea, atypical pain for AP, etc.) that should trigger the performance of a CT scan.

3 Predicting the Severity of Acute Pancreatitis

One of the most important issues when caring for patients with AP is the prediction of severity, but this remains a challenge. It is important because it helps in triaging a patient and making early decisions about whether a patient with predicted severe AP needs to be transferred (e.g., to a tertiary center or into an intensive care unit) or whether the patient requires further investigation (e.g., CT scan) or specific treatment (e.g., antibiotics, ERCP, or drainage). On the other hand, early and accurate prediction of mild AP allows for early discharge and reduced costs.

As most AP patients will ultimately experience a mild disease course, in an individual patient, the pretest probability of severe AP is usually not higher than 20%. The purpose of prediction is to generate a post-test probability that is as high as possible, in the order of 85% or more.

Many different approaches have been developed to improve the accuracy of predicting severity of acute pancreatitis including:

- Clinical features (comorbidities, symptoms, and signs)
- Laboratory tests
- Scoring systems from combining laboratory tests and clinical features

3.1 Clinical Features to Predict Severity

The clinical assessment of an experienced clinician can be helpful, but sensitivity has been shown to be no more than 50% [6]. Clinical signs and symptoms are not usually incorporated into prediction scoring systems. While it would be reasonable to suggest that age and comorbidities impact the severity of AP, this has not been proven. In a large multicenter study, age was not associated with persistent organ failure, but patients aged >85 years had a higher risk of death [7]. This study also demonstrated that comorbidities and obesity were not independently associated with the severity of AP.

Data on body weight are controversial, as a recent meta-analysis reported that BMI >25 is associated with severe AP and BMI >30 with mortality [8]. In another large multicenter prospective cohort study, pre-existing diabetes was not a risk factor for severe AP [9].

Another interesting issue is the impact of the etiology of AP on its severity. Acute biliary pancreatitis has been reported to present a more severe course compared with alcoholic AP and post-ERCP AP [10]. On the other hand, patients with hypertriglyceridemia (HTG) AP tend to present with a more pronounced inflammatory response, and the levels of serum triglyceride are correlated with severe disease [11].

3.2 Scoring Systems to Predict Severity

The characteristics of most scoring systems in current use are summarized in Table 2. These include some that were specifically developed for AP, such as *Ranson score* and the *Bedside Index for Severity in Acute Pancreatitis* (BISAP). There are others that are not specific for AP such as the *Acute Physiology and Chronic Health Examination* (APACHE) II and the *Systemic Inflammatory Response Syndrome* (SIRS) [12]. These and other scoring systems that use combi-

Table 2 Features of the most employed clinical score systems to predict the severity of acute pancreatitis

Score	Year	Specific for AP	Parameters	User-friendly	Clinical use	Pros	Cons
Ranson	1974	Yes	At admission: Age (_55 years), WBC (_16,000/mL), glucose (_200 mg/dL), LDH (_350 IU/mL), AST (_250 IU/mL) At 48 h: Hematocrit (decrease _10%), BUN (increase _5 mg/dL), calcium (_8 mg/dL), PaO$_2$ (_60 mmHg), base deficit (_4 mEq/L), fluid sequestration (_6 L)	No	To predict a severe disease course	Good specificity	Low sensitivity
Glasgow	1984	Yes	At admission and at 48 h Age (_55 years), WBC (_15,000/mL), glucose (_180 mg/dL), BUN (_45 mg/dL), PaO$_2$ (_60 mmHg), calcium (_8 g/dL), albumin (_3.2 g/dL), LDH (_600 IU/L)	No	To predict a severe disease course	Good specificity	Low sensitivity
Apache II	1989	No	At admission and at 48 h Temperature, MAP, heart rate, respiratory rate, PaO$_2$, arterial pH, HCO$_3$, sodium, potassium, creatinine, hematocrit, WBC, Glasgow Coma Scale score, age, chronic health points	No	To predict a severe disease course	Good sensitivity	Low specificity
SIRS	2006	No	At admission and at 48 h Temperature (_36 °C or _38 °C), heart rate (_90/min), respiratory rate (_20/min or PaCO$_2$ _32 mmHg), WBC (_4000/mm^3, _12,000/mm^3, or _10% bands)	Yes	To predict a severe disease course	Simple	Low accuracy
BISAP	2008	Yes	At admission and at 48 h BUN (_25 mg/dL), impaired mental status (Glasgow coma score _15), SIRS (_2), age (_60 years), pleural effusion	Yes	To predict a severe disease course	Simple	Low sensitivity
HAPS	2009	Yes	At admission and at 48 h Abdominal tenderness, hematocrit (_43 mg/dL for men or _39.6 mg/dL for women), creatinine (_2 mg/dL)	Yes	To predict a non-severe disease course	Simple	Not useful to predict severe course
PASS		Yes	During disease course (to be repeated) Organ failure, SIRS, abdominal pain, need of opiates, and ability to tolerate oral diet	Yes	To measure trajectories during disease course	Can be measured during event or used to predict posthospital outcomes	Low accuracy for early prediction of severe course

nations of physiologic, laboratory, and radiographic parameters have been developed and validated, but they all show only moderate accuracy and positive predictive value.

Another approach is to predict mild AP (rather than severe AP) to allow de-escalation of care and early discharge. The *Harmless Acute Pancreatitis Score* (HAPS) is a validated and readily available score that only requires the absence of abdominal tenderness or rebound, normal hematocrit, and normal creatinine level to be scored as positive. The score has a high positive predictive value of 97% to identify patients with harmless acute pancreatitis defined as the absence of pancreatic necrosis, no need for artificial ventilation or dialysis, and no mortality. When the HAPS is positive, the post-test probability of a non-severe course of 86% increases to 97%. However, the test is not accurate if used in different contexts or to predict a severe course [13].

Another different approach is not to predict a rare outcome, such as persistent organ failure or mortality, but rather to monitor the dynamic evolution of AP during its course. To this end the *Pancreatitis Activity Scoring System* (PASS) was developed and takes into consideration organ failure, SIRS, abdominal pain, the need of opiates, and ability to tolerate oral diet [14]. PASS is useful in tracking the clinical trajectories of an AP episode, anticipating deterioration, and identifying the risk of complication and need for rehospitalization. But as with other scores, PASS is not accurate for the early prediction of severe AP, especially when scored at a single timepoint.

One of the limitations of scoring systems is that they were developed and validated in groups of patients, but the clinician needs to make a prediction in the individual patient they are caring for. There are several ways that sensitivity and specificity can be combined into a single score. The most commonly used method is the receiver operator characteristic curve which plots sensitivity against 1-specificity, and the performance of the scoring system is expressed as a unitless

"area under the curve." While this helps in comparing the performance of different scoring systems in groups of patients, it has little clinical relevance for the individual patient. A better approach is to derive a post-test probability for the individual patient by (1) knowing the pretest probability for the patient's population, (2) calculating the positive and negative likelihood ratios, and (3) using a nomogram to read the post-test probability (or severe or not severe AP) for that patient [15]. The probability of severe AP is a clinically meaningful outcome for prediction in the individual patient. But these approaches do not overcome limitations with the laboratory tests and scoring systems themselves, but rather provide a more useful outcome for clinical decision-making.

3.3 New Tools to Predict Severity

As mentioned, most of the approaches to prediction of severity have an acceptable negative predictive value but usually a lower positive predictive value. For this reason many alternative approaches have been explored including radiological imaging with a canonical methodology or with the use of artificial intelligence.

The approach to radiological imaging for prediction has been most often based on the use of computed tomography (CT) to derive a Balthazar score that combines inflammatory signs and peripancreatic liquid collections with the extent of glandular necrosis in a total 10-point severity scale [16]. CT scans can provide much additional information, which has been used more recently to develop alternative scores to predict severity in an elegant manner. Sternby et al. investigated the relevance of adipose and muscle tissue parameters and demonstrated that a low muscle attenuation level at the first CT scan is associated with severe AP [17]. Gupta et al. employed seven variables (pancreatic necrosis, number of collections, size of collections, ascites, pleural effusion, celiac artery involvement, and liver steatosis) to develop a nomogram-based index that has reasonable accuracy [18]. The most obvious limitation of radiological approaches to prediction is that a CT scan is not required on admission in the majority of patients and would expose patients to unnecessary radiation and cost. Further, the performance of radiology-based scoring has not been shown to be superior to other scoring system.

The development of severe AP is associated with a transition from SIRS to organ failure, the development of a capillary leak syndrome leading to third space fluid loss [19]. This phenomenon has been investigated by examining the trajectories of biomarkers which suggest that the initial pro-inflammatory cytokine storm causes an increase in epithelial permeability leading to a loss of plasma oncotic pressure, tissue edema, and eventually organ failure. Interleukin-6 and other cytokines have been shown to be a strong predictor of severe AP, but these are not generally available for routine clinical use.

As multiple factors interact in complex ways to determine risk of developing severe AP, there has been a move to develop algorithms that improve the accuracy of predicting severe AP. The first study to use artificial neural networks and to show the superiority of this approach to the Glasgow and APACHE II scores was published by Mofidi et al. [20]. Artificial intelligence and machine learning platforms will become increasingly important for the integration of complex data to continue improving the accuracy of severity prediction [21]. More recently, a sophisticated methodology combined machine learning models to examine the data from a large cohort of over 1100 AP patients. They derived an approach with an accuracy of 89% using simple variables such as the respiratory rate, body temperature, abdominal rebound tenderness, gender, age, and glucose levels. The authors also created a web application ("EASY") for wider application [22]. Using artificial intelligence to improve the accuracy of prediction will become a more common, if not standard, approach, for rapid, early, and accurate prediction of AP severity and outcomes, which will outperform scoring systems in current use.

4 Classifying the Severity of Acute Pancreatitis

Severity classifications are useful to describe patients with similar patterns of the clinical course of AP, for research purposes, to compare patients from different centers, and for recording the severity of an episode of AP in the clinical record. Definitive severity classification is usually performed at discharge once complications have been diagnosed or ruled out, and the maximum severity during the episode is applied.

The Atlanta Classification [23], widely adopted after its publication in 1993, described two severity categories, mild (absence of complications) and severe (presence of complications: pancreatic necrosis, abscess, pseudocyst, or organ failure). The Atlanta Classification provided clear definitions for those complications, including organ failure (although it was not based on a validated organ failure scale). It soon became clear that patients classified as having severe disease were in fact heterogeneous, so more categories of severity were needed [24]. In particular, patients with an increased risk of death were not specifically recognized in the 1993 Atlanta Classification. Many articles were published, describing the determinants of the disease course. Local complications (acute peripancreatic fluid collections, necrosis of the pancreatic gland, and/or peripancreatic fat) were linked to morbidity and organ failure to increased risk of mortality. Then, different types of organ failure were recognized. Observational studies showed that transient (lasting less than 48 h) or single organ failure had a lower risk of mortality, but persistent (lasting more than 48 h) or multiple organ failure had up to 50% risk of mortality. Furthermore, it was described that persistent organ failure associated with infection of pancreatic and/or peripancreatic fat necrosis had the highest risk of death [25]. Two new severity classifications were published in 2012 (Determinant-Based Classification, DBC) and 2013 (Revised Atlanta Classification, RAC) [5, 26]. Both used validated scales to define organ failure, SOFA, and Marshall classification, respectively. The

DBC classifies patients into four categories with increasing severity (mild, moderate, severe, and critical) according to the presence of pancreatic and/or peripancreatic fat necrosis, if the necrosis is infected, and the presence and type (transient or persistent) of organ failure (Table 3). The RAC grades patients into three groups, mild, moderately severe, and severe, based on the presence of local complications (acute peripancreatic fluid collections, pancreatic and/or peripancreatic fat necrosis), exacerbation of previous comorbidity, and presence and type (transient or persistent) of organ failure (Table 3). In both classifications, the mild category is associated with excellent outcome, the moderate category is associated with increased morbidity but negligible mortality, the severe category is associated with a high risk of mortality and maximum morbidity, and the critical category in DBC is associated with even higher risk of mortality. In Table 4 hospital stay (as a measure of morbidity) and mortality are shown for the three classifications, based on a multicenter prospective nationwide validation study [2]. As shown in that study, severity classifications are useful in categorizing different groups of patients with similar outcomes. More recently a modified DBC has been published from a multicenter intensive care study, and it

Table 3 Classifications of severity

Definitions of severity: Atlanta Classification, Revised Atlanta Classification, and Determinant-Based Classification				
Classification	Mild	Moderate/moderately severe	Severe	Critical
Atlanta classification	No OF and no local complications	N/A	OF and/or local complications (necrosis, abscess, and/or pseudocyst)	N/A
Revised Atlanta classification	No OF, no local nor systemic complications	OF that resolves within 48 h (transient OF) and/or local or systemic complications without persistent OF	Persistent OF (>48 h)	N/A
Determinant-based classification	No (peri)pancreatic necrosis and no OF	Sterile (peri)pancreatic necrosis and/or transient (<48 h) OF	IPN or persistent (≥48 h) OF	IPN and persistent (≥48 h) OF

OF organ failure, *N/A* not applicable, *(Peri)pancreatic necrosis* necrosis of the pancreas and/or peripancreatic tissue, *IPN* infected (peri)pancreatic necrosis

Table 4 Outcomes according to the different severity classifications according to a multicenter prospective study (Sternby et al., Annals of Surgery 2019)

Classification	Severity category	Hospital stay median (IQR) days	Mortality n (%)
Atlanta	Mild $n = 1175$	6.2 (4.1–8.7)	1 (0.1%)
	Severe $n = 480$	13.8 (7.9–25.5)	69 (14.4%)
	p	<0.001	<0.001
Revision of Atlanta	Mild $n = 1076$	5.9 (4–8.2)	1 (0.1%)
	Moderately severe $n = 466$	11.4 (7.4–18.3)	10 (2.1%)
	Severe $n = 113$	39.1 (16.4–69.9)	59 (52.2%)
	p	<0.001	<0.001
Determinant-based	Mild $n = 1247$	6.3 (4.2–9.1)	1 (0.1%)
	Moderate $n = 274$	12.9 (7.6–19.2)	11 (4%)
	Severe $n = 97$	34.3 (16.5–66)	38 (39.2%)
	Critical $n = 37$	88 (54.4–119.7)	20 (54.1%)
	p	<0.001	<0.001

IQR interquartile range
p Statistical significance according to the linear-by-linear association test (dichotomous outcome variables) or Jonckheere–Terpstra test (quantitative outcome variables)

demonstrated that the severe category is best divided into two: infected pancreatic necrosis without persistent organ failure (which had high morbidity but low mortality) and persistent organ failure without infected pancreatic necrosis (with low morbidity but high mortality) [27]. The approach to the classification of severity should reflect the setting. In secondary hospitals the decision needed is whether patients should be transferred or not. This binary decision only requires the identification of patients with predicted severe AP. In tertiary hospital settings and particularly in the context of clinical trials, greater granularity is required, and the modified DBC is recommended.

5 Conclusion

Acute pancreatitis is a complex disease, with a broad clinical spectrum ranging from mild to severe/critical disease, with prolonged symptoms and high risk of morbidity and mortality. The diagnosis is usually straightforward and severe disease is usually due to organ dysfunction/failure. The prediction of severe pancreatitis is important in both the clinical and research setting, but the suboptimal accuracy of current predictive tools limits their value in managing individual patients.

References

1. Garcia-Rayado G, Cardenas-Jaen K, de-Madaria E. Towards evidence-based and personalised care of acute pancreatitis. United Eur Gastroenterol J. 2020;8:403–9.
2. Sternby H, Bolado F, Canaval-Zuleta HJ, et al. Determinants of severity in acute pancreatitis: a nation-wide multicenter prospective cohort study. Ann Surg. 2019;270:348–55.
3. de-Madaria E, Sanchez-Marin C, Carrillo I, et al. Design and validation of a patient-reported outcome measure scale in acute pancreatitis: the PAN-PROMISE study. Gut. 2021;70:139–47.
4. Rompianesi G, Hann A, Komolafe O, Pereira SP, Davidson BR, Gurusamy KS. Serum amylase and lipase and urinary trypsinogen and amylase for diagnosis of acute pancreatitis. Cochrane Database Syst Rev. 2017;4:CD012010.
5. Banks PA, Bollen TL, Dervenis C, et al. Classification of acute pancreatitis—2012: revision of the Atlanta classification and definitions by international consensus. Gut. 2013;62:102–11.
6. Wilson C, Heath DI, Imrie CW. Prediction of outcome in acute pancreatitis: a comparative study of APACHE II, clinical assessment and multiple factor scoring systems. Br J Surg. 1990;77:1260–4.
7. Moran RA, Garcia-Rayado G, de la Iglesia-Garcia D, et al. Influence of age, body mass index and comorbidity on major outcomes in acute pancreatitis, a prospective nation-wide multicentre study. United Eur Gastroenterol J. 2018;6:1508–18.
8. Dobszai D, Matrai P, Gyongyi Z, et al. Body-mass index correlates with severity and mortality in acute pancreatitis: a meta-analysis. World J Gastroenterol. 2019;25:729–43.
9. Paragomi P, Papachristou GI, Jeong K, et al. The relationship between pre-existing diabetes mellitus and the severity of acute pancreatitis: report from a large international registry. Pancreatology. 2022;22:85–91.
10. Kamal A, Akshintala VS, Kamal MM, et al. Does etiology of pancreatitis matter? Differences in outcomes among patients with post-endoscopic retrograde cholangiopancreatography, acute biliary, and alcoholic pancreatitis. Pancreas. 2019;48:574–8.
11. Pothoulakis I, Paragomi P, Tuft M, et al. Association of serum triglyceride levels with severity in acute pancreatitis: results from an international, multicenter cohort study. Digestion. 2021;102:809–13.
12. Mounzer R, Langmead CJ, Wu BU, et al. Comparison of existing clinical scoring systems to predict persistent organ failure in patients with acute pancreatitis. Gastroenterology. 2012;142:1476–82.
13. Maisonneuve P, Lowenfels AB, Lankisch PG. The harmless acute pancreatitis score (HAPS) identifies non-severe patients: a systematic review and meta-analysis. Pancreatology. 2021;21:1419–27.
14. Buxbaum J, Quezada M, Chong B, et al. The Pancreatitis Activity Scoring System predicts clinical outcomes in acute pancreatitis: findings from a prospective cohort study. Am J Gastroenterol. 2018;113:755–64.
15. Windsor JA. Assessment of the severity of acute pancreatitis: no room for complacency. Pancreatology. 2008;8:105–9.
16. Nordestgaard AG, Wilson SE, Williams RA. Early computerized tomography as a predictor of outcome in acute pancreatitis. Am J Surg . 1986;152(1):127–32. https://doi.org/10.1016/0002-9610(86)90162-5. PMID: 3728806.
17. Sternby H, Mahle M, Linder N, et al. Mean muscle attenuation correlates with severe acute pancreatitis unlike visceral adipose tissue and subcutaneous adipose tissue. United Eur Gastroenterol J. 2019;7:1312–20.
18. Gupta P, Kumar MP, Verma M, et al. Development and validation of a computed tomography index for assessing outcomes in patients with acute pancre-

atitis: "SMART-CT" index. Abdom Radiol (NY). 2021;46:1618–28.

19. de-Madaria E, Banks PA, Moya-Hoyo N, et al. Early factors associated with fluid sequestration and outcomes of patients with acute pancreatitis. Clin Gastroenterol Hepatol. 2014;12:997–1002.

20. Mofidi R, Duff MD, Madhavan KK, Garden OJ, Parks RW. Identification of severe acute pancreatitis using an artificial neural network. Surgery. 2007;141:59–66.

21. Qiu Q, Nian YJ, Guo Y, et al. Development and validation of three machine-learning models for predicting multiple organ failure in moderately severe and severe acute pancreatitis. BMC Gastroenterol. 2019;19:118.

22. Kui B, Pinter J, Molontay R, et al. EASY-APP: an artificial intelligence model and application for early and easy prediction of severity in acute pancreatitis. Clin Transl Med. 2022;12:e842.

23. Bradley EL 3rd. A clinically based classification system for acute pancreatitis. Summary of the International Symposium on Acute Pancreatitis, Atlanta, GA, September 11 through 13, 1992. Arch Surg. 1993;128:586–90.

24. de-Madaria E, Soler-Sala G, Lopez-Font I, et al. Update of the Atlanta Classification of severity of acute pancreatitis: should a moderate category be included? Pancreatology. 2010;10:613–9.

25. Petrov MS, Shanbhag S, Chakraborty M, Phillips AR, Windsor JA. Organ failure and infection of pancreatic necrosis as determinants of mortality in patients with acute pancreatitis. Gastroenterology. 2010;139:813–20.

26. Dellinger EP, Forsmark CE, Layer P, et al. Determinant-based classification of acute pancreatitis severity: an international multidisciplinary consultation. Ann Surg. 2012;256:875–80.

27. Zubia-Olaskoaga F, Maravi-Poma E, Urreta-Barallobre I, et al. Comparison between revised Atlanta Classification and determinant-based classification for acute pancreatitis in intensive care medicine. Why do not use a modified determinant-based classification? Crit Care Med. 2016;44:910–7.

Acute Pancreatitis: Pain and Analgesia

Sanjay Pandanaboyana and Asbjørn Mohr Drewes

Key Points

1. In patients with mild acute pancreatitis, opioid-sparing strategies should be used whenever possible.
2. In patients with moderate AP, nonsteroidal anti-inflammatory drugs and paracetamol can provide equivalent pain relief when compared with opioids.
3. In patients with severe AP, opioids are often needed, and a step-down approach may be appropriate to which adjuvant and experimental analgesics might be added.
4. Epidural analgesia provides optimum pain relief in the first 24 h of onset of AP with the potential to improve pancreatic perfusion.
5. Acupuncture and several experimental analgesics have potential in management of pain in acute pancreatitis.

S. Pandanaboyana
HPB and Transplant Unit, Freeman Hospital, Newcastle Upon Tyne, United Kingdom

Population Health Sciences, Newcastle University, Newcastle Upon Tyne, United Kingdom

A. M. Drewes (✉)
Department of Gastroenterology and Hepatology, Centre for Pancreatic Diseases and Mech-Sense, Aalborg University Hospital, Aalborg, Denmark
e-mail: amd@rn.dk

1 Introduction

Abdominal pain is the presenting and dominating symptom in almost all patients with acute pancreatitis (AP) and is a diagnostic criterion [1]. This requires that the abdominal pain is typical of AP and that there is either a significant elevation ($\geq$3-fold) of pancreatic enzymes (lipase or amylase) or evidence of pancreatic inflammation on cross-sectional imaging [1]. The assessment of pain is usually confined to pain intensity and a 1–10 visual analogue scale is typically used [2]. There are no specific and validated scales for pain assessment in AP, although these are available for patients with chronic pancreatitis [3]. Furthermore guidelines and recommendations for the management of pain in patients with AP are not consistent meaning that pain management strategies are often extrapolated from management of other painful abdominal conditions [4]. In fact, the IAP/APA guidelines for management of AP [5] do not mention pain management, and no recommendations were given in the AGA guidelines from 2018 [6]. In a recent *The Lancet* review [4], it was only mentioned that no analgesics are superior and that opioids may decrease the need for supplementary analgesics. As pain is the most important symptom in AP, it is astonishing that there are no specific recommendations for management in the international literature, reflecting the urgent need for research.

© The Author(s), under exclusive license to Springer Nature Singapore Pte Ltd. 2024
J. A. Windsor et al. (eds.), *Acute Pancreatitis*, https://doi.org/10.1007/978-981-97-3132-9_9

2 Management of Acute Pain in General

Acute pain perception in individual patients involves sensory, emotional, cognitive and social dimensions [7]. Management of acute pain should be tailored for individual patients and take into account these dimensions for effective treatment and to avoid transition to chronic pain [8]. In contrast, chronic pain often leads to reorganization of central nervous structures and neuroplastic changes. When such central pain pathways become maladaptive and self-perpetuating with spontaneous firing of the neurones, pain can become independent of the initial nociceptive drive [9, 10]. This difference between acute and chronic pain ought to be reflected in differences in pain management.

Management of pain often follows the WHO pain ladder [11], which is a 'step-up' approach that was originally developed for cancer-related pain. Patients with AP often present with sudden onset severe pain associated with autonomic symptoms, and a WHO pain ladder pathway may not be as effective under such conditions. Furthermore, this approach has not been tested in randomized controlled trials, and studies often compare one pain modality against another rather than specifically testing the step-up strategy [12]. And this may not be appropriate in patients with severe acute pain where a step-down approach (where the most potent analgesics are used first to gain rapid control of pain) may be more appropriate.

A recent systematic review of randomized controlled trials assessing the effect of treatment for acute pain has shown that opioids are not superior to nonsteroidal anti-inflammatory drugs (NSAIDs) for several common acute pain conditions such as dental pain and renal stones and in some cases may be inferior [13]. Furthermore, current evidence for pain management in general is focused on pain outcomes in <1 week and often <1 day with lack of data on function and quality of life. There is often little consideration of demographic, clinical or genetic factors and their impact on pain management.

3 Management of Pain in Acute Pancreatitis

The selection of the best strategy for analgesia in a patient with AP requires consideration of a number of factors (such as age, comorbidity, gender and social status) and might also include existing treatment for other painful condition, risk of dependency, other medication, interactions and most importantly the predicted severity of AP and the severity of pain on presentation.

As shown in Fig. 1, it is recommended that management is stratified based on pain intensity and predicted severity of disease. The latter is described in the previous chapter and will not be repeated here, but it is obvious that actual pain intensity dominates the patient's experience and is a crucial focus of the early management strategy. In acute pain, the intensity is the dominant domain of pain, but cognitive and psychological aspects are also part of the complex clinical picture. There is no validated comprehensive pain assessment tool for pain with AP. It is recommended that pain intensity is rated on a 0–10 numeric rating scale as the visual analogue scale may be more difficult to use, especially for the elderly [14].

The optimal and effective pain management for patients with AP is not clear from published data, but emerging evidence is now starting to inform current practice, as in Fig. 1.

3.1 Simple Analgesics and Weak Opioids

The majority of RCTs assessing the efficacy of simple analgesics were undertaken prior to 2020. Only one RCT has been published since then and this compared IV diclofenac and tramadol [15]. This study found no difference in visual analogue scores (VAS) or in number of painful days but the time to significant reduction in VAS (>33%) was shorter for diclofenac. The trial concluded that diclofenac and tramadol were equally effective treatments of pain in AP. This is in contrast to a recent meta-analysis, which suggested

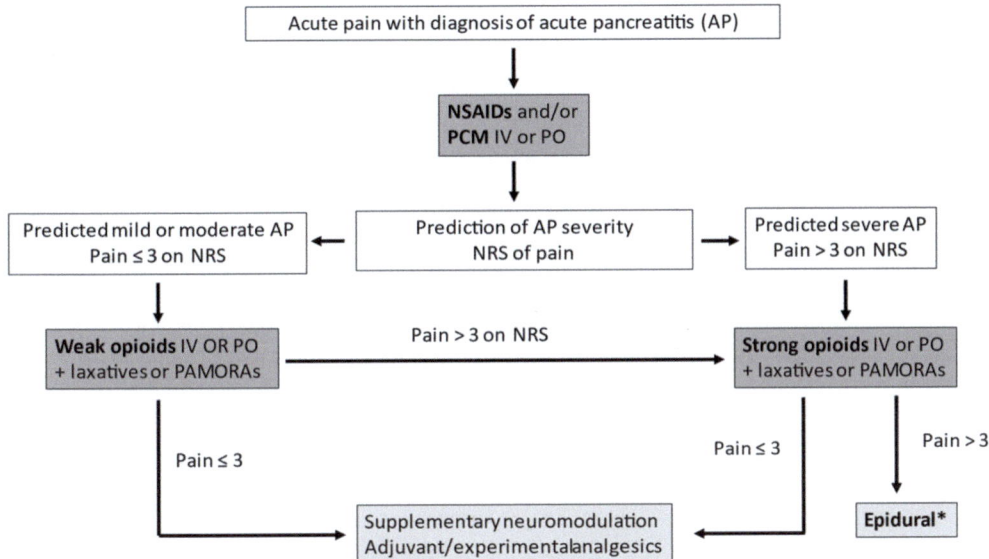

Fig. 1 Pragmatic approach to pain management in AP based on WHO ladder and recent evidence [Figure adapted with permission from Pandanaboyana et al. (2022). Copyright Wolters Kluwer Health]. *NRS* 0–10 numerical rating scale for pain intensity, *PCM* paracetamol, *NSAIDs* nonsteroidal anti-inflammatory drugs, *PAMORA* peripherally acting μ-opioid receptor antagonist, *neuromodulation* acupuncture and transcutaneous electrical nerve stimulation. Epidural anaesthesia can be used instead of strong opioids where available. See Table 1 for dosages

Table 1 Recommended analgesics for treatment of acute pancreatitis pain

Drug class	Examples[a]	Comments
Non-opioid analgesics	Paracetamol oral 1 g × every 6 h *or* i.v. 650 mg every 4 h	Used for milder pain. May be combined with NSAIDs
NSAIDs	Ibuprofen: 2–400 mg every 6–8 h. Can be used rectally or i.v.	In long-term use, gastrointestinal and cardiovascular side-effects shall be considered
Weak opioids	Tramadol PR oral 50–200 mg × 2	Codeine and tramadol potentiate the effect of non-opioid analgesics. Both are prodrugs, metabolized to active opioids
Strong opioids	Oxycodone PR starting at 10 mg × 2 Morphine or oxycodone 5 mg s.c. or i.v. as starting dose with adjustment depending on effect	Addiction is not of major concern in acute pancreatitis and short-term usage. Drugs without active metabolites are often preferred. Laxatives are needed, but still many patients develop opioid induced bowel function
Anticonvulsants	Pregabalin oral 75–150 mg × 2 daily	Likely not very effective in acute pain
Anxiolytics	Diazepam 5 mg × 3	Have limited analgesic effect but may dampen anxiety
NMDA inhibitors	Ketamine oral titrated up to 50 mg × 3 daily. Magnesium i.v. as 30–50 mg/kg bolus and maintained at 6–20 mg/kg/h	As the strongest NMDA inhibitor, ketamine may be effective, but side-effects are often severe. Absorption following oral use is variable but can be used
Cannabinoids	Nabilone oral 1–2 mg, up to 6 mg daily	Mostly used as adjunctive pain medication and useful for nausea, appetite and sleep

[Table adapted with permission from Pandanaboyana et al. (2022). Copyright Wolters Kluwer Health]
The authors own suggestions reflecting their normal practice. The availability of medications varies between countries and regions and is dependent on traditions. For details see text
NSAID nonsteroidal anti-inflammatory drugs, *BZD* benzodiazepines, *NMDA* N-methyl-D-aspartate, *PR* prolonged release
[a]Dosage reduced to 12.5 mg/kg every 4 h in patients weighing <50 kg

NSAID to be more effective at suppressing proin-flammatory cytokines, relieving pain, ameliorating systematic complications and reducing mortality [16]. The most recent meta-analysis performed a pooled analysis of pain management in the first 24 h and confirmed that NSAIDS and opioids were equally effective in achieving pain relief. Another recent meta-analysis compared non-opioid and opioid analgesia in AP and showed equivalent efficacy [17]. Data for pain management beyond the first 24 h and whether opioid use is more effective in patients who are readmitted is lacking.

3.2   Strong Opioids

There has been an increased awareness of opioid overuse, and especially in the USA. The so-called opioid crises have tipped the balance at times into opiophobia [18]. Although a relevant discussion, the problems with opioids (especially addiction) when used for chronic pain cannot be translated to the acute settings. Optimal pain management is an ethical and clinical priority to ensure patients are as comfortable as possible, to reduce the risk of complications with suboptimal pain relief (e.g. atelectasis, pneumonia, DVT) and to avoid central sensitization [10]. When pain is severe opioids are the most effective analgesic and have a reasonable safety profile. Recent US guidelines recommend the lowest effective dose in acute pain and opioids should not be prescribed for longer than the expected duration of pain [19]. This balanced view is in line with European guidelines for opioid treatment [20, 21].

A retrospective study from the USA in 2019 showed that 80% of AP patient received opioids during initial stages, and this was influenced by age, gender, race/culture, disease severity/pain score, comorbidity and alcohol use [22]. Another recent study from 2020 showed that opioid-treated patients with AP are unlikely to receive narcotics after discharge unless there was evidence of chronic pancreatitis [23]. The risk of readmission following AP was not related to opioid use at discharge [24]. When used carefully it would appear that opioids are effective analgesics for severe pain associated with AP, and

unless patients have recurrent AP or acute on chronic pancreatitis, the risk for addiction appears negligible.

A recent meta-analysis of RCTs assessing pain management in AP [25], opiates were featured in 10 of 12 studies using a total of 6 different opiate analgesics. While the meta-analysis indicates improved pain relief with opiates when compared to local analgesics and NSAIDS, overall comparison (using VAS) between opiates and non-opiates found no significant difference in analgesic effect. Whether this holds out when a more comprehensive assessment of pain is used, awaits further research. But it does serve as a reminder to consider non-opiate alternatives when possible.

Many patients treated with opioids (weak and strong) experience some side-effects including respiratory depression, sedation and pruritus. Opioid use also carries a risk of addiction [18]. Other side-effects include opioid-induced bowel dysfunction with dysmotility, decreased fluid secretion and increased sphincter tone. These may manifest as nausea, vomiting, bloating, gastrooesophageal reflux-related symptoms and constipation [26]. Opioid-induced intestinal dysmotility is managed with laxatives although it is unknown which laxative is most effective. There may be a role for peripherally acting μ-opioid receptor antagonists (PAMORA) such as methylnaltrexone which have been shown to be effective in treating postoperative ileus and chronic constipation that share common mechanisms to that seen in opioid-induced intestinal dysmotility [27]. New opioids such as oliceridine mainly activate G-protein signalling, and there is some evidence that it may have a better safety profile than commonly used opioids [28].

An important unresolved issue is whether opioids worsen outcomes from AP. The sphincter of Oddi is sensitive to all opiates with an increased biliary sphincter pressure seen with higher doses of morphine. It is unclear, however, if this increased pressure worsens severity of AP. Bacterial overgrowth may also be promoted with opiate-induced ileus and decreased motility. Recent animal studies suggest that morphine may worsen the disease severity by increasing gut barrier permeability and may delay pancreatic epithelial regeneration in response to injury [29]. There is no data on the effect of opioids on local and systemic complications in patients with AP due to lack of detailed reporting and trials. This means that comparing different analgesic classes with severity and outcome from AP is not possible from the available data.

Pain intensity typically wanes when inflammation and tissue pressure decrease, and analgesics should be tapered accordingly. It is recommended to monitor pain intensity at least twice daily and adjust the medication accordingly. In acute pain, opioid dependency seldomly becomes an issue [30], and tapering can be done fast (within 24 h) without physical withdrawal symptoms unless treatment has been ongoing for weeks and/or high dosages are used.

In summary, non-opioid analgesic can be used to manage pain in many patients with AP. Opioids can be considered in patients with high pain intensity and predicted severe disease but should be tapered as soon as pain vanishes. To avoid central sensitization, it is important that pain is treated promptly and optimally.

3.3 Acupuncture and Transcutaneous Electrical Nerve Stimulation

Acupuncture has been widely used in China and elsewhere as a non-pharmacological treatment for a range of diseases, and there is emerging evidence regarding the neuroanatomical basis for the efficacy of this as an analgesic [31]. There are many randomized controlled trials demonstrating safety and efficacy in migraine prophylaxis [32, 33], cancer pain [34], osteoarthritis [35], dyspepsia [36], postprandial distress syndrome [37] and other diseases. It is also effective in reducing abdominal pain in patients with AP, attested to by two systematic reviews and meta-analyses [38, 39]. Results from the latest meta-analysis [38] showed that acupuncture was effective in reducing pain intensity, the time to relief, abdominal distension and the time to relief of distension compared with routine treatment of AP pain. Two studies noted that acupuncture reduced intestinal permeability and the local inflammatory response

[40, 41]. Taken together there is now sufficient evidence to state that acupuncture reduces the need for opioids, reduces inflammation and promotes gastrointestinal motility. However, it will be important to standardize acupuncture techniques to ensure predictable benefit and to ensure optimal training for practitioners. Thus, acupuncture should be more widely considered as a strategy for pain management in AP patients.

Transcutaneous electrical nerve stimulation (TENS) is another non-pharmacological treatment for pain [42] that has been widely used for neuropathic pain [43], cancer pain [44], fibromyalgia [45] and other painful conditions. Because of its safety, it can be used in selected cases, but there is a lack of clinical trials investigating the efficacy of TENS in relieving AP pain.

3.4 Epidural Analgesia

There is strong evidence to support the use of epidural analgesia in the postoperative setting. It provides excellent pain control, reduces the risk of cardiovascular, thrombotic and pulmonary complications, enables early mobilization, and decreases the rate of ileus [46, 47]. Another potential benefit of epidural analgesia in patients with AP is that it improves pancreatic perfusion and may reduce ischemic injury and inflammation by selective segmental sympathectomy [48]. There have been two small underpowered randomized controlled trials testing the safety and efficacy of epidural analgesia in AP patients. The first showed an improvement in pancreatic perfusion and better pain relief in the first 24 h, but no difference in length of hospital stay or mortality [49]. The other one showed that epidural analgesia significantly decreased serum procalcitonin, with a nonsignificant trend towards improved organ function and decreased mortality [50]. These results are encouraging and provide the justification for high-quality and well-powered clinical trials in AP patients that will provide definitive evidence for the benefit of epidural analgesia on pain intensity, pain duration, organ dysfunction and mortality. A recent randomized trial, however, was not able to reproduce the encouraging results on outcome, although epidural analgesia was effective to treat the pain associated with AP [51].

3.5 Acute on Chronic Pancreatitis and Recurrent Acute Pancreatitis

In patients with acute on chronic pancreatitis, pain is often an exacerbation of the existing pain syndrome related to the chronic pancreatitis [52]. These patients often receive analgesics and can therefore be more difficult to treat due to tachyphylaxis to opioids and psychosocial comorbidity, for example. Pain management can therefore be challenging and is outside the scope of this chapter, but often parenteral opioids are needed to dampen the pain. It is important to inform the patient that this increase in dosage is temporary and as soon as pain intensity decreases, tapering should be initiated with the clear goal not to exceed the usual daily dose of opioids [20, 21]. This is also in keeping with recently published Centers for Disease Control and Prevention (CDC) recommendations on opioid use in non-cancer pain [53].

Patients with acute recurrent pancreatitis are treated as those with AP and seldomly need special considerations. However, if the time interval between the acute attacks is narrow and decreasing, the concern is the development of central sensitisation and the development of a constant background pain. In this situation the patient the management of pain should be as for chronic pancreatitis.

3.6 Pragmatic Approach to Pain Management in Acute Pancreatitis

The recommended analgesics in AP, routes of administration and side-effects are summarized in Table 1. Opioids and NSAIDS currently form the mainstay of pain management in AP (Fig. 1). Severity of pain and clinical severity of AP should both be considered when planning the analgesic strategy. In patients with mild AP and mild pain

[numerical rating scale (NRS) 1–3], the initial pain management with NSAIDs (as an opioid-sparing strategy) and paracetamol is appropriate. With increasing pain, escalation or step-up to a weaker and then stronger opioid is often required. In patients with predicted moderately severe and severe AP with moderate to severe pain on the NRS scale, a step-down approach with a stronger opioid to get on top of to get on top of the pain, and then stepping down a weaker opioid or opioid alternative when possible Epidural analgesia should be considered in selected patients, especially in those with cardiorespiratory comorbidities and those who do not respond well to stronger opioids.

4 Conclusion

The current published data on pain management of AP suggests there is significant scope for improvement. Current practice is varied, recommendations from guidelines are conflicting, and we are too often reliant on evidence from the postoperative pain setting. New knowledge about the mechanisms of AP pain will undoubtedly reveal new and specific treatment targets. Until then we need to make better use of the analgesic options available to our patients.

References

1. Banks PA, Bollen TL, Dervenis C, et al. Classification of acute pancreatitis—2012: revision of the Atlanta classification and definitions by international consensus. Gut. 2013;62:102–11.
2. Streiner DL, Norman GR, Cairney J. Health measurement scales, vol. 1. Oxford University Press; 2015. https://doi.org/10.1093/med/9780199685219.001.0001.
3. Drewes AM, van Veldhuisen CL, Bellin MD, et al. Assessment of pain associated with chronic pancreatitis: an international consensus guideline. Pancreatology. 2021;21(7):1256–8.
4. Boxhoorn L, Voermans RP, Bouwense SA, et al. Acute pancreatitis. Lancet (London, England). 2020;396(10252):726–34.
5. Working Group IAP/APA Acute Pancreatitis Guidelines. IAP/APA evidence-based guidelines for the management of acute pancreatitis. Pancreatology.

2013;13(4 Suppl 2):e1–15. https://doi.org/10.1016/j.pan.2013.07.063.

6. Crockett SD, Wani S, Gardner TB, Falck-Ytter Y, Barkun AN, American Gastroenterological Association Institute Clinical Guidelines Committee. American Gastroenterological Association Institute guideline on initial management of acute pancreatitis. Gastroenterology. 2018;154(4):1096–101.

7. Hooten WM, Brummett CM, Sullivan MD, et al. A conceptual framework for understanding unintended prolonged opioid use. Mayo Clin Proc. 2017;92(12):1822–30.

8. Gan TJ. Poorly controlled postoperative pain: prevalence, consequences, and prevention. J Pain Res. 2017;10:2287–98.

9. Drewes AM, Olesen AE, Farmer AD, et al. Gastrointestinal pain. Nat Rev Dis Prim. 2020;6(1):1.

10. Arendt-Nielsen L, Morlion B, Perrot S, et al. Assessment and manifestation of central sensitisation across different chronic pain conditions. Eur J Pain. 2018;22(2):216–41.

11. Ventafridda V, Saita L, Ripamonti C, De Conno F. WHO guidelines for the use of analgesics in cancer pain. Int J Tissue React. 1985;7(1):93–6.

12. Vargas-Schaffer G. Is the WHO analgesic ladder still valid? Twenty-four years of experience. Can Fam Physician. 2010;56(6):514–7.

13. Chou R, Wagner J, Ahmed AY, et al. Treatments for acute pain: a systematic review. Rockville: Agency for Healthcare Research and Quality (US); 2020. https://effectivehealthcare.ahrq.gov/products/treatments-acute-pain/research.

14. Drewes AM, van Veldhuisen CL, Bellin MD, Besselink MG, Bouwense SA, Olesen SS, van Santvoort H, Vase L, Windsor JA. Assessment of pain associated with chronic pancreatitis: an international consensus guideline. Pancreatology. 2021;21(7):1256–84.

15. Kumar NS, Muktesh G, Samra T, et al. Comparison of efficacy of diclofenac and tramadol in relieving pain in patients of acute pancreatitis: a randomized parallel group double blind active controlled pilot study. Eur J Pain (United Kingdom). 2020;24(3):639–48.

16. Wu D, Bai X, Lee P, et al. A systematic review of NSAIDs treatment for acute pancreatitis in animal studies and clinical trials. Clin Res Hepatol Gastroenterol. 2020;44:100002.

17. Nelson AD, Lugo-Fagundo NS, Mahapatra SJ, et al. A systematic review and meta-analysis of opioids vs nonopioids in acute pancreatitis. Gastro Hep Adv. 2022;1(1):83–92.

18. The Lancet Public Health. Opioid overdose crisis: time for a radical rethink. Lancet Public Health. 2022;7(3):e195. https://doi.org/10.1016/S2468-2667(22)00043-3.

19. Dowell D, Ragan KR, Jones CM, Baldwin GT, Chou R. CDC clinical practice guideline for prescribing opioids for pain—United States, 2022. MMWR Recomm Rep. 2022;71(3):1–95.

20. Häuser W, Morlion B, Vowles KE, Bannister K, Buchser E, et al. European clinical practice recommendations on opioids for chronic noncancer pain—Part 1: role of opioids in the management of chronic noncancer pain. Eur J Pain. 2021;25(5):949–68.

21. Krčevski Škvarč N, Morlion B, Vowles KE, Bannister K, Buchsner E, et al. European clinical practice recommendations on opioids for chronic noncancer pain—Part 2: special situations. Eur J Pain. 2021;25(5):969–85.

22. Wu BU, Butler RK, Chen W. Factors associated with opioid use in patients hospitalized for acute pancreatitis. JAMA Netw open. 2019;2(4):e191827.

23. Ahmed A, Yakah W, Freedman SD, et al. Evaluation of opioid use in acute pancreatitis in absence of chronic pancreatitis: absence of opioid dependence an important feature. Am J Med. 2020;133(10):1209–18.

24. Yang AL, Jin DX, Rudder M, et al. Opiate prescriptions at discharge are not associated with early readmissions in acute pancreatitis. Dig Dis Sci. 2020;65(2):611–4.

25. Thavanesan N, White S, Lee S, et al. Analgesia in the initial management of acute pancreatitis: a systematic review and meta-analysis of randomised controlled trials. World J Surg. 2022;46(4):878–90.

26. Farmer AD, Drewes AM, Chiarioni G, et al. Pathophysiology and management of opioid-induced constipation: European expert consensus statement. United Eur Gastroenterol J. 2019;7(1):7–20.

27. Knoph CS, Cook ME, Fjelsted CA, et al. Effects of the peripherally acting μ-opioid receptor antagonist methylnaltrexone on acute pancreatitis severity: study protocol for a multicentre double-blind randomised placebo-controlled interventional trial, the PAMORA-AP trial. Trials. 2021;22(1):940.

28. Xu L-L, Zhou X-Q, Yi P-S, et al. Alvimopan combined with enhanced recovery strategy for managing postoperative ileus after open abdominal surgery: a systematic review and meta-analysis. J Surg Res. 2016;203(1):211–21.

29. Barlass U, Dutta R, Cheema H, George J, Sareen A, et al. Morphine worsens the severity and prevents pancreatic regeneration in mouse models of acute pancreatitis. Gut. 2018;67(4):600–2.

30. Ahmed A, Yakah W, Freedman SD, Kothari DJ, Sheth SG. Evaluation of opioid use in acute pancreatitis in absence of chronic pancreatitis: absence of opioid dependence an important feature. Am J Med. 2020;133(10):1209–18.

31. Liu S, Wang Z, Su Y, et al. A neuroanatomical basis for electroacupuncture to drive the vagal-adrenal axis. Nature. 2021;598(7882):641–5.

32. Zhao L, Chen J, Li Y, et al. The long-term effect of acupuncture for migraine prophylaxis: a randomized clinical trial. JAMA Intern Med. 2017;177(4):508–15.

33. Xu S, Yu L, Luo X, et al. Manual acupuncture versus sham acupuncture and usual care for prophylaxis of episodic migraine without aura: multicentre, randomised clinical trial. BMJ. 2020;368:m697.

34. Mao JJ, Liou KT, Baser RE, et al. Effectiveness of electroacupuncture or auricular acupuncture vs usual care for chronic musculoskeletal pain among can-

cer survivors: the PEACE randomized clinical trial. JAMA Oncol. 2021;7(5):720–7.

35. Tu J-F, Yang J-W, Shi G-X, et al. Efficacy of intensive acupuncture versus sham acupuncture in knee osteoarthritis: a randomized controlled trial. Arthritis Rheumatol (Hoboken, NJ). 2021;73(3):448–58.

36. Zeng F, Qin W, Ma T, et al. Influence of acupuncture treatment on cerebral activity in functional dyspepsia patients and its relationship with efficacy. Am J Gastroenterol. 2012;107(8):1236–47. http://www.ncbi.nlm.nih.gov/pubmed/22641307.

37. Yang J-W, Wang L-Q, Zou X, et al. Effect of acupuncture for postprandial distress syndrome: a randomized clinical trial. Ann Intern Med. 2020;172(12):777–85.

38. Zhu F, Yin S, Zhu X, et al. Acupuncture for relieving abdominal pain and distension in acute pancreatitis: a systematic review and meta-analysis. Front Psychiatry. 2021;12:786401.

39. Zhang K, Gao C, Li C, et al. Acupuncture for acute pancreatitis: a systematic review and meta-analysis. Pancreas. 2019;48(9):1136–47.

40. Wang X. Electroacupuncture for treatment of acute pancreatitis and its effect on the intestinal permeability of the patient. Zhongguo Zhen Jiu. 2007;27(6):421–3.

41. Zhu S-F, Guo H, Zhang R-R, et al. Effect of electroacupuncture on the inflammatory response in patients with acute pancreatitis: an exploratory study. Acupunct Med. 2015;33(2):115–20.

42. Gibson W, Wand BM, Meads C, et al. Transcutaneous electrical nerve stimulation (TENS) for chronic pain—an overview of Cochrane reviews. Cochrane Database Syst Rev. 2019;4:CD011890.

43. Gibson W, Wand BM, O'Connell NE. Transcutaneous electrical nerve stimulation (TENS) for neuropathic pain in adults. Cochrane Database Syst Rev. 2017;9:CD011976.

44. Hurlow A, Bennett MI, Robb KA, et al. Transcutaneous electric nerve stimulation (TENS) for cancer pain in adults. Cochrane Database Syst Rev. 2012;3:CD006276.

45. Johnson MI, Claydon LS, Herbison GP, et al. Transcutaneous electrical nerve stimulation (TENS) for fibromyalgia in adults. Cochrane Database Syst Rev. 2017;10:CD012172.

46. Nimmo SM, Harrington LS. What is the role of epidural analgesia in abdominal surgery? Contin Educ Anaesth Crit Care Pain. 2014;14(5):224–9.

47. Rodgers A, Walker N, Schug S, et al. Reduction of postoperative mortality and morbidity with epidural or spinal anaesthesia: results from overview of randomised trials. BMJ. 2000;321(7275):1493.

48. Windisch O, Heidegger C-P, Giraud R, et al. Thoracic epidural analgesia: a new approach for the treatment of acute pancreatitis? Crit Care. 2016;20(1):116.

49. Sadowski SM, Andres A, Morel P, et al. Epidural anesthesia improves pancreatic perfusion and decreases the severity of acute pancreatitis. World J Gastroenterol. 2015;21(43):12448–56.

50. Tyagi A, Gupta YR, Das S, et al. Effect of segmental thoracic epidural block on pancreatitis induced organ dysfunction: a preliminary study. Indian J Crit Care Med. 2019;23(2):89–94.

51. Jabaudon M, Genevrier A, Jaber S, Windisch O, Bulyez S, Laterre PF, Escudier E, Sossou A, Guerci P, Bertrand PM, Danin PE, Bonnassieux M, Bühler L, Heidegger CP, Chabanne R, Godet T, Roszyk L, Sapin V, Futier E, Pereira B, Constantin JM, EPIPAN Study Group. Thoracic epidural analgesia in intensive care unit patients with acute pancreatitis: the EPIPAN multicenter randomized controlled trial. Crit Care. 2023;27(1):213. https://doi.org/10.1186/s13054-023-04502-w.

52. Drewes AM, Bouwense SAW, Campbell CM, Ceyhan GO, Delhaye M, Working group for the International (IAP—APA—JPS—EPC) Consensus Guidelines for Chronic Pancreatitis, et al. Guidelines for the understanding and management of pain in chronic pancreatitis. Pancreatology. 2017;17(5):720–31.

53. CDC guidance on opioid use in non cancer pain. https://www.cdc.gov/mmwr/volumes/71/rr/pdfs/rr7103a1-H.pdf.

Fluids and Resuscitation

Jorge D. Machicado and Georgios I. Papachristou

Key Points

1. Fluids should be initiated as soon as the diagnosis of acute pancreatitis is suspected or made, using an intravenous route, and with lactated Ringer's as the preferred fluid.
2. Aggressive fluid resuscitation increases the risk of volume overload with potentially. Adverse clinical consequences, including pulmonary oedema.
3. Moderate fluid resuscitation is recommended for patients with acute pancreatitis of any severity at a rate of 1.5 mL/kg/h. Fluid boluses of 10 mL/kg should be administered when hypovolemia is present.
4. Objective clinical assessment of volume status should be performed frequently during the first 24 h and at least every 24 h thereafter. These assessments aim to detect and correct any fluid excess or deficits.

J. D. Machicado
Division of Gastroenterology and Hepatology, University of Michigan, Ann Arbor, MI, USA
e-mail: machicad@med.umich.edu

G. I. Papachristou (✉)
Division of Gastroenterology, Hepatology, and Nutrition, The Ohio State University Wexner Medical Center, Columbus, OH, USA
e-mail: georgios.papachristou@osumc.edu

1 Introduction

Intravenous fluid resuscitation is considered the cornerstone in the early management of acute pancreatitis (AP) [1]. Although practice guidelines have recommended fluid therapy in AP for decades, it's not until recently that a number of randomized controlled trials (RCTs) have emerged to better delineate what type of fluid and rate of administration are beneficial. In this chapter, we will review the rationale of intravenous fluid therapy, provide guidance on appropriate fluid resuscitation, and discuss methods to guide resuscitation efforts during the inpatient management of patients with AP.

2 Rationale of Fluid Therapy in AP

The onset of AP is associated with the release of proinflammatory cytokines and vasoactive mediators that increase vascular permeability, interstitial fluid extravasation, capillary vasoconstriction, and microthrombi formation [2–4]. These pathophysiologic alterations can impair pancreatic microcirculation, which can lead to local ischemia and ultimately pancreatic necrosis [5]. In addition, patients with AP can develop capillary leak syndrome, tissue edema, and intravascular volume depletion, which can result in hypotension, acute kidney injury, noncardiogenic pulmo-

© The Author(s), under exclusive license to Springer Nature Singapore Pte Ltd. 2024
J. A. Windsor et al. (eds.), *Acute Pancreatitis*, https://doi.org/10.1007/978-981-97-3132-9_10

nary edema, and acute respiratory distress syndrome (ARDS) [6, 7]. Thus, the goal of fluid therapy in AP is to improve pancreatic and systemic perfusion and to potentially reduce pancreatitis severity and the risk of complications.

Evidence supporting the role of fluid therapy in AP started to emerge in the 1980s. In preclinical animal models with AP, vigorous intravenous fluid resuscitation was shown to improve pancreatic microcirculation, systemic perfusion, and overall survival [8–11]. The effect of fluids in humans with AP was unknown until the late 1990s, when two pivotal observational studies reported that hemoconcentration and/or failure to decrease admission hematocrit at 24 h was significantly associated with pancreatic necrosis [12, 13]. As hemoconcentration is a surrogate marker for systemic hypovolemia and was strongly associated with pancreatic necrosis, these studies suggested early, aggressive fluid resuscitation to reduce the risk of pancreatic necrosis and severity of AP. Since then, society guidelines have unanimously recommended early fluid resuscitation in AP. However, the details of how to most effectively administer intravenous fluids to patients with AP in clinical practice remain uncertain, translating to significant variations in guideline recommendations and clinical practice [14–18].

3 Principles of Fluid Therapy

Fluids should be prescribed as any other drug, with a clear understanding of the composition (type of fluid), dosing (rate of administration), endpoints, potential harms, and contraindications. An international working group has proposed a conceptual model that distinguishes four distinct dynamic phases of fluid therapy: rescue, optimization, stabilization, and de-escalation [19]. This framework provides guidance to rationally administer fluid therapy, although not specifically in patients with AP (Table 1). Studies are required to demonstrate that this framework results in improved outcomes in AP patients. During the rescue phase, rapid infusion of fluid boluses is given within minutes to correct hypovolemia. In the optimization phase, fluid infusion is administered cautiously and titrated in a "goal-directed" fashion to optimize tissue perfusion and minimize volume overload. The duration of this phase in AP usually lasts 24–72 h, during which time patients may require more or less fluid. During the stabilization phase, patients are in a steady state and maintenance fluids are used for replacement of normal fluid losses. This phase can be skipped if patients have resumed normal oral intake. In the last phase, fluids are discontinued, and a negative

Table 1 Stages of fluid resuscitation in acute pancreatitis (adapted from [19])

	Rescue	Optimization	Stabilization	De-escalation
Intervention	Fluid infusion and bolus	Fluid infusion and close monitoring	Maintenance fluids	Stopping fluids
Goals	Correct hypovolemia	Optimize tissue perfusion and prevent volume overload	Reach zero or negative fluid balance	Mitigate volume overload
Setting	Emergency department	Inpatient wards or intensive care unit	Inpatient wards	Inpatient wards
Duration	1–2 h	24–72 h	Variable based on oral tolerance	Hours to days
Notes	Bolus when hypovolemia is present	If hypovolemia, need fluid bolus. If hypervolemia, decrease or stop fluids	Maintenance IV fluids when patients do not tolerate oral diet within 72 h	In addition to stopping IV fluids, may require diuretics

balance is promoted, sometimes by using diuretics, or rarely renal dialysis. Healthcare providers administering fluid therapy to AP patients are often from different hospital units and subspecialties and should be mindful of these phases to meet individual patient goals rather than using a "one-size-fits-all" fluid therapy protocol.

4   Setting and Timing of Initial Fluid Resuscitation

Fluid therapy is usually initiated in the Emergency Department and rarely in the inpatient wards or intensive care unit. Fluid therapy should be initiated as soon as the diagnosis of AP has been established or when there is a high clinical suspicion of AP while awaiting for tests to confirm the diagnosis. In most published studies, fluids were initiated within 4–8 h of hospital presentation and/or diagnosis of AP [20, 21]. A multidisciplinary expert panel has recently proposed that fluid resuscitation should be initiated within 2 h of diagnosis and this should be used as a quality indicator to monitor hospitals and physicians managing patients with AP [22]. It's important to acknowledge that patients may present to the hospital over a range of times since the onset of symptoms and this can make a difference to their fluid requirements. Also some patients may be transferred to tertiary care hospitals after fluids have been commenced and are more likely to be in the second phase of resuscitation ("optimization") rather than the first phase ("rescue").

5   Route of Fluid Resuscitation

Fluids are typically administered intravenously because patients with AP are not able to take sufficient fluids by mouth, especially with abdominal pain, bloating, nausea, and/or vomiting. A small RCT has shown that it is feasible and effective to deliver fluid enterally through a nasojejunal feeding tube [23]. This approach is not preferred by patients and it fails in the majority of patients.

6   Type of Fluids

Early animal studies suggested that colloids were superior to crystalloids because they reduced capillary leak and improved tissue perfusion [11, 12]. However, in a RCT of 120 patients with severe AP, colloids were associated with higher rate of adverse events and organ failure when compared with crystalloids, and there was no difference in survival [24]. In critically ill patients, hydroxyethyl starch has consistently been found to increase mortality and renal injury when compared with crystalloid solutions [25]. In addition to the safety concerns with colloids, these solutions are more expensive and less available worldwide than crystalloids. Therefore, crystalloids are preferred over colloids for fluid resuscitation in AP.

Crystalloids, apart from dextrose solutions, contain sodium, chloride, and other anions. The chemical properties of each solution determine its efficacy, tonicity, and potential toxicity (Table 2). Normal saline (NS, 0.9% sodium chloride) has equal concentrations of sodium and chloride, and its rapid high-volume infusion can cause hyperchloremic metabolic acidosis. The concerns with the high chloride content of NS resulted in the introduction of balanced crystalloids, in which chloride is substituted for alternative anions such as lactate (lactated Ringer's solution [LR], Hartmann's solution), acetate (Ringer's acetate), or gluconate/malate (PlasmaLyte) [26]. Rapid administration of solutions containing lactate can result in hyperlactataemia, metabolic alkalosis, and hypotonicity.

There have been five RCTs comparing NS and LR in patients with AP [27–31]. A recent meta-analysis of four RCTs ($n = 248$) showed that, compared to NS, LR reduced the risk of ICU admissions (RR, 0.42; 95% CI, 0.20, 0.89) and shortened the hospital stay (mean difference, −1.10; 95% CI, −1.92, −0.28), but there was no difference in mortality or systemic inflammatory response syndrome (SIRS) [32]. In another meta-analysis of the same RCTs, LR was found to be associated with less severe adverse events than NS (RR, 0.48; 95% CI, 0.29, 0.81) [33]. Some of the theoretical advantages of LR over other crystalloids include anti-inflammatory properties,

Table 2 Characteristics of commonly used crystalloids for fluid resuscitation

	Normal saline (NS)	Lactated Ringer's solution (LR)	Hartmann's solution
Osmolarity	308 mOsm/L	273 mOsm/L	280.6 mOsm/L
pH	5.0	6.5	5.0–7.0
Sodium	154 mmol	130 mmol	131 mmol
Chloride	154 mmol	109 mmol	111 mmol
Other ions	None	Lactate: 28 mmol Potassium: 4 mmol Calcium: 2.7 mmol	Lactate: 29 mmol Potassium: 5.4 mmol Calcium: 2 mmol
Potential risks	Hyperchloremic metabolic acidosis Higher risk of pancreatic necrosis Renal vasoconstriction and acute kidney injury Coagulopathy	Metabolic alkalosis Hyperlactataemia Hypotonicity Relative contraindication in liver failure	
Potential benefits	In hypochloremic metabolic alkalosis (e.g., upper GI fluid losses, diabetic ketoacidosis) Universally available	Anti-inflammatory properties Reduces trypsin activity Provides extracellular calcium Lowers pancreatic acidosis	
Clinical data in AP	LR reduces ICU admission, length of stay, and adverse events in AP, compared to NS. Although RCTs have not evaluated Hartmann's solution, it has a similar composition to LR and could be used as an alternative when LR is not available		

reduced trypsin activity, increased extracellular calcium, and decreased pancreatic acidosis [29, 34, 35]. For all these reasons, LR is the crystalloid of choice in AP, and this is supported by societal guidelines and recently proposed quality indicators [16, 17, 22, 36]. In countries where LR is not available, Hartmann's solution with a similar composition can be used as an alternative.

7   Rate of Fluid Administration

One of the major areas of uncertainty in the management of patients with AP is about the volume and rate of fluid administration. Early observational studies found that the administration of ≥33% of the total fluid volume within the first 24 h was associated with lower rates of mortality and organ failure, supporting the view that early aggressive fluid resuscitation was beneficial [37, 38]. Subsequent observational studies raised concerns about the safety of early aggressive fluid resuscitation (>4 L within the first 24 h), because of higher rates of respiratory failure [39–41], acute kidney injury [40, 42], and local pancreatic complications [40, 43].

Data from RCTs have also produced conflicting results (Table 3). Two initial RCTs conducted by Mao et al. in patients with severe AP showed that rapid volume expansion (10–15 mL/kg/h) or rapid hemodilution (hematocrit <35% at 48 h) protocols were more harmful than controlled or slow hemodilution protocols, resulting in higher rates of sepsis and mortality [44, 45]. Three small RCTs comparing aggressive (20 mL/kg bolus, followed by 3 mL/kg/h) vs. nonaggressive (either determined by physician or 1.5 mL/kg/h with or without bolus) fluid resuscitation protocols in patients of any AP severity found no difference in surrogate outcomes (SIRS, C-reactive protein, hemoconcentration) [27, 46, 47]. Only a RCT by Buxbaum et al. conducted in 60 patients with predicted mild AP revealed that an aggressive fluid protocol (20 mL/kg bolus, followed by 3 mL/kg/h) was superior to nonaggressive fluids (15 mL/kg bolus, followed by 1.5 mL/kg/h) in reducing the composite surrogate outcome of SIRS and hemoconcentration [48]. Although none of these RCTs were sufficiently powered for clinically relevant outcomes, data from a recent meta-analysis of RCTs indicated that aggressive fluid resuscitation increased the risk

Table 3 Summary of RCTs comparing aggressive vs. nonaggressive fluid resuscitation in acute pancreatitis

Author (year), country	Design	N	Participants	Randomization[a]	Aggressive resuscitation	Nonaggressive resuscitation	Effect of early aggressive resuscitation
Mao et al. (2009) [45], China	Superiority	76	Severe AP	72 h	Rapid volume expansion (10–15 mL/kg/h)	Controlled volume expansion (5–10 mL/kg/h)	Harmful, more sepsis, mortality, mechanical ventilation and ACS
Mao et al. (2010) [44], China	Superiority	115	Severe AP	24 h	Rapid hemodilution with goal Hct <35% at 48 h	Slow hemodilution with goal Hct ≥35% at 48 h	Harmful, more sepsis and mortality
Wu et al. (2011) [27], USA	Factorial	40	Any severity	6 h	LR or NS bolus 20 mL/kg, followed by 3 mL/kg/h and then 1.5 mL/kg/h	LR or NS fluid therapy determined by treating physician	Similar, SIRS and CRP at 24 h
Buxbaum et al. (2017) [48], USA	Superiority	60	Predicted mild AP	4 h	LR bolus 20 mL/kg, then 3 mL/kg/h	LR bolus 15 mL/kg, then 1.5 mL/kg/h	Beneficial, less composite outcome, SIRS, and hemoconcentration
Cuellar-Monterrubio et al. (2020) [46], Mexico	Superiority	88	Any severity	>24 h from symptom onset	Bolus 20 mL/kg, then 3 mL/kg/h × 24 h, then 30 mL/kg × 24 h	No bolus, 1.5 mL/kg/h × 24 h, then 30 mL/kg × 24 h	Similar, SIRS, pancreatic necrosis, organ failure, and length of stay
Angsubhakorn et al. (2021) [47], Thailand	Superiority	44	Mild AP	<4 h from diagnosis	LR bolus 20 mL/kg, then 3 mL/kg/h	LR bolus 10 mL/kg, then 1.5 mL/kg/h	Similar, SIRS and hemoconcentration at 36 h
de Madaria et al. (2022) [21], Spain	Superiority	249	AP without moderately severe or severe AP	<8 h from diagnosis, <24 h from symptom onset	LR bolus 20 mL/kg, then 3 mL/kg/h	LR bolus 10 mL/kg only if hypovolemia was present, 1.5 mL/kg/h of LR	Harmful, more fluid overload, and similar progression to moderately severe or severe AP

Hct hematocrit, *ACS* abdominal compartment syndrome, *SIRS* systemic inflammatory response syndrome, *CRP* C-reactive protein, *LR* lactated Ringer's solution

[a] Maximal time interval allowed from time of initial hospital presentation to randomization

of mortality, adverse events, and sepsis [33]. However, these findings cannot be considered conclusive because some of the RCTs only included patients with severe AP while others only included patients with predicted mild AP.

A recent RCT by de-Madaria et al. (WATERFALL trial) has helped clarify the question about the rate of fluid administration in patients with AP [21]. This study was conducted at 18 centers across 4 countries (Spain, Italy, Mexico, India) and randomly assigned patients with AP of any severity to aggressive (20 mL/kg bolus, followed by 3 mL/kg/h) or moderate (1.5 mL/kg/h, with a bolus of 10 mL/kg only if hypovolemia was present) fluid resuscitation protocols. The study was powered to detect a difference in the development of moderately severe or severe AP (primary endpoint) with a sample size of 744 patients. The study also evaluated fluid overload as the main safety outcome and defined this on the basis of symptoms, physical signs, or imaging evidence of hypervolemia. The first planned interim analysis of 249 patients found that the odds of fluid overload in the aggressive-resuscitation group were 2.85 greater than with moderate resuscitation (20.5% vs. 6.5%, $p = 0.004$), but the incidence of moderately severe or severe AP was similar across treatment arms (22.1% in aggressive vs. 17.3% in moderate fluid protocol, $p = 0.32$). The results did not differ in subgroup analysis of patients with or without baseline hypovolemia or SIRS. Given that aggressive fluid resuscitation increased the rate of adverse events without any clinical benefits, the data and safety monitoring board terminated the trial early. The authors concluded that moderate fluid rate is more safe and as effective as aggressive fluid resuscitation.

To summarize, all patients with AP require early and adequate fluid resuscitation. IVFs need to be initiated at the time of diagnosis without delays. Based on the protocol used by the WATERFALL trial, most patients don't need a bolus at time of initiation of fluid therapy and should receive continuous fluids at a rate of 1.5 mL/kg/h, which is around 100 mL/h for an average patient weighing 70 kg. Patients with evidence of dehydration or hypovolemia should receive a fluid bolus of 10 mL/kg bolus over 1–2 h at time of fluid initiation, meaning around 700 mL for an average patient. Patients with predicted severe AP may require higher fluid rate as they are prone to capillary leak and greater third spacing. However, future studies are needed to determine what fluid rate is appropriate in this subset of patients with AP.

8   Optimization of Fluids and De-escalation

Following the initiation of fluid therapy aimed at restoring blood volume in the rescue phase, clinicians need to regularly assess the patients' ongoing fluid needs. This approach aims to assess the patient's volume status and correct fluid excess or deficits when detected. The appropriate frequency and methods to monitor volume status in AP are not well defined [49]. Even outside of AP, the quality of evidence for noninvasive tools to monitor fluid therapy is scant [50]. In well-conducted RCTs, volume status was monitored three times during the first 24 h and every 24 h thereafter [21, 27]. In the WATERFALL trial, checkpoints were conducted at 3, 12, and 24 h after fluid initiation, and this is a reasonable framework for the clinical management of most patients with AP. The frequency of these checkpoints may vary according to severity of the disease, duration of AP, and volume status. More frequent assessments will be necessary in patients with hypovolemia who respond poorly to initial fluid bolus, those with predicted severe and severe AP, or those at high risk for volume overload (e.g., heart failure, chronic kidney disease, cirrhosis).

Objective clinical assessment of volume status is required during each checkpoint (Table 4). Bedside markers of hypovolemia include hypotension (systolic blood pressure [BP] <90 mmHg or mean arterial pressure < 65 mmHg), signs and/or symptoms of dehydration (intense thirst, dehydrated oral mucosa, decreased skin turgor–skin pinch), and low urine output (<5 mL/kg/h). But there are limitations with clinical signs for the assessment of volume status. Hypotension is often compensated and delayed, tachycardia and

Table 4 Parameters of volume status and management during fluid optimization phase of AP

	Hypovolemia	Fluid overload*
Signs	Hypotension (systolic blood pressure <90 mmHg or mean arterial pressure <65 mmHg) Signs and/or symptoms of dehydration (intense thirst, dehydrated oral mucosa, decreased skin turgor–skin pinch) Low urine output (<5 mL/kg/h)	Dyspnea Peripheral edema Pulmonary rales Increased jugular venous pressure or hepatojugular reflux Oxygen saturation <92%
Ancillary tests	Elevated creatinine >1.1 mg/d High blood urea nitrogen (BUN) >20 mg/dL Increase in creatinine/BUN from prior value Hemoconcentration (hematocrit >44%)	Pulmonary congestion on chest X-ray
Management strategies	Fluid bolus of 10 mL/kg over 1–2 h Mini-bolus of 250 mL within 10–30 min Vasopressors when severe	Decrease or stop fluids Diuretics as needed Mechanical ventilation and/or hemofiltration when severe
Alternative methods to monitor volume status	Blood pressure monitoring with an arterial line Central venous pressure measurements Invasive stroke volume monitoring with a transducer or echocardiography Noninvasive cardiac output monitoring Passive leg raising test Artificial intelligence platforms	

In patients with fluid overload, acute respiratory distress syndrome (ARDS) has to be ruled out based on the presence of at least of two criteria:
A. Prompt response to diuretics and/or decrease in fluid rate and/or hemofiltration
B. Absence of ARDS criteria. Patients have ARDS if they meet the following four criteria: (1) onset within 1 week of the pancreatitis onset; (2) bilateral opacities not fully explained by effusions, lobar collapse, or nodules; (3) respiratory failure not fully explained by cardiac failure or fluid overload; (4) partial pressure of arterial oxygen (PaO_2)/fraction of inspired oxygen (FIO_2) ≤300

tachypnea are expected responses to pain, and anxiety and oliguria are a physiological response to stress. Laboratory tests that reflect hypovolemia include elevated creatinine >1.1 mg/d, high blood urea nitrogen (BUN) >20 mg/dL, increase in creatinine/BUN from prior value, or hemoconcentration (hematocrit >44%). More invasive methods of volume status, such as continuous BP monitoring with an arterial line, central venous pressure measurements, invasive stroke volume monitoring with a transducer or echocardiography, or noninvasive cardiac output monitoring, are feasible but not routinely used in clinical practice [51]. Recently, the passive leg raising test was successfully utilized in patients with predicted severe AP to assess the fluid response (by a change in stroke volume) and whether a patient required additional fluids between checkpoints, and this had advantages over objective clinical assessment [52]. Commonly used indicators of fluid overload include the presence of dyspnea, peripheral edema, pulmonary rales, increased jugular venous pressure or hepatojugular reflux,

pulmonary congestion on chest X-ray, and oxygen saturation of <92% [21]. Other markers such as S3–S4 heart sounds and pleural effusions are less reliable for diagnosis of fluid overload.

Patients with hypovolemia may benefit from a fluid bolus or mini-bolus. In the WATERFALL trial, patients with hypovolemia were given a fluid bolus of 10 mL/kg over 1–2 h [21]. An alternative approach would be administering a mini-bolus challenge of 250 mL within 10–30 min and assessing hemodynamic response before giving additional fluids; however, this may need more invasive monitoring for accuracy [52]. When mild fluid overload is suspected, intravenous fluids should be decreased or stopped. In severe fluid overload, patients may require diuretics and even ICU admission, mechanical ventilation, and/or hemofiltration. A more systemic method of determining volume status that uses widely available parameters and defined thresholds is urgently needed [51]. Fluid therapy in AP should be discontinued when patients are able to tolerate their fluid requirements orally for at least 4 h.

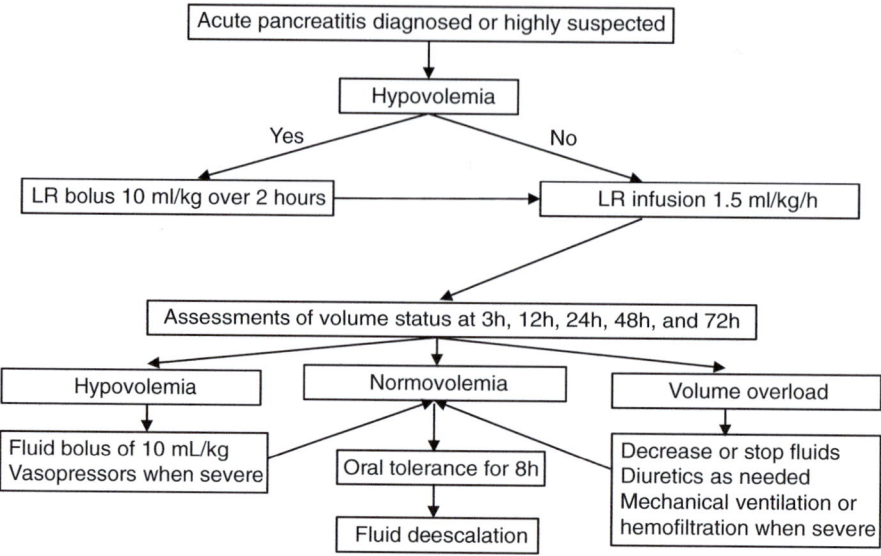

Fig. 1 Algorithm of fluid therapy in acute pancreatitis

9 Fluid Management Algorithm

Based on the available evidence and recommendations on fluid resuscitation described in this chapter, we propose a practical algorithm for fluid therapy in AP (Fig. 1).

10 Conclusion

Fluid resuscitation is critical to the management of patients with AP, but their needs vary greatly, and there is a need to develop goal-directed protocols that are sensitive to individual patient requirements. It is helpful to consider the four stages of fluid resuscitation (Table 1). Intravenous fluids should be started as soon as the diagnosis of AP is suspected or made. The fluid of choice is lactated Ringer's solution (LR). On balance, the available evidence indicates that aggressive fluid therapy (>10 mL/kg/h) is not appropriate and associated with increased risk of mortality (Table 2). And there is evidence that it is safer to normalize the hematocrit over 48–72 h. The WATERFALL randomized controlled trial in mainly mild AP indicates that moderate fluid resuscitation at 1.5 mL/kg/h is appropriate and

that this should be supplemented with fluid boluses of 10 mL/kg over 1–2 h if hypovolemia is present. It is less clear whether this is appropriate for patients with severe AP. Frequent assessment of patients to detect signs of hypovolemia or fluid overload is important and goes some way toward individualizing fluid resuscitation.

Acknowledgments None.

Financial Support and SponsorshipNone.

Conflicts of Interest None.

References

1. Machicado JD, Papachristou GI. Pharmacologic management and prevention of acute pancreatitis. Curr Opin Gastroenterol. 2019;35:460–7.
2. Sanfey H, Cameron JL. Increased capillary permeability: an early lesion in acute pancreatitis. Surgery. 1984;96:485–91.
3. Klar E, Messmer K, Warshaw AL, et al. Pancreatic ischaemia in experimental acute pancreatitis: mechanism, significance and therapy. Br J Surg. 1990;77:1205–10.
4. Kusterer K, Poschmann T, Friedemann A, et al. Arterial constriction, ischemia-reperfusion, and leukocyte adherence in acute pancreatitis. Am J Phys. 1993;265:G165–71.

5. Knoefel WT, Kollias N, Warshaw AL, et al. Pancreatic microcirculatory changes in experimental pancreatitis of graded severity in the rat. Surgery. 1994;116:904–13.

6. Cuthbertson CM, Christophi C. Disturbances of the microcirculation in acute pancreatitis. Br J Surg. 2006;93:518–30.

7. Komara NL, Paragomi P, Greer PJ, et al. Severe acute pancreatitis: capillary permeability model linking systemic inflammation to multiorgan failure. Am J Physiol Gastrointest Liver Physiol. 2020;319:G573–83.

8. Niederau C, Crass RA, Silver G, et al. Therapeutic regimens in acute experimental hemorrhagic pancreatitis. Effects of hydration, oxygenation, peritoneal lavage, and a potent protease inhibitor. Gastroenterology. 1988;95:1648–57.

9. Knol JA, Inman MG, Strodel WE, et al. Pancreatic response to crystalloid resuscitation in experimental pancreatitis. J Surg Res. 1987;43:387–92.

10. Martin DT, Steinberg SM, Kopolovic R, et al. Crystalloid versus colloid resuscitation in experimental hemorrhagic pancreatitis. Surg Gynecol Obstet. 1984;159:445–9.

11. Schmidt J, Fernandez-del Castillo C, Rattner DW, et al. Hyperoncotic ultrahigh molecular weight dextran solutions reduce trypsinogen activation, prevent acinar necrosis, and lower mortality in rodent pancreatitis. Am J Surg. 1993;165:40–4. discussion 45

12. Klar E, Foitzik T, Buhr H, et al. Isovolemic hemodilution with dextran 60 as treatment of pancreatic ischemia in acute pancreatitis. Clinical practicability of an experimental concept. Ann Surg. 1993;217:369–74.

13. Brown A, Baillargeon JD, Hughes MD, et al. Can fluid resuscitation prevent pancreatic necrosis in severe acute pancreatitis? Pancreatology. 2002;2:104–7.

14. Hamada S, Masamune A, Shimosegawa T. Transition of early-phase treatment for acute pancreatitis: an analysis of nationwide epidemiological survey. World J Gastroenterol. 2017;23:2826–31.

15. Matta B, Gougol A, Gao X, et al. Worldwide variations in demographics, management, and outcomes of acute pancreatitis. Clin Gastroenterol Hepatol. 2020;18(7):1567–1575.e2.

16. Tenner S, Baillie J, DeWitt J, et al. American College of Gastroenterology guideline: management of acute pancreatitis. Am J Gastroenterol. 2013;108:1400–15; 1416

17. Working Group IAPAPAAPG. IAP/APA evidence-based guidelines for the management of acute pancreatitis. Pancreatology. 2013;13:e1–15.

18. Crockett SD, Wani S, Gardner TB, et al. American gastroenterological association institute guideline on initial management of acute pancreatitis. Gastroenterology. 2018;154:1096–101.

19. Hoste EA, Maitland K, Brudney CS, et al. Four phases of intravenous fluid therapy: a conceptual model. Br J Anaesth. 2014;113:740–7.

20. Machicado JD, Papachristou GI. Intravenous fluid resuscitation in the management of acute pancreatitis. Curr Opin Gastroenterol. 2020;36:409–16.

21. de Madaria E, Buxbaum JL, Maisonneuve P, et al. Aggressive or moderate fluid resuscitation in acute pancreatitis. N Engl J Med. 2022;387:989–1000.

22. Vivian E, Cler L, Conwell D, et al. Acute pancreatitis task force on quality: development of quality indicators for acute pancreatitis management. Am J Gastroenterol. 2019;114:1322–42.

23. Sharma V, Rana SS, Sharma R, et al. Naso-jejunal fluid resuscitation in predicted severe acute pancreatitis: randomized comparative study with intravenous Ringer's lactate. J Gastroenterol Hepatol. 2016;31:265–9.

24. Zhao G, Zhang JG, Wu HS, et al. Effects of different resuscitation fluid on severe acute pancreatitis. World J Gastroenterol. 2013;19:2044–52.

25. Zarychanski R, Abou-Setta AM, Turgeon AF, et al. Association of hydroxyethyl starch administration with mortality and acute kidney injury in critically ill patients requiring volume resuscitation: a systematic review and meta-analysis. JAMA. 2013;309:678–88.

26. Finfer S, Myburgh J, Bellomo R. Intravenous fluid therapy in critically ill adults. Nat Rev Nephrol. 2018;14:541–57.

27. Wu BU, Hwang JQ, Gardner TH, et al. Lactated Ringer's solution reduces systemic inflammation compared with saline in patients with acute pancreatitis. Clin Gastroenterol Hepatol. 2011;9:710–7. e1

28. Choosakul S, Harinwan K, Chirapongsathorn S, et al. Comparison of normal saline versus lactated Ringer's solution for fluid resuscitation in patients with mild acute pancreatitis, A randomized controlled trial. Pancreatology. 2018;18:507–12.

29. de Madaria E, Herrera-Marante I, Gonzalez-Camacho V, et al. Fluid resuscitation with lactated Ringer's solution vs normal saline in acute pancreatitis: a triple-blind, randomized, controlled trial. United European Gastroenterol J. 2018;6:63–72.

30. Lee A, Ko C, Buitrago C, et al. Lactated ringers vs normal saline resuscitation for mild acute pancreatitis: a randomized trial. Gastroenterology. 2021;160:955–7. e4

31. Karki B, Thapa S, Khadka D, et al. Intravenous ringers lactate versus normal saline for predominantly mild acute pancreatitis in a Nepalese tertiary hospital. PLoS One. 2022;17:e0263221.

32. Guzman-Calderon E, Diaz-Arocutipa C, Monge E. Lactate ringer's versus normal saline in the management of acute pancreatitis: a systematic review and meta-analysis of randomized controlled trials. Dig Dis Sci. 2022;67:4131–9.

33. Di Martino M, Van Laarhoven S, Ielpo B, et al. Systematic review and meta-analysis of fluid therapy protocols in acute pancreatitis: type, rate and route. HPB (Oxford). 2021;23:1629–38.

34. Khatua B, Yaron JR, El-Kurdi B, et al. Ringer's lactate prevents early organ failure by providing extracellular calcium. J Clin Med. 2020;9

35. Hoque R, Farooq A, Ghani A, et al. Lactate reduces liver and pancreatic injury in toll-like receptor- and inflammasome-mediated inflammation via

GPR81-mediated suppression of innate immunity. Gastroenterology. 2014;146:1763–74.

36. Ketwaroo G, Sealock RJ, Freedman S, et al. Quality of care indicators in patients with acute pancreatitis. Dig Dis Sci. 2019;64:2514–26.

37. Gardner TB, Vege SS, Chari ST, et al. Faster rate of initial fluid resuscitation in severe acute pancreatitis diminishes in-hospital mortality. Pancreatology. 2009;9:770–6.

38. Warndorf MG, Kurtzman JT, Bartel MJ, et al. Early fluid resuscitation reduces morbidity among patients with acute pancreatitis. Clin Gastroenterol Hepatol. 2011;9:705–9.

39. Eckerwall G, Olin H, Andersson B, et al. Fluid resuscitation and nutritional support during severe acute pancreatitis in the past: what have we learned and how can we do better? Clin Nutr. 2006;25:497–504.

40. de Madaria E, Soler-Sala G, Sanchez-Paya J, et al. Influence of fluid therapy on the prognosis of acute pancreatitis: a prospective cohort study. Am J Gastroenterol. 2011;106:1843–50.

41. Li L, Jin T, Wen S, et al. Early rapid fluid therapy is associated with increased rate of noninvasive positive-pressure ventilation in hemoconcentrated patients with severe acute pancreatitis. Dig Dis Sci 2020, 65, 2700–2711.

42. Ye B, Mao W, Chen Y, et al. Aggressive resuscitation is associated with the development of acute kidney injury in acute pancreatitis. Dig Dis Sci. 2019;64:544–52.

43. Singh VK, Gardner TB, Papachristou GI, et al. An international multicenter study of early intravenous fluid administration and outcome in acute pancreatitis. United European Gastroenterol J. 2017;5:491–8.

44. Mao EQ, Fei J, Peng YB, et al. Rapid hemodilution is associated with increased sepsis and mortality among patients with severe acute pancreatitis. Chin Med J. 2010;123:1639–44.

45. Mao EQ, Tang YQ, Fei J, et al. Fluid therapy for severe acute pancreatitis in acute response stage. Chin Med J. 2009;122:169–73.

46. Cuellar-Monterrubio JE, Monreal-Robles R, Gonzalez-Moreno EI, et al. Nonaggressive versus aggressive intravenous fluid therapy in acute pancreatitis with more than 24 hours from disease onset: a randomized controlled trial. Pancreas. 2020;49:579–83.

47. Angsubhakorn A, Tipchaichatta K, Chirapongsathorn S. Comparison of aggressive versus standard intravenous hydration for clinical improvement among patients with mild acute pancreatitis: a randomized controlled trial. Pancreatology. 2021;21:1224–30.

48. Buxbaum JL, Quezada M, Da B, et al. Early aggressive hydration hastens clinical improvement in mild acute pancreatitis. Am J Gastroenterol. 2017;112:797–803.

49. Haydock MD, Mittal A, Wilms HR, et al. Fluid therapy in acute pancreatitis: anybody's guess. Ann Surg. 2013;257:182–8.

50. Wilms H, Mittal A, Haydock MD, et al. A systematic review of goal directed fluid therapy: rating of evidence for goals and monitoring methods. J Crit Care. 2014;29:204–9.

51. Froghi F, Soggiu F, Ricciardi F, et al. Ward based goal directed fluid therapy (GDFT) in acute pancreatitis (GAP) trial: a feasibility randomised controlled trial. Int J Surg. 2022;104:106737.

52. Jin T, Li L, Zhu P, et al. Optimising fluid requirements after initial resuscitation: a pilot study evaluating mini-fluid challenge and passive leg raising test in patients with predicted severe acute pancreatitis. Pancreatology. 2022;22:894.

Nutritional Support

Jenifer Barrie and Dileep N. Lobo

Key Points

1. Patients with severe acute pancreatitis should be considered to be at moderate to high nutritional risk, because of the catabolic nature of the disease and the impact of the patient's nutritional status for disease development.
2. The majority of patients with acute pancreatitis will experience a mild clinical course with a short hospital stay and do not need artificial nutritional support unless malnourished.
3. All patients with acute pancreatitis should be screened for nutritional risk using validated screening methods. Those found to be at nutritional risk should have a formal nutritional assessment.
4. Enteral nutrition is useful in the treatment or prevention of malnutrition in patients with severe acute pancreatitis when the gut is functional.
5. Parenteral nutrition, including fat, is well tolerated, does not stimulate pancreatic secretion and can minimise malnutrition when gastrointestinal dysfunction is prolonged.
6. A combination of enteral and parenteral nutrition is a reasonable way to meet metabolic demands in these patients, and the amount of nutrients delivered parenterally can be progressively reduced as larger volumes are tolerated enterally.
7. Particular attention should be paid to prevent refeeding syndrome.

Jenifer Barrie and Dileep N. Lobo contributed equally with all other contributors.

J. Barrie
Nottingham Digestive Diseases Centre, Division of Translational Medical Sciences, School of Medicine, University of Nottingham, Queen's Medical Centre, Nottingham, UK
e-mail: j.barrie@nhs.net

D. N. Lobo (✉)
National Institute for Health Research (NIHR) Nottingham Biomedical Research Centre, Nottingham University Hospitals NHS Trust and University of Nottingham, Queen's Medical Centre, Nottingham, UK

MRC Versus Arthritis Centre for Musculoskeletal Ageing Research, School of Life Sciences, University of Nottingham, Queen's Medical Centre, Nottingham, UK
e-mail: Dileep.Lobo@nottingham.ac.uk

© The Author(s), under exclusive license to Springer Nature Singapore Pte Ltd. 2024
J. A. Windsor et al. (eds.), *Acute Pancreatitis*, https://doi.org/10.1007/978-981-97-3132-9_11

1 Introduction

Patients with acute pancreatitis, particularly the severe form, should be considered to be at moderate to high nutritional risk, because of the catabolic nature of the disease and the impact of the patient's nutritional status for disease development [1, 2]. The principles of nutritional management of patients with acute pancreatitis have evolved over several decades. Traditionally the concept of 'pancreatic rest' (which is perhaps the oldest dogma in the management of acute pancreatitis) was used, and it was considered that enteral nutrition (EN), delivered into any part of the upper gastrointestinal tract other than the jejunum, stimulates pancreatic enzyme secretion, leading to increased pancreatic autodigestion and, consequently, exacerbation of the severity of acute pancreatitis [1, 3]. This concept is based on only physiologic assumption and is not supported by good-quality scientific evidence [1, 4]. Further studies have found that pancreatic enzyme secretion is significantly reduced in acute pancreatitis and the secretion was inversely related to the severity of pancreatitis [4]. A lower secretion of trypsin, amylase and lipase was found in severe pancreatitis [5], and these data suggest that the injured acinar cells cannot fully respond to physiologic stimuli, and may explain why enteral feeding is safe and does not worsen autodigestion during an attack of pancreatitis [4]. This chapter outlines the current principles of nutritional support of patients with acute pancreatitis.

The majority of patients with acute pancreatitis will experience a mild clinical course with a short hospital stay, whereas 10–20% of patients will develop severe acute pancreatitis with organ failure [6]. In severe acute pancreatitis, with the systemic inflammatory response syndrome (SIRS), the body enters a state of hypermetabolism and high protein breakdown, and during the course of the disease, the patient's energy and muscle reserves are depleted rapidly [7].

2 Assessment of Nutritional Requirements

Approximately one-third to two-thirds of patients with pancreatic diseases are at risk of malnutrition [8], but the incidence of malnutrition in patients with acute pancreatitis has not been specifically quantified. Patients with increased alcohol consumption and those with chronic substance misuse are more likely to have preexisting malnutrition and, in addition, may be depleted in micronutrients and vitamins [9].

Although there is no direct evidence that nutritional screening has an impact on outcome in acute pancreatitis, it is good clinical practice to screen all patients for nutritional risk at admission using validated screening methods such as the Nutritional Risk Screening 2002 (NRS-2002) [10] or the Malnutrition Universal Screening Tool (MUST) [11]. However, patients with predicted severe acute pancreatitis should always be considered at nutritional risk because of SIRS and the catabolic nature of the disease [2]. If patients are found to be at nutritional risk, nutritional assessment can be done using a variety of approaches, such as anthropometric and body composition measurements, food and nutrition-related history, clinical signs, biochemical data and functional assessment [12]. More recently, the Global Leadership Initiative on Malnutrition (GLIM) criteria have been advocated to diagnose malnutrition [13]. The GLIM criteria are a two-step approach for the diagnosis of malnutrition: first, screening to identify 'at risk' status by the use of any validated screening tool and, second, assessment for diagnosis and grading the severity of malnutrition [13]. The current approach to screening for and diagnosis of malnutrition is summarised in Fig. 1 [14].

Step 1: screening for nutritional risk

Use of validated screening tool (NRS)				
	Impaired nutritional status	**Points**	**Severity of the disease**	**Points**
Absent	Normal nutritional status	0	Normal nutritional requirements	0
Mild	Weight loss >5% of bodyweight in 3 months or food intake <50–75% of normal in the preceding week	1	Patients admitted to hospital due to complications associated with chronic diseases	1
Moderate	Weight loss >5% in 2 months; BMI 18·5–20·5 kg/m² and impaired general condition; or food intake 25–50% of normal in the preceding week	2	Patients confined to bed due to illness	2
Severe	Weight loss >5% in 1 month; BMI <18·0 kg/m² and impaired general condition; or food intake 0–25% of normal preceding week	3	Patients on intensive care units	3

+1 point if the patient is aged ≥70 years

If NRS score is ≥3 then patient is nutritionally at risk

Step 2: diagnosis of malnutrition

GLIM criteria

Phenotypic criteria		
Weight loss	**Low BMI**	**Reduced muscle mass**
>5% of bodyweight in the past 6 months or >10% of body weight in >6 months	<20 kg/m² (<18·5 kg/m² for Asian patients) for patients <70 years or <22 kg/m² (<20 kg/m² for Asian patients) for patients ≥70 years	Validated with body composition measuring techniques (eg, DXA, BIA, CT, and MRI)

Aetiological criteria	
Reduced food intake or assimilation	**Inflammation**
≤50% of energy requirement met by food intake for >1 week; any reduction in food intake for >2 weeks; or any chronic gastroenterological condition that adversely affects food assimilation or absorption	Acute disease (or injury) or chronic disease-related inflammation

Diagnosis of malnutrition if the patient has ≥1 from the phenotypic criteria and ≥1 from the aetiological criteria

Fig. 1 Current approach to screening and diagnosis. Approach to screening is according to NRS-2002 [8] and diagnosis is according to GLIM [11]. *BIA* bioelectrical impedance analysis, *BMI* body mass index, *DXA* dual-energy X-ray absorptiometry, *GLIM* global leadership initiative on malnutrition, *NRS* nutritional risk screening. Reproduced from Schuetz P et al. [14], with permission

3   Malnutrition in Pancreatitis

Resting energy expenditure (REE) in patients with acute pancreatitis is generally higher than in healthy individuals [15] because of a combination of inflammation-induced hypermetabolism and septic complications. It is also imperative that sepsis is dealt with, both to treat the disease and to achieve nutritional gains [15]. In fact, almost 60% of patients with severe acute pancreatitis have an increase in resting energy expenditure, and this increases when complicated by infection. Approximate net nitrogen losses are 20–40 g per day, and proteolysis of skeletal muscle can increase by up to 80% [16]. The circulating pool of amino acids decreases to as low as 40% of normal levels, while circulating and skeletal muscle glutamine levels drop to as low as 55% and 15%, respectively [17]. In one study it was found that muscle mass and function (measured by grip strength and respiratory muscle strength) rapidly decreased within 5 days without nutritional support in healthy men suffering from acute pancreatitis [18].

Energy requirements should be estimated with indirect calorimetry (IC) if possible, or 25 kcal/kg/d can be used as energy goal. A number of variables affect energy expenditure in severe pancreatitis, such as body temperature, volume status and medications, making predictive equations inaccurate and of limited value. Nevertheless, IC remains the gold standard to determine energy expenditure, helping to prevent over- or underfeeding [19]. It is recommended that energy requirements are re-evaluated more than once per week in order to ensure accurate energy balance [4].

4   Gut Factors in Acute Pancreatitis

Micro-organisms responsible for pancreatic infection and septic complications are generally common enteric bacteria normally present in the gut [20]. Gut barrier dysfunction may occur in up to 60% of patients with acute pancreatitis, mostly in severe acute pancreatitis. It is thought to lead to bacterial translocation and infection of necrosis [21]. The mechanisms in gut barrier dysfunction includes microcirculatory injury and hypovolemia, leading to gut mucosal ischaemia and reperfusion injury resulting in loss of gut barrier integrity [22]. Vulnerable ischaemic gut is also subject to the digestive action of activated pancreatic enzymes in the proximal small bowel [23], and this is, perhaps, an overlooked mechanism of injury.

The use of probiotics containing live micro-organisms of healthy gut flora has been shown to be detrimental in acute pancreatitis [24], and until an acceptable safety profile can be proven, their use should be avoided [25]. However, it is possible that the increased intestinal ischaemic events in the PROPATRIA study [24] had little to do with probiotics themselves but the aggressive approach to EN in patients who still had splanchnic vasoconstriction and were under-resuscitated.

Acute pancreatitis is also associated with deficiency of various vitamins and micronutrients including vitamins B_1, B_2, B_3, B_{12}, C, A, folic acid and zinc [26]. This could be pre-existing (as in the case of some patients with alcohol-induced pancreatitis) or could develop during the course of the disease. This may be both a cause and effect of gut dysfunction.

5   Obesity

Obesity has long been considered a risk factor for mortality in pancreatitis, as well as a risk factor for local and systemic complications [27, 28]. Excessive proinflammatory cytokines derived from visceral adipose tissue can promote the development of SIRS, which is thought to progress to organ failure and lead to death in patients with severe acute pancreatitis [29]. Obese patients have increased intra-pancreatic fat [30], and evidence suggests that the release of nonesterified fatty acids from pancreatic adipocytes may potentiate local pancreatic injury during acute pancreatitis [31]. Emerging evidence suggests that an obesity paradox also exists in patients with acute pancreatitis [32] and the presence of obesity may be protective.

At present there is a paucity of literature on feeding in obese patients with acute pancreatitis. However, in one recent study, it took longer for class III obese (BMI > 40 kg/m^2) patients to reach goal rate of jejunal feeding than non-class III obese patients, and this correlated with mortality [33]. It has been found in the laboratory that obesity aggravates acute pancreatitis via damage to the intestinal mucosal barrier and changing the composition of microbiota [34]. It is, thus, thought that obese patients have altered intestinal mucosal reactions to EN [33].

6 Evolution of Nutritional Support in Acute Pancreatitis

The contemporary evidence for nutritional support in patients with acute pancreatitis has been summarised in Table 1 [35–38], and an overview of the twentieth-century literature can be found here [1].

6.1 Oral Nutrition

The European Society of Parenteral and Enteral Nutrition (ESPEN) recommends that oral feeding with low-fat diet may be offered as soon as it is clinically tolerated in patients with predicted mild acute pancreatitis, independent of serum lipase (or amylase) concentrations [2]. The proven benefits of early oral feeding in patients with mild to moderate acute pancreatitis are now well recognised and have been translated into clinical practice. Patients are able to tolerate this, and it correlates with a shorter length of stay when compared with conventional oral feeding practices (traditionally introduced after resolution of symptoms or decrease in serum lipase or amylase) [39]. It is acceptable to start an oral diet without waiting for abdominal pain to abate, peristalsis to begin or appetite to recover. There is no benefit to applying restrictions based on biochemical results such as serum lipase or amylase concentrations, leukocyte counts or C-reactive protein concentrations in order to commence diet in patients with mild or moderate acute pancreatitis [40]. Oral feeding in the literature has classically been defined as immediate and early. More recently, immediate oral feeding and hunger-based feeding [41] have been studied.

Table 1 Contemporary evidence for current management of nutritional support in patients with acute pancreatitis

Author	Year	Type of study	Clinical question	Conclusions
Al-Omran et al. [35]	2010	Cochrane systematic review	PN vs. EN effect on mortality, morbidity and length of hospital stay in patients with acute pancreatitis	Enteral nutrition significantly reduced mortality, multiple organ failure, systemic infections and the need for operative interventions compared to those who received PN
Bakker et al. [36]	2014	Multicentre, randomised clinical trial	Early nasoenteral tube feeding vs. oral diet at 72 h after presentation with acute pancreatitis	Early nasoenteral tube feeding was not superior to oral diet in patients with acute pancreatitis at high risk for complications
Dutta et al. [37]	2020	Cochrane systematic review	NJ vs. NG in severe acute pancreatitis effect on mortality, morbidity and nutritional status	Insufficient evidence to conclude that there is superiority, inferiority or equivalence between the nasogastric and nasojejunal mode of enteral tube feeding in people with severe acute pancreatitis
Jiang et al. [38]	2020	Systematic review and meta-analysis	Clinical benefit of glutamine-supported early EN in patients with severe acute pancreatitis	Glutamine-supported early EN is beneficial in severe acute pancreatitis management

EN enteral nutrition, *PN* parenteral nutrition, *NJ* nasojejunal, *NG* nasogastric

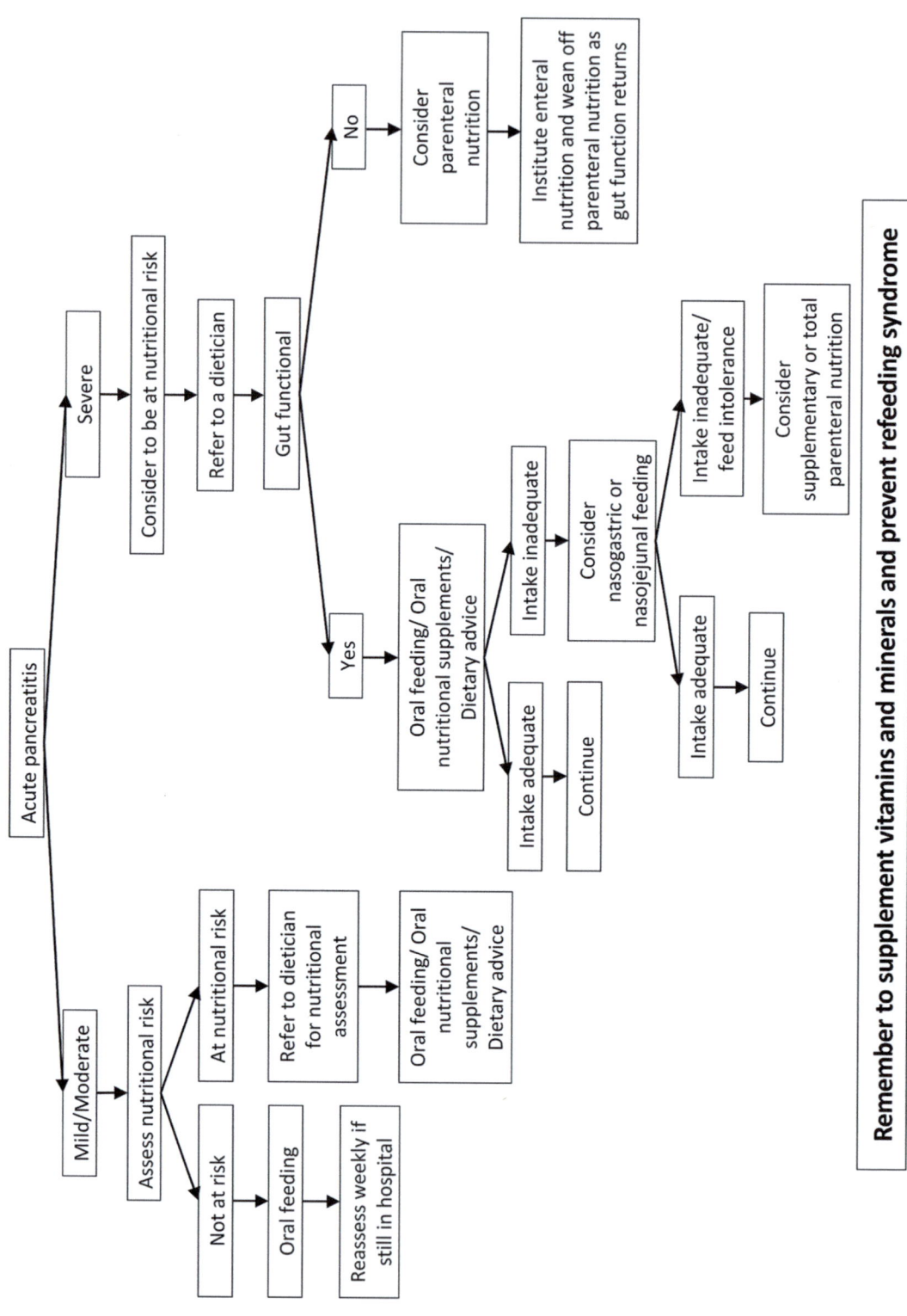

Fig. 2 Suggested algorithm for nutritional support in patients with acute pancreatitis

Hunger-based feeding is established on the physiology of hunger and the fact that experiencing hunger in acute pancreatitis demonstrates recovery of the gut [41]. The ESPEN guidelines recommend using low-fat, oral diet when reinitiating oral feeding in patients with mild acute pancreatitis [2]. Figure 2 demonstrates the role of oral feeding in acute pancreatitis.

Around 16% of patients with mild or moderate acute pancreatitis may have intolerance to oral feeding [25]. Oral feeding intolerance (OFI) is characterised by recurrent gastrointestinal symptoms on resuming an oral diet, such as abdominal pain, nausea and vomiting [42]. This is often accompanied by biochemical abnormalities and increased opioid requirements [42]. Relapse of pain can occur in 20% of patients after oral refeeding, which may, in turn, suggest severe acute pancreatitis [43]. Risk factors for OFI are summarised in Table 2. The timing of initiation of an oral diet does not appear to be related with the development of OFI, but OFI has been found to be associated with worse clinical outcomes including longer hospital length of stay and increased risk of admission to intensive care [42]. Oral food intake in patients undergoing minimally invasive necrosectomy is safe and feasible and may be initiated in the first 24 h after the procedure, if the clinical state (haemodynamic stability, septic parameters, gastric emptying) of the patients allows it [2]. Patients with acute pancreatitis who are discharged with gastrointestinal symptoms, or without having tolerated solid diet during their hospital stay, are at higher risk of early readmission [44]. Nausea and vomiting

Table 2 Risk factors associated with oral feeding intolerance (OFI) in patients with acute pancreatitis

Risk factors
Younger age
Male sex
Smoking
Active alcohol use
Elevated admission blood urea nitrogen
High admission haematocrit
Non-biliary pathology
Systemic inflammatory response at 48 h after admission
Pancreatic necrosis

may be due to gut dysmotility. Strategies to reduce this include the use of prokinetic agents and, in a recent study, soluble dietary fibre [45].

6.2 Enteral Nutrition

Oral feeding is sometimes not appropriate in patients with acute pancreatitis due to OFI often associated with significant symptoms of pain, nausea and vomiting, gastrointestinal dysmotility and severe or necrotising disease. The severity of pancreatitis is in itself not a contraindication to oral feeding. The preferred primary feeding route in patients with severe acute pancreatitis is enteral, as there are benefits over parenteral feeding [2]. For example, recent studies have found more than a twofold reduction in rates of multi-organ failure and almost a fourfold reduction in pancreatic necrosis with EN compared with parenteral nutrition (PN) across all severities of acute pancreatitis [46]. According to the ESPEN guidelines, EN should be started early, within 24–72 h of admission, in case of intolerance to oral feeding [2]. EN carries a lower potential for hyperglycaemia than PN [47]. The benefits of enteral over PN are most observable when EN is started within 48 h of admission [48].

However, aggressive EN in critically ill patients is not without risk. Abdominal distension caused by aggressive enteral feeding can compromise ventilation and respiratory function [49] and can also lead to an increase in intra-abdominal pressure and compartment syndrome. A multicentre study in critically ill patients showed that one or more gastrointestinal complications occurred in 62.8% of patients receiving EN, necessitating the withdrawal in 15.2% of patients [50]. Patients with gastrointestinal complications had a longer hospital stay (20.6 vs. 15.2 days, $P < 0.01$) and a higher mortality rate (31 vs. 16.1%, $P < 0.001$) than those without gastrointestinal complications [50]. The metabolic stress of aggressive enteral feeding in the under-resuscitated patient and in some critically ill patients can increase the risk of non-occlusive mesenteric ischaemia or enteral feeding intolerance (EFI) [51].

EN comprises nutritional preparations in liquid form, which are absorbed by the intestines. Typically, it involves the administration of nutrients directly into the stomach or small intestine. This can be done with either a nasogastric tube (NG) or a nasojejunal tube (NJ). NG feeding carries the advantages of ease of commencement due to the simplicity of bedside placement compared with the need for fluoroscopic or endoscopic placement of a NJ tube. There is a known aspiration risk with NG feeding, particularly in patients with a reduced Glasgow Coma Score. Any degree of gastroparesis or gastric outlet or duodenal obstruction resulting from retroperitoneal inflammation in severe pancreatitis is a contraindication to nasogastric feeding [37]. These patients will have early satiety, nausea and vomiting. In this case, insertion of a NJ tube should be considered, and a NG tube may be left in situ for gastric decompression. In a recent meta-analysis, post-pyloric feeding had a lower incidence rate of pulmonary aspiration, gastric reflux and pneumonia. It has also been attributed with a reduced incidence of gastrointestinal complications such as vomiting, nausea, diarrhoea, abdominal distension, high gastric residual volume and constipation. It has been associated with more optimal nutrition as measured by the percentage of total nutrition provided to the patient, the time to tolerate EN and the time required to reach nutritional targets. Shorter length of mechanical ventilation, critical care and hospital stay have also been attributed to post-pyloric feeding [52]. However, in an up-to-date Cochrane systematic review looking at severe acute pancreatitis, there was not sufficient evidence to conclude that there is superiority, inferiority or equivalence between the NG and NJ mode of enteral tube feeding [37]. In practical terms it would be beneficial to insert the NG and start feeding into the stomach and then change to post-pyloric feeding if there were any early signs of gastric outlet obstruction or impaired gastric emptying.

In patients who need tube feeding, current guidelines recommend continuous feeding over bolus feeding [53]. Better feeding tolerance and fewer interruptions of delivery of EN due to elevated residuals and vomiting were found with continuous infusion of feed [54].

A wide range of supplemental feeds are available, but the main categories of feed are broadly subdivided into oligomeric feeds, polymeric feeds and immunonutrition [25]. EN can also be given orally, most often as a supplement to oral intake (oral nutritional supplements—ONS) [20].

Oligomeric, also termed semi-elemental, formulations contain small peptides, medium chain fatty acids and simple polysaccharides. Polymeric feeds contain full proteins, complex lipids and carbohydrates. Oligomeric formulations do not require digestion by pancreatic enzymes, so, in theory, these offer a greater degree of pancreatic rest than the polymeric feeds [25] and, although more expensive, they are better tolerated in patients with acute pancreatitis. Having said that, there has been no demonstrable clinical advantage with the use of oligomeric formulations, so relatively inexpensive polymeric formulations should be used [25]. Other specialised formulations are also available for clinical use.

Immunonutrition refers to specialised formulations composed of immunomodulatory supplements that are believed to enhance the immune response. These formulations are enhanced by specific amino acids such as glutamine or arginine, ω3FAs and nucleotides with the potential to modify the immune response [37]. Data from experimental studies have demonstrated that marine ω-3 polyunsaturated fatty acids (ω3FAs) have anti-inflammatory properties [55]. ω3FA administration in the early phase of acute pancreatitis and sepsis appears safe and has the potential to reduce the incidence of acute organ dysfunction, infectious complications and mortality [56]. Glutamine improves lymphocyte function and contributes to antioxidative defences. It can also support the intestinal integrity and decrease bacterial translocation, hence reducing systemic inflammatory responses and sepsis, which are important in critical illnesses such as acute pancreatitis [57]. Glutamine-supplemented EN has been shown to improve outcomes in pancreatitis in terms of mortality, multi-organ failure and length of hospital stay in initial studies. It has also been found that supplementing PN but not EN with glutamine may be of value [58]. Additional high-quality, large-scale RCTs or multi-centre collaborative research is required to confirm these findings [38].

When EN is not feasible (EFI) or contraindicated and PN is indicated, parenteral glutamine should be supplemented at 0.20 g/kg/day of L-glutamine [2]. The advantages of glutamine supplementation include reduced mortality [59], rate of infections and length of hospital stay [59–61], but large-scale high-quality trials are necessary before glutamine can be recommended in routine clinical practice.

Other specialised formulations include fibre-enhanced formulations that can stimulate the growth of normal enteral micro-organisms, probiotic-enhanced formulations containing live bacteria or yeasts and symbiotic formulations that contain probiotics and prebiotic fibres. There is not enough evidence to support any of these formulations as a preferred feeding method [37, 62].

EN can be given safely even in severe acute pancreatitis complicated by fistulae, ascites or pseudocysts [63] unless there is EFI. In cases of ileus, it is still suggested to administer EN in reduced amounts [63]. Common complications in patients receiving EN include EFI, abdominal distension, diarrhoea and tube displacement or blockage [7]. In the event of EFI, patients should be started on PN within 72 h [64]. Trophic feeding, defined as a small volume of balanced EN insufficient for the patient's nutritional needs, has been recommended as it may help maintain gastrointestinal mucosal integrity and produce some positive gastrointestinal or systemic benefit [65]. There is, however, no specific evidence for the benefit of trophic feeding in patients with severe acute pancreatitis.

In patients who require nasoenteral tube feeding for an extended period (typically beyond 30 days), other feeding options should be considered. Complications of prolonged duration of NG or NJ feeding include sinusitis and nasal passage trauma, malpositioning or inadvertent removal of the tube [66]. Complications of EN are listed in Table 3. In these patients, a percutaneous endoscopic gastrostomy, surgical jejunostomy or gastrojejunostomy (by an endoscopic, laparoscopic or open approach) should be considered. There is a paucity of literature regarding extended enteral feeding and further studies are required to clarify the optimal method for long-term EN.

6.3   Parenteral Nutrition

PN is the intravenous administration of nutrients that a patient receives via a catheter inserted directly into a major central or via a smaller peripheral vein [20]. PN is indicated in patients with severe acute pancreatitis who do not tolerate EN over 72 h, where a NG or NJ tube cannot be placed, or patients who are unable to achieve targeted requirements (Fig. 2).

Increased mortality has been demonstrated in a subset of patients with severe acute pancreatitis receiving PN. This is thought to reflect the severity of disease rather than due to a complication of PN, including catheter-related infections, sepsis, metabolic derangements and gut barrier dysfunction (Table 3). The lack of stimulus for peristalsis can result in hypomotility of the gut, and stagnant bowel contents can lead to significant changes in the intestinal microflora, including bacterial overgrowth and dysbiosis [63]. Patients receiving PN have been shown to require a significantly higher dose of insulin in order to achieve normoglycaemia than those having EN [47]. It is worth noting that it is believed that hyperglycaemia influences the risk of infectious complications and mortality [47] through a number of potential mechanisms including oxidative stress, cytokine activation and hypercoagulability [47].

In some patients, a combination of EN and PN is a reasonable way to meet metabolic and nutrient demands, and the amount of nutrients delivered parenterally can be progressively reduced as larger volumes are tolerated enterally. Complications of EN are listed in Table 3.

Table 3 Some complications of artificial nutrition

Enteral nutrition	Parenteral nutrition
Tube insertion • Nasal/oesophageal injury • Oesophagitis • Oesophageal erosions • Oesophageal stricture • Tube misplacement • Tube displacement/withdrawal • Tube blockage	Catheter-related or catheter insertion-related • Pneumothorax • Haemothorax • Hydrothorax (intrapleural infusion of feed) • Arterial injuries • Nerve injuries • Air embolism • Catheter/central venous thrombosis • Arrhythmias
Regurgitation and aspiration	Catheter-related sepsis
Gastrointestinal • Diarrhoea • Abdominal distension • Abdominal pain	Gastrointestinal • Increased gastric acid secretion • Intestinal stasis • Bacterial overgrowth
Metabolic • Hyperglycaemia • Hypokalaemia • Hypomagnesaemia • Hypocalcaemia • Hypophosphataemia • Low zinc • Low RBC folate • Refeeding syndrome	Metabolic • Hyperglycaemia • Rebound hypoglycaemia and hyperkalaemia • Hypokalaemia • Hyponatraemia • Hypomagnesaemia • Hypocalcaemia • Hypophosphataemia • Low zinc • Low RBC folate • Vitamin/trace element deficiencies • Osteomalacia • Metabolic acidosis • Hyperammonaemia • Refeeding syndrome
Abnormal liver function tests	Hepatic dysfunction • Abnormal liver function tests • Jaundice • Intrahepatic cholestasis • Biliary sludge • Fatty liver
Intravenous administration of enteral feed	Fluid and electrolyte abnormalities

7　Refeeding Syndrome

Refeeding syndrome is a life-threatening metabolic complication that results from rapid feeding in combination with inadequate provision of micronutrients and electrolytes (e.g. phosphate, potassium, magnesium and vitamin B_1) [14]. The syndrome can occur with oral, enteral or PN [67], and is often not recognised or treated appropriately [68]. The National Institute for Health and Care Excellence (NICE) criteria (low BMI; significant unintentional weight loss; insufficient nutritional intake; low concentrations of potassium, phosphate or magnesium prior to feeding;

or a history of alcohol abuse or drugs including insulin, chemotherapy, antacids or diuretics) are helpful for identification of patients at high risk of refeeding syndrome, with starvation being the predominant risk factor [69].

Patients with acute pancreatitis who have not been fed, particularly those with alcohol-induced pancreatitis and pre-existing malnutrition, are at high risk of developing refeeding syndrome. Diagnostic criteria for imminent refeeding syndrome have been defined as decrease in phosphate concentrations from baseline by >30% or to <0.6 mmol/L or any two other electrolyte shifts below the normal range (phosphate, magnesium, potassium) within 72 h of starting nutritional therapy [70]. In addition, manifest refeeding syndrome is diagnosed when any electrolyte shifts occur in combination with clinical symptoms (e.g. oedema, tachycardia, tachypnoea, neurological symptoms, etc.) [70]. Risk assessment, establishment of a care plan and monitoring of patients throughout nutritional therapy are important to reduce refeeding syndrome-related morbidity. Patients at risk should receive generous prophylactic provision of electrolytes unless plasma concentrations are high (potassium 2–4 mmol/kg/day, phosphate 0.3–0.6 mmol/kg/day, magnesium 0.2–0.4 mmol/kg/day) [69]. Patients should also receive vitamin B_1 (thiamine, 200–300 mg daily) and multivitamin supplements immediately before and during the first 10 days of feeding [69]. There are also dangers of excess provision of sodium and fluid in patients at risk of the refeeding syndrome, and an intake of <1 mmol/kg/day sodium and 20 ml/kg/day fluid is recommended in the early phase of refeeding [67, 71]. Nutritional therapy should be started with reduced energy goals and increased slowly to the full caloric requirements over 5–10 days according to the individual risk classification [70]. Electrolyte concentrations should be monitored daily during the vulnerable refeeding period alongside additional clinical examination, with special attention to hydration status as well as vital parameters to detect signs and symptoms of fluid overload and/or micronutrient deficiency.

8   Conclusion

Nutritional therapy in patients with acute pancreatitis is generally safe, with low risk of complications. EN is useful in the treatment or prevention of malnutrition in patients with acute pancreatitis when the gut is functional and when nutritional requirements cannot be met by oral feeding. PN, including fat, is well tolerated, does not stimulate pancreatic secretion and can minimise malnutrition when gastrointestinal dysfunction is prolonged. A diagnosis of acute pancreatitis alone is not an indication for instituting artificial nutrition as most patients with mild or moderate acute pancreatitis can tolerate an oral diet. Nevertheless, in severe disease in patients who are hypercatabolic and/or unable to eat normally, it is prudent to begin early artificial nutrition either parenterally or via the jejunum, or both, in order to prevent the clinical consequences of malnutrition. The establishment and maintenance of jejunal access in patients with severe acute pancreatitis may be problematic, and it may be difficult to achieve the targeted intrajejunal nutrient delivery within the first few days. A combination of EN and PN is, therefore, a reasonable way to meet metabolic demands in these patients, and the amount of nutrients delivered parenterally can be progressively reduced as larger volumes are tolerated enterally. Particular attention should be paid to prevent refeeding syndrome.

Declarations
Conflict of Interest None of the authors have a direct conflict of interest to declare.

Funding No external funding was received for this book chapter.

References

1. Lobo DN, Memon MA, Allison SP, Rowlands BJ. Evolution of nutritional support in acute pancreatitis. Br J Surg. 2000;87(6):695–707.
2. Arvanitakis M, Ockenga J, Bezmarevic M, Gianotti L, Krznarić Ž, Lobo DN, et al. ESPEN guideline on clinical nutrition in acute and chronic pancreatitis. Clin Nutr. 2020;39(3):612–31.
3. Petrov MS. Moving beyond the 'pancreatic rest' in severe and critical acute pancreatitis. Crit Care. 2013;17(4):1–2.
4. Lakananurak N, Gramlich L. Nutrition management in acute pancreatitis: clinical practice consideration. World J Clin Cases. 2020;8(9):1561.
5. O'Keefe SJ, Lee RB, Li J, Stevens S, Abou-Assi S, Zhou W. Trypsin secretion and turnover in patients with acute pancreatitis. Am J Physiol Gastrointest Liver Physiol. 2005;289(2):G181–G7.
6. Mofidi R, Duff M, Wigmore S, Madhavan K, Garden O, Parks R. Association between early systemic inflammatory response, severity of multiorgan dysfunction and death in acute pancreatitis. Br J Surg. 2006;93(6):738–44.

7. Liu M, Gao C. A systematic review and meta-analysis of the effect of total parenteral nutrition and enteral nutrition on the prognosis of patients with acute pancreatitis. Ann Palliat Med. 2021;10(10):10779–88.

8. Tangvik RJ, Tell GS, Guttormsen AB, Eisman JA, Henriksen A, Nilsen RM, et al. Nutritional risk profile in a university hospital population. Clin Nutr. 2015;34(4):705–11.

9. Ross LJ, Wilson M, Banks M, Rezannah F, Daglish M. Prevalence of malnutrition and nutritional risk factors in patients undergoing alcohol and drug treatment. Nutrition. 2012;28(7–8):738–43.

10. Kondrup J, Rasmussen HH, Hamberg O, Stanga Z, Ad Hoc ESPEN Working Group. Nutritional risk screening (NRS 2002): a new method based on an analysis of controlled clinical trials. Clin Nutr. 2003;22(3):321–36.

11. Weekes CE, Elia M, Emery PW. The development, validation and reliability of a nutrition screening tool based on the recommendations of the British Association for Parenteral and Enteral Nutrition (BAPEN). Clin Nutr. 2004;23(5):1104–12.

12. Prado C, Ford K, Gonzalez M, Murnane L, Gillis C, Wischmeyer P, et al. Nascent to novel methods to evaluate malnutrition and frailty in the surgical patient. JPEN J Parenter Enter Nutr. 2023; 47(Suppl1):S54–68.

13. Cederholm T, Jensen GL, Correia M, Gonzalez MC, Fukushima R, Higashiguchi T, et al. GLIM criteria for the diagnosis of malnutrition—A consensus report from the global clinical nutrition community. Clin Nutr. 2019;38(1):1–9.

14. Schuetz P, Seres D, Lobo DN, Gomes F, Kaegi-Braun N, Stanga Z. Management of disease-related malnutrition for patients being treated in hospital. Lancet. 2021;398(10314):1927–38.

15. Chandrasegaram MD, Plank LD, Windsor JA. The impact of parenteral nutrition on the body composition of patients with acute pancreatitis. JPEN J Parenter Enter Nutr. 2005;29(2):65–73.

16. Dickerson RN, Vehe KL, Mullen JL, Feurer ID. Resting energy expenditure in patients with pancreatitis. Crit Care Med. 1991;19(4):484–90.

17. Arutla M, Raghunath M, Deepika G, Jakkampudi A, Murthy H, Rao G, et al. Efficacy of enteral glutamine supplementation in patients with severe and predicted severe acute pancreatitis—a randomized controlled trial. Ind J Gastroenterol. 2019;38(4):338–47.

18. Hill GL, Jonathan E, Lecture R. Body composition research: implications for the practice of clinical nutrition. JPEN J Parenter Enter Nutr. 1992;16(3):197–218.

19. Bendavid I, Lobo DN, Barazzoni R, Cederholm T, Coeffier M, de van der Schueren M, et al. The centenary of the Harris-Benedict equations: how to assess energy requirements best? Recommendations from the ESPEN expert group. Clin Nutr. 2021;40(3):690–701.

20. Poropat G, Giljaca V, Hauser G, Štimac D. Enteral nutrition formulations for acute pancreatitis. Cochrane Database Syst Rev. 2015;(3):CD010605.

21. Wu L, Sankaran S, Plank L, Windsor J, Petrov M. Meta-analysis of gut barrier dysfunction in patients with acute pancreatitis. Br J Surg. 2014;101(13):1644–56.

22. Akshintala VS, Talukdar R, Singh VK, Goggins M. The gut microbiome in pancreatic disease. Clin Gastroenterol Hepatol. 2019;17(2):290–5.

23. Schmid-Schonbein GW, Hugli TE. A new hypothesis for microvascular inflammation in shock and multiorgan failure: self-digestion by pancreatic enzymes. Microcirculation. 2005;12(1):71–82.

24. Besselink MG, van Santvoort HC, Buskens E, Boermeester MA, van Goor H, Timmerman HM, et al. Probiotic prophylaxis in predicted severe acute pancreatitis: a randomised, double-blind, placebo-controlled trial. Lancet. 2008;371(9613):651–9.

25. Kanthasamy KA, Akshintala VS, Singh VK. Nutritional management of acute pancreatitis. Gastroenterol Clin N Am. 2021;50(1):141–50.

26. Jabłońska B, Mrowiec S. Nutritional support in patients with severe acute pancreatitis-current standards. Nutrients. 2021;13(5):1498.

27. Martinez J, Johnson C, Sanchez-Paya J, De Madaria E, Robles-Diaz G, Pérez-Mateo M. Obesity is a definitive risk factor of severity and mortality in acute pancreatitis: an updated meta-analysis. Pancreatology. 2006;6(3):206–9.

28. Hall T, Stephenson J, Jones M, Ngu W, Horsfield M, Rajesh A, et al. Is abdominal fat distribution measured by axial CT imaging an indicator of complications and mortality in acute pancreatitis? J Gastrointest Surg. 2015;19(12):2126–31.

29. Higaki Y, Nishida T, Matsumoto K, Yamaoka S, Osugi N, Sugimoto A, et al. Effect of abdominal visceral fat on mortality risk in patients with severe acute pancreatitis. JGH Open. 2021;5(12):1357–62.

30. Saisho Y, Butler A, Meier J, Monchamp T, Allen-Auerbach M, Rizza R, et al. Pancreas volumes in humans from birth to age one hundred taking into account sex, obesity, and presence of type-2 diabetes. Clin Anat. 2007;20(8):933–42.

31. Navina S, Acharya C, DeLany JP, Orlichenko LS, Baty CJ, Shiva SS, et al. Lipotoxicity causes multisystem organ failure and exacerbates acute pancreatitis in obesity. Sci Transl Med. 2011;3(107):107ra110.

32. Premkumar R, Phillips AR, Petrov MS, Windsor JA. The clinical relevance of obesity in acute pancreatitis: targeted systematic reviews. Pancreatology. 2015;15(1):25–33.

33. Hegazi R, Raina A, Graham T, Rolniak S, Centa P, Kandil H, et al. Early jejunal feeding initiation and clinical outcomes in patients with severe acute pancreatitis. JPEN J Parenter Enteral Nutr. 2011;35(1):91–6.

34. Ye C, Liu L, Ma X, Tong H, Gao J, Tai Y, et al. Obesity aggravates acute pancreatitis via damaging intestinal mucosal barrier and changing microbiota composition in rats. Sci Rep. 2019;9(1):1–9.

35. Al-Omran M, AlBalawi ZH, Tashkandi MF, Al-Ansary LA. Enteral versus parenteral nutrition

for acute pancreatitis. Cochrane Database Syst Rev. 2010;(1):CD002837.

36. Bakker OJ, van Brunschot S, van Santvoort HC, Besselink MG, Bollen TL, Boermeester MA, et al. Early versus on-demand nasoenteric tube feeding in acute pancreatitis. N Engl J Med. 2014;371(21):1983–93.

37. Dutta AK, Goel A, Kirubakaran R, Chacko A, Tharyan P. Nasogastric versus nasojejunal tube feeding for severe acute pancreatitis. Cochrane Database Syst Rev. 2020;3(3):CD010582.

38. Jiang X, Pei L-Y, Guo W-X, Qi X, Lu X-G. Glutamine supported early enteral therapy for severe acute pancreatitis: a systematic review and metaanalysis. Asia Pac J Clin Nutr. 2020;29(2):253–61.

39. Arvanitakis M, Gkolfakis P, Viesca MFY. Nutrition in acute pancreatitis. Curr Opin Clin Nutr Metab Care. 2021;24(5):428–32.

40. Ramírez-Maldonado E, López Gordo S, Pueyo EM, Sanchez-Garcia A, Mayol S, Gonzalez S, et al. Immediate oral refeeding in patients with mild and moderate acute pancreatitis: a multicenter, randomized controlled trial (PADI trial). Ann Surg. 2021;274(2):255–63.

41. Rai A, Anandhi A, Sureshkumar S, Kate V. Hunger-based versus conventional oral feeding in moderate and severe acute pancreatitis: a randomized controlled trial. Dig Dis Sci. 2022;67(6):2535–42.

42. Pothoulakis I, Nawaz H, Paragomi P, Jeong K, Talukdar R, Kochhar R, et al. Incidence and risk factors of oral feeding intolerance in acute pancreatitis: results from an international, multicenter, prospective cohort study. UEG J. 2021;9(1):54–62.

43. Petrov MS, Van Santvoort HC, Besselink MG, Cirkel GA, Brink MA, Gooszen HG. Oral refeeding after onset of acute pancreatitis: a review of literature. Am J Gastroenterol. 2007;102(9):2079–84.

44. Whitlock TL, Repas K, Tignor A, Conwell D, Singh V, Banks PA, et al. Early readmission in acute pancreatitis: incidence and risk factors. Am J Gastroenterol. 2010;105(11):2492–7.

45. Chen T, Ma Y, Xu L, Sun C, Xu H, Zhu J. Soluble dietary fiber reduces feeding intolerance in severe acute pancreatitis: a randomized study. JPEN J Parenter Enteral Nutr. 2021;45(1):125–35.

46. Vege SS, DiMagno MJ, Forsmark CE, Martel M, Barkun AN. Initial medical treatment of acute pancreatitis: American Gastroenterological Association Institute technical review. Gastroenterology. 2018;154(4):1103–39.

47. Petrov MS, Zagainov VE. Influence of enteral versus parenteral nutrition on blood glucose control in acute pancreatitis: a systematic review. Clin Nutr. 2007;26(5):514–23.

48. Petrov M, Loveday B, Pylypchuk R, McIlroy K, Phillips A, Windsor J. Systematic review and meta-analysis of enteral nutrition formulations in acute pancreatitis. Br J Surg. 2009;96(11):1243–52.

49. Watters JM, Kirkpatrick SM, Norris SB, Shamji FM, Wells GA. Immediate postoperative enteral feed-

ing results in impaired respiratory mechanics and decreased mobility. Ann Surg. 1997;226(3):369–77; discussion 77–80

50. Montejo JC. Enteral nutrition-related gastrointestinal complications in critically ill patients: a multicenter study. The Nutritional and Metabolic Working Group of the Spanish Society of Intensive Care Medicine and Coronary Units. Crit Care Med. 1999;27(8):1447–53.

51. Al-Diery H, Phillips A, Evennett N, Pandanaboyana S, Gilham M, Windsor JA. The pathogenesis of nonocclusive mesenteric ischemia: implications for research and clinical practice. J Intensive Care Med. 2019;34(10):771–81.

52. Liu Y, Wang Y, Zhang B, Wang J, Sun L, Xiao Q. Gastric-tube versus post-pyloric feeding in critical patients: a systematic review and meta-analysis of pulmonary aspiration-and nutrition-related outcomes. Eur J Clin Nutr. 2021;75(9):1337–48.

53. Tenner S, Baillie J, DeWitt J, Vege SS. American College of Gastroenterology guideline: management of acute pancreatitis. Am J Gastroenterol. 2013;108(9):1400–15.

54. Van Dyck L, Casaer MP. Intermittent or continuous feeding: any difference during the first week? Curr Opin Crit Care. 2019;25(4):356–62.

55. Aldoori J, Cockbain AJ, Toogood GJ, Hull MA. Omega-3 polyunsaturated fatty acids: moving towards precision use for prevention and treatment of colorectal cancer. Gut. 2022;71(4):822–37.

56. Wolbrink DR, Grundsell JR, Witteman B, van de Poll M, van Santvoort HC, Issa E, et al. Are omega-3 fatty acids safe and effective in acute pancreatitis or sepsis? A systematic review and meta-analysis. Clin Nutr. 2020;39(9):2686–94.

57. O'Riordain M, De Beaux A, Fearon K. Effect of glutamine on immune function in the surgical patient. Nutrition. 1996;12(11–12 Suppl):S82–4.

58. Asrani V, Chang WK, Dong Z, Hardy G, Windsor JA, Petrov MS. Glutamine supplementation in acute pancreatitis: a meta-analysis of randomized controlled trials. Pancreatology. 2013;13(5):468–74.

59. Yong L, Lu QP, Liu SH, Fan H. Efficacy of glutamine-enriched nutrition support for patients with severe acute pancreatitis: a meta-analysis. JPEN J Parenter Enteral Nutr. 2016;40(1):83–94.

60. Jafari T, Feizi A, Askari G, Fallah AA. Parenteral immunonutrition in patients with acute pancreatitis: a systematic review and meta-analysis. Clin Nutr. 2015;34(1):35–43.

61. Jeurnink S, Nijs M, Prins H, Greving J, Siersema P. Antioxidants as a treatment for acute pancreatitis: a meta-analysis. Pancreatology. 2015;15(3):203–8.

62. Sharma B, Srivastava S, Singh N, Sachdev V, Kapur S, Saraya A. Role of probiotics on gut permeability and endotoxemia in patients with acute pancreatitis: a double-blind randomized controlled trial. J Cin Gastroenterol. 2011;45(5):442–8.

63. Oláh A, Romics L Jr. Enteral nutrition in acute pancreatitis: a review of the current evidence. World J Gastroenterol. 2014;20(43):16123.

64. Mederos MA, Reber HA, Girgis MD. Acute pancreatitis: a review. JAMA. 2021;325(4):382–90.

65. Sondheimer JM. A critical perspective on trophic feeding. J Pediatr Gastroenterol Nutr. 2004;38(3): 237–8.

66. Ramanathan M, Aadam AA. Nutrition management in acute pancreatitis. Nutr Clin Pract. 2019;34(Suppl1):S7–S12.

67. Stanga Z, Brunner A, Leuenberger M, Grimble RF, Shenkin A, Allison SP, et al. Nutrition in clinical practice-the refeeding syndrome: illustrative cases and guidelines for prevention and treatment. Eur J Clin Nutr. 2008;62(6):687–94.

68. Schuetz P, Zurfluh S, Stanga Z. Mortality due to refeeding syndrome? You only find what you look for, and you only look for what you know. Eur J Clin Nutr. 2018;72(2):307–8.

69. National Collaborating Centre for Acute Care. Nutrition support in adults: oral nutrition support, enteral tube feeding and parenteral nutrition. 2006. https://www.nice.org.uk/guidance/cg32/evidence/full-guideline-194889853. Accessed 9 Jan 2023.

70. Friedli N, Stanga Z, Culkin A, Crook M, Laviano A, Sobotka L, et al. Management and prevention of refeeding syndrome in medical inpatients: an evidence-based and consensus-supported algorithm. Nutrition. 2018;47:13–20.

71. Nightingale J, Turner P, De Silva A, and the BIFA Committee. Top tips for preventing and managing refeeding syndrome https://www.bapen.org.uk/pdfs/bifa/bifa-top-tips-series-7.pdf. Accessed 9 Jan 2023.

Antibiotics and Probiotics

Rupjyoti Talukdar

Key Points

1. Increase in the total leucocyte count and fever in the first week of acute pancreatitis (AP) are usually due to non-septic systemic inflammatory response syndrome (SIRS).
2. Prophylactic antibiotics have not shown consistent benefit in the higher-quality studies and are not recommended.
3. Empirical antibiotics in patients with acute necrotizing pancreatitis should be started based on clinical and radiological.
4. Choice of empirical antibiotics should be those which penetrate the necrotic pancreas.
5. Probiotics, prebiotics, and synbiotics are currently not recommended in AP.

1 Introduction

Acute pancreatitis (AP) begins as a sterile inflammation within the pancreatic parenchyma, triggered by acinar cell injury. Around 15–20% of the patients with AP develop pancreatic and/or extrapancreatic fat necrosis, out of which a proportion of susceptible patients get primary infected pancreatic necrosis (IPN). The other potential and occasionally underrecognized infections seen in patients with AP are urinary tract infection (UTI), pneumonia, including ventilator-associated pneumonia (VAP), cholangitis, sepsis, intravenous (IV) catheter site infections, and secondary IPN [1, 2]. Antibiotics have a role in the management of complications of AP. While there is no debate about the use of therapeutic antibiotics for the septic indications stated above, there are varying opinions about the use of prophylactic and empirical antibiotics. There remains a tendency toward the early use of prophylactic antibiotics in real-world clinical practice despite most guidelines recommending the contrary.

This chapter discusses the current pattern of antibiotic and probiotic use in AP, rationale for its use, evidence, guidelines, and future perspectives.

2 Real-World Practice of Prophylactic Antibiotic Usage in AP

Several studies that have addressed the subject of antibiotic usage in AP report a high prevalence of prophylactic antibiotic usage. Table 1 illustrates this practice based on global data. Prophylactic antibiotics were used not only in patients with moderately severe AP (MSAP) and severe AP (SAP) but also in patients with mild AP (MAP) [13, 14]. Evaluation of the

R. Talukdar (✉)
Pancreas Research Group and Division of Gut Microbiome Research, Asian Institute of Gastroenterology Hospitals, Institute of Translational Research, Asian Healthcare Foundation, Hyderabad, Telangana, India

© The Author(s), under exclusive license to Springer Nature Singapore Pte Ltd. 2024
J. A. Windsor et al. (eds.), *Acute Pancreatitis*, https://doi.org/10.1007/978-981-97-3132-9_12

Table 1 Prophylactic antibiotic usage in different parts of the world

Author (year)	Country/continent	Proportion of use of prophylactic antibiotics
Powell et al. (1999) [3]	United Kingdom; Ireland	• 24% used prophylactic antibiotics for all patients with AP • 81% used prophylactic antibiotics for severe disease • 65% used prophylactic antibiotics for pancreatic necrosis
King et al. (2004) [4]	Pan-Europe	• 73% used antibiotic prophylaxis
Lankisch et al. (2005) [5]	Germany	• 47% used antibiotic prophylaxis
Foitzik et al. (2007) [6]	Germany	• 44% prescribe prophylactic antibiotics in all patients with SAP • 34% selectively prescribed prophylactic antibiotics in SAP
Sekimoto et al. (2010) [7]	Japan	*Before guidelines* • 59% received for MAP and 98% for SAP *After guidelines* • 43% received for MAP and 100% for SAP
Hutan et al. (2010) [8]	Slovak Republic	• 41.2% of wards use prophylactic antibiotics
Murata et al. (2011) [9]	Japan	• 80% with MAP received • 91% with SAP received
Rebours et al. (2012) [10]	France	*In 2001* • 19% used for all patients and 57% used for pancreatic necrosis *In 2008* • 8% used for all patients and 20% used for pancreatic necrosis
Sun et al. (2013) [11]	North America	• 1% use in >75% of all AP • 69% use in >50% of SAP
Talukdar et al. (2014) [12]	India	• 66.4% patients overall received prophylactic antibiotics • 46.1% of MAP patients received prophylactic antibiotics • 55.8% of MSAP patients received prophylactic antibiotics • 34.5% of SAP patients received prophylactic antibiotics
Thong et al. (2020) [13]	Vietnam	• 31.1% of MAP patients received antibiotics • 73.6% of MSAP patients received antibiotics • 100% of SAP patients received antibiotics

Abbreviations: *AP* acute pancreatitis, *MAP* mild acute pancreatitis, *MSAP* moderately severe acute pancreatitis, *SAP* severe acute pancreatitis

type of antibiotics used for prophylaxis revealed carbapenems, third- and fourth-generation cephalosporins, nitroimidazoles, and quinolones alone, or in combinations [12]. Further international surveys reported varied indications for starting antibiotics in the first week, the most frequent being high total leucocyte count (TLC) and C-reactive protein (CRP), fever, and presence of necrosis on contrast-enhanced computed tomography (CECT). There exist geographic differences in the use of prophylactic antibiotics (higher frequency of prophylactic antibiotic use in Asia/Oceania), including differences in physician characteristics (for instance, higher proportion of surgeons, clinicians from nonacademic institution, and those from institutions with lower case volume opting to use prophylactic antibiotics) [15, 16].

3 Is there a Rationale for Early Antibiotic Use in AP?

The vast majority of studies on the early pathophysiology of AP were conducted in animal models. Recent studies using human pancreatic tissue have shown that biliary and alcohol-related acinar injuries result in the release of proinflammatory cytokines from the acinar cells to the local pancreatic milieu [17, 18]. These cytokines activate circulating mononuclear cells that traverse the pancreas which then disseminate into the systemic circulation, releasing cytokines. This results in a cascade that eventually leads to elevation of the TLC, and/or an increase in heart and respiratory rates, and/or increase in body temperature, all of which are components of systemic inflammatory response syndrome (SIRS). Other potential factors that could contribute to

SIRS are the damage-associated molecular patterns (DAMPs) that are liberated in response to acinar injury/necrosis. This explains that fever and high TLC during this stage of the disease are related to sterile systemic inflammation and not bacterial infection (Fig. 1). Hence, there is no rationale for using prophylactic or empirical antibiotics in this early stage of AP.

Therapeutic antibiotics in the early stage of the disease (first week) will find rationale only in the presence of documented extrapancreatic infection including UTI, pneumonia, cholangitis, and IV catheter site infections, which will produce infection and organ-specific signs.

4 Evidence and Pitfalls of Prophylactic Antibiotic Usage

Several observational studies and randomized controlled trials have so far been conducted to determine the efficacy of prophylactic systemic antibiotics in AP. Though many of these RCTs were unblinded, four were double-blinded placebo-controlled studies. These showed no reduction in the incidence of IPN and extrapancreatic infections (Table 2) [19–22]. The antibiotics used in these randomized controlled trials (RCTs) were meropenem, imipenem-cilastatin, ciprofloxacin, and ciprofloxacin with metronidazole. Meta-analysis of RCTs have failed to demonstrate a role for prophylactic antibiotics in the prevention of IPN, mortality, and intervention, while there were variable results in relation to the prevention of extrapancreatic infections. In an earlier meta-analysis, a subgroup analysis performed appeared to suggest that carbapenems may have a role in mortality prevention.

Subsequently, it was shown that there was an inverse relationship of the quality of the study and the efficacy of prophylactic antibiotics [23–25].

Despite studies demonstrating the futility of antibiotic prophylaxis in AP, a closer look into the meta-analyses reveals substantial heterogeneity among the individual studies. Table 3 illustrates the areas of heterogeneity among the studies. This could be one of the reasons for the varying recommendations on the use of prophylactic antibiotics in the first week of AP. For instance, the American Gastroenterological Association (AGA) 2018 guidelines provide a conditional recommendation based on low-quality evidence, while the American College of Gastroenterology (ACG) 2019 guidelines suggest a strong recommendation based on moderate-quality evidence against the use of prophylactic antibiotics [26, 27].

It is now clearly shown from experimental and clinical research that there is an alteration in the intestinal permeability barrier which supports bacterial translocation and colonization in the necrotic tissue, thereby resulting in IPN. Studies conducted on experimental models and patients over the past few years have also demonstrated gut microbial dysbiosis in patients with AP [28, 29]. For instance, studies have reported an increase in the phylum Bacteroidetes, *Escherichia-Shigella* complex, and the genus *Enterococcus*, with a reduction in the abundance of beneficial organisms such as *Bifidobacterium*. Dysbiosis correlated with inflammation [interleukin-6 (IL-6)], multiorgan failure, infectious complications, and intestinal barrier function. Therefore, it is plausible that selective gut decontamination with antibiotics could be another form of prophylactic approach. Unfortunately, results from studies performed in

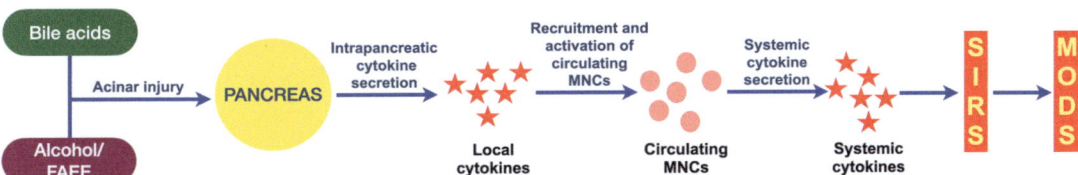

Fig. 1 Schematic representation of the events on how initial acinar injury leads to sterile inflammation in the first week of acute pancreatitis. Abbreviations: *FAEE* fatty acid ethyl ester, *MNC* mononuclear cell, *SIRS* systemic inflammatory response syndrome, *MODS* multiorgan dysfunction syndrome. (Adapted from references [17, 18])

Table 2 Double-blind randomized placebo-controlled studies that evaluated the role of prophylactic antibiotics for acute pancreatitis

Study details			Outcomes (treated vs. placebo)		
Author (year)	N	Antibiotics used	Infected necrosis	Need for surgery	Mortality
Isenmann et al. (2004) [19]	114	Ciprofloxacin + metronidazole	12 vs. 14%	23 vs. 15%	36 vs. 42%
Dellinger et al. (2007) [20]	100	Meropenem	17 vs. 11%	23 vs. 24%	50 vs. 42%
Garcia-Barrasa et al. (2009) [21]	41	Ciprofloxacin	12 vs. 9%	20 vs. 18%	18 vs. 11%
Poropat et al. (2019) [22]	98	Imipenem-cilastatin	6.1 vs. 4.8%		14.2 vs. 16.3%

Table 3 Areas of heterogeneity in clinical trials evaluating the role prophylactic antibiotics

1. Variable methodology (single-blind, double-blind, single/multicenter)
2. Nonuniform selection criteria
3. Sample size variation
4. Different treatment duration
   (1 week or less to 3 weeks)
5. Selection of antibiotics
   (Imipenem, meropenem, ciprofloxacin, ofloxacin, cefuroxime, metronidazole)
6. Outcome measures
   (Infected necrosis, extrapancreatic infection, fungal infections, need for interventions, mortality)

this regard over the past several years have been unclear. While a multicenter randomized study from Netherlands in 1995 demonstrated significant reduction of gram-negative bacterial colonization and infected pancreatic necrosis by selective decontamination with norfloxacin, amphotericin, and colistin, a subsequent study from 2007 failed to show any benefit [30, 31]. On the contrary, a more recent study reported a significant reduction in the hospitalization duration and IPN with selective decontamination by rifaximin [32]. However, this was a non-randomized retrospective study, and patients with different modalities were enrolled over different time periods. Therefore, in the absence of supportive data from large and high-quality RCTs, there is no role for selective gut decontamination in the current management armamentarium of AP [33]. However it would be prudent to hold off on a definitive position regarding selective gut decontamination until more evidence is available from adequately powered RCTs.

Since only a proportion of patients with acute necrotizing pancreatitis (ANP) develop IPN, it is plausible that there could be susceptibility factors that determine the development of infections. Identification of these susceptibility factors could result in a rational use of prophylactic antibiotic in targeted populations that might show potential beneficial effects. A few earlier studies that attempted to identify predictors of IPN reported that procalcitonin [34], low admission systolic blood pressure [35], rising blood urea nitrogen [36], and low lymphocyte count [37] could be potential predictors of IPN. However, it was not clear what cutoff values of procalcitonin and measurement in which timepoint was predictive of IPN, the other markers were not specific for infections. Another recent study demonstrated that persistent downregulation of HLA-DR, which is a marker of immunosuppression, till the second week of illness increases the risk of developing IPN by 4.5 (1.2–16.9) [38]. However, this study had a small sample size and a larger multicenter study is required. Studies have also implicated the altered kynurenine pathway metabolites, including reduction of circulating tryptophan with organ failure and development of IPN [39, 40]. The predictive capability of these also needs to be validated in large multicenter cohorts of patients.

In conclusion, there is lack of substantial evidence and the use of prophylactic antibiotics in AP is not recommended.

5   Use of Therapeutic Antibiotics in AP

Infected pancreatic necrosis should ideally be treated with therapeutic antibiotics based on culture sensitivity from the necrotic fluid collection. However, it may be difficult to confirm the presence of infection in necrotic pancreatic tissue until a drainage procedure is conducted. Fine needle aspiration (FNA) used to be advised to confirm IPN. However, it is no longer used in routine clinical practice due to false negative results of 12–25% and the risk of secondary infection of pancreatic necrosis. Therefore, empirical antibiotics can be started in these patients with an indication of infection, including clinical markers such as persistent fever in the second week of illness or beyond, progressive increase in the TLC, increased inflammatory markers, and imaging evidence of free air within the necrotic collections/WON [27]. Another recent study has suggested that empirical antibiotics can be started/continued or stopped based on a serum procalcitonin value of greater than or equal to 1.0 ng/mL or lower, respectively [41]. It is important to select antibiotics that have been shown to have good penetration into necrotic pancreatic tissue such as imipenem, ciprofloxacin, ofloxacin, metronidazole, and cefoperazone [42, 43]. Once drainage of the infected pancreatic necrosis is done, then therapeutic antibiotics can be directed according to the culture and sensitivity of the drained fluid. Blood culture- and sensitivity-directed therapeutic antibiotics can be used if the patient develops secondary sepsis resulting from IPN.

(PROPATRIA trial) from the Dutch Pancreatitis Research Group, mortality was significantly higher in the probiotics group compared to that in the placebo group [44]. It was subsequently reported that even though the probiotic strains used in this trial reduced bacterial translocation overall, there were increased enterocyte damage and bacterial translocation in the patients with organ failure [45]. There was also a significant increase in gastrointestinal ischaemia and mortality. It was argued that the elevated lactic acid level due to the bacterial fermentation of carbohydrates was the primary factor responsible for higher mortality [46]. While this is still a subject of scrutiny, it can also be inferred that probiotic therapy could still have a place if the appropriate strain is used, treatment is initiated at the correct time, and diet is modified to include a lower volume of fermentable carbohydrates. A subsequent meta-analysis confirmed divergent results, i.e., failed to show neither benefit of probiotics, prebiotics, and synbiotics in preventing IPN nor any harm to the patients sufficient to result in an increased frequency of organ failure and hospital stay [47]. Nevertheless, in the absence of high-quality evidence and potential harm, means there is no role for probiotics and/or synbiotics in patients with ANP/IPN.

6 Use of Probiotics in AP

Probiotics with, or without, prebiotics, in general, have been shown to confer immunomodulatory, anti-inflammatory, and gut mucosal health benefits. In the context of AP, since the alteration in the gut barrier integrity and bacterial translocation are established pathophysiologic events, treating patients especially with ANP with prophylactic probiotics or synbiotics appears to be a plausible option. However, RCTs that evaluated the protective role of probiotics against IPN failed to demonstrate a protective role. In a well-designed and adequately powered RCT

7 Conclusion

In view of the absence of high-quality studies and the heterogeneous data from the existing studies, prophylactic antibiotics and probiotics/synbiotics should not be used in patients with AP. Figure 2 depicts the current approach to antibiotic therapy in patients with AP. Empirical pancreas-penetrating antibiotics should be used when the patient is suspected to have an IPN based on clinical and radiological criteria. Further placebo-controlled RCTs examining the roles of prophylactic antibiotics and probiotics using targeted predictors of IPN are warranted.

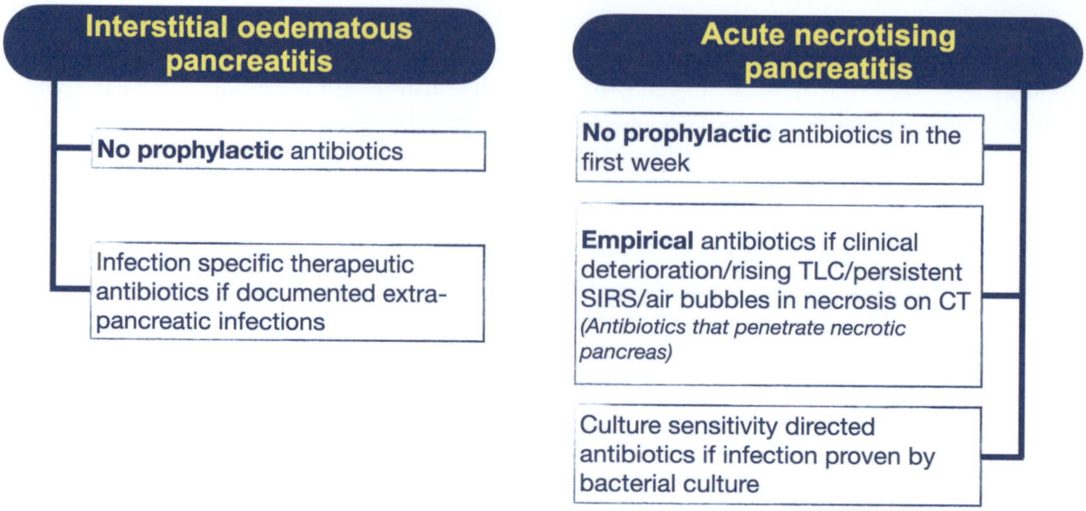

Fig. 2 Schematic representation of the current approach, antibiotic therapy, in acute pancreatitis. Interstitial acute pancreatitis is characterized by diffuse (or occasionally localized) enlargement of the pancreas due to inflammatory edema, with peripancreatic stranding, with or without some peripancreatic fluid, but without pancreatic or extrapancreatic necrosis. Most often this is described as mild acute pancreatitis (MAP) unless there is organ dysfunction [48]. Acute necrotizing pancreatitis can be moderately severe AP (MSAP) or severe AP (SAP) if there is associated persistent (>48 h) organ failure as per modified Marshall's criteria [49]. Abbreviations: *TLC* total leucocyte count, *CT* computed tomography, *SIRS* systemic inflammatory response syndrome

References

1. Wu BU, Johannes RS, Kurtz S, Banks PA. The impact of hospital-acquired infection on outcome in acute pancreatitis. Gastroenterology. 2008;135(3):816–20.
2. Talukdar R, Bhattacharrya A, Rao B, Sharma M, Nageshwar Reddy D. Clinical utility of the revised Atlanta classification of acute pancreatitis in a prospective cohort: have all loose ends been tied? Pancreatology. 2014;14(4):257–62.
3. Powell JJ, Campbell E, Johnson CD, Siriwardena AK. Survey of antibiotic prophylaxis in acute pancreatitis in the UK and Ireland. Br J Surg. 1999;86(3):320–2. https://doi.org/10.1046/j.1365-2168.1999.01052.x.
4. King NKK, Siriwardena AK. European survey of surgical strategies for the management of severe acute pancreatitis. Am J Gastroenterol. 2004;99(4):719–28. https://doi.org/10.1111/j.1572-0241.2004.04111.x.
5. Lankisch PG, Weber-Dany B, Lerch MM. Clinical perspectives in pancreatology: compliance with acute pancreatitis guidelines in Germany. Pancreatology. 2005;5(6):591–3. https://doi.org/10.1159/000087501. Epub 2005 Aug 16
6. Foitzik T, Klar E. Non-compliance with guidelines for the management of severe acutepancreatitis among German surgeons. Pancreatology. 2007;7(1):80–5. https://doi.org/10.1159/000101882.
7. Sekimoto M, Shikata S, Takada T, Hirata K, Yoshida M, Hirota M, Kitamura N, Shirai K, Kimura Y, Wada K, Amano H, Kiriyama S, Arata S, Gabata T. Changes in management of acute pancreatitis before and after the publication of evidence-based practice guidelines in 2003. J Hepatobiliary Pancreat Sci. 2010;17(1):17–23. https://doi.org/10.1007/s00534-009-0212-5. Epub 2009 Dec 15
8. Hutan M Sr, Hutan M Jr, Payer J Jr. Selected indicators of care in patients with acute pancreatitis in the Slovak Republic. Bratisl Lek Listy. 2010;111(11):599–603.
9. Murata A, Matsuda S, Mayumi T, Yokoe M, Kuwabara K, Ichimiya Y, Fujino Y, Kubo T, Fujimori K, Horiguchi H. A descriptive study evaluating the circumstances of medical treatment for acute pancreatitis before publication of the new JPN guidelines based on the Japanese administrative database associated with the Diagnosis Procedure Combination system. J Hepatobiliary Pancreat Sci. 2011;18(5):678–83. https://doi.org/10.1007/s00534-011-0375-8.
10. Rebours V, Lévy P, Bretagne J-F, Bommelaer G, Hammel P, Ruszniewski P. Do guidelines influence medical practice? Changes in management of acute pancreatitis 7 years after the publication of the French guidelines. Eur J Gastroenterol Hepatol. 2012;24(2):143–8. https://doi.org/10.1097/MEG.0b013e32834d864f.
11. Sun E, Tharakan M, Kapoor S, Chakravarty R, Salhab A, Buscaglia JM, Nagula S. Poor compliance with ACG guidelines for nutrition and antibiotics in the management of acute pancreatitis: a North American survey of gastrointestinal specialists and primary care physicians. JOP. 2013;14(3):221–7. https://doi.org/10.6092/1590-8577/871.

12. Talukdar R, Ingale P, Choudhury HP, Dhingra R, Shetty S, Joshi H, et al. Antibiotic use in acute pancreatitis: an Indian multicenter observational study. Indian J Gastroenterol. 2014;33(5):458–65.

13. Thong VD, Anh TTH, Quynh BTH, Quyt NTT. Investigation of antibiotic use in patients with acute pancreatitis in a Vietnamese hospital. JGH Open. 2020;5(1):128–32. https://doi.org/10.1002/jgh3.12461. eCollection 2021 Jan.

14. Baltatzis M, Jegatheeswaran S, O'Reilly DA, Siriwardena AK. Antibiotic use in acute pancreatitis: global overview of compliance with international guidelines. Pancreatology. 2016;16(2):189–93.

15. Párniczky A, Lantos T, Tóth EM, Szakács Z, Gódi S, Hágendorn R, et al. Antibiotic therapy in acute pancreatitis: from global overuse to evidence based recommendations. Pancreatology. 2019;19(4):488–99.

16. Talukdar R, Tsuji Y, Jagtap N, Pradeep R, Rao GV, Reddy DN. Non-compliance to practice guidelines still exist in the early management of acute pancreatitis: time for reappraisal? Pancreatology. 2021;S1424-3903(21):00471–3.

17. Jakkampudi A, Jangala R, Reddy R, Mitnala S, Rao GV, Pradeep R, et al. Acinar injury and early cytokine response in human acute biliary pancreatitis. Sci Rep. 2017;7(1):15276.

18. Jakkampudi A, Jangala R, Reddy R, Reddy B, Venkat Rao G, Pradeep R, et al. Fatty acid ethyl ester (FAEE) associated acute pancreatitis: an ex-vivo study using human pancreatic acini. Pancreatology. 2020;20(8):1620–30.

19. Isenmann R, Rünzi M, Kron M, Kahl S, Kraus D, Jung N, et al. Prophylactic antibiotic treatment in patients with predicted severe acute pancreatitis: a placebo-controlled, double-blind trial. Gastroenterology. 2004;126(4):997–1004.

20. Dellinger EP, Tellado JM, Soto NE, Ashley SW, Barie PS, Dugernier T, et al. Early antibiotic treatment for severe acute necrotizing pancreatitis: a randomized, double-blind, placebo-controlled study. Ann Surg. 2007;245(5):674–83.

21. García-Barrasa A, Borobia FG, Pallares R, Jorba R, Poves I, Busquets J, et al. A double-blind, placebo-controlled trial of ciprofloxacin prophylaxis in patients with acute necrotizing pancreatitis. J Gastrointest Surg. 2009;13(4):768–74.

22. Poropat G, Radovan A, Peric M, Mikolasevic I, Giljaca V, Hauser G, et al. Prevention of infectious complications in acute pancreatitis: results of a single-center, randomized, controlled trial. Pancreas. 2019;48(8):1056–60.

23. Heinrich S, Schäfer M, Rousson V, Clavien PA. Evidence-based treatment of acute pancreatitis: a look at established paradigms. Ann Surg. 2006;243(2):154–68.

24. Villatoro E, Bassi C, Larvin M. Antibiotic therapy for prophylaxis against infection of pancreatic necrosis in acute pancreatitis. Cochrane Database Syst Rev. 2006;4:CD002941.

25. Yao L, Huang X, Li Y, Shi R, Zhang G. Prophylactic antibiotics reduce pancreatic necrosis in acute necrotizing pancreatitis: a meta-analysis of randomized trials. Dig Surg. 2010;27(6):442–9.

26. Crockett SD, Wani S, Gardner TB, Falck-Ytter Y, Barkun AN, American Gastroenterological Association Institute Clinical Guidelines Committee. American Gastroenterological Association Institute Guideline on Initial Management of Acute Pancreatitis. Gastroenterology. 2018;154(4):1096–101.

27. Vivian E, Cler L, Conwell D, Coté GA, Dickerman R, Freeman M, et al. Acute pancreatitis task force on quality: development of quality indicators for acute pancreatitis management. Am J Gastroenterol. 2019;114(8):1322–42.

28. Zhu Y, He C, Li X, Cai Y, Hu J, Liao Y, et al. Gut microbiota dysbiosis worsens the severity of acute pancreatitis in patients and mice. J Gastroenterol. 2019;54(4):347–58.

29. Akshintala VS, Talukdar R, Singh VK, Goggins M. The gut microbiome in pancreatic disease. Clin Gastroenterol Hepatol. 2019;17(2):290–5.

30. Sawa H, Ueda T, Takeyama Y, Yasuda T, Shinzeki M, Matsumura N, et al. Treatment outcome of selective digestive decontamination and enteral nutrition in patients with severe acute pancreatitis. J Hepato-Biliary-Pancreat Surg. 2007;14(5):503–8.

31. Luiten EJ, Hop WC, Lange JF, Bruining HA. Controlled clinical trial of selective decontamination for the treatment of severe acute pancreatitis. Ann Surg. 1995;222(1):57–65.

32. Tatur J, Lipiński M, Sznurkowska M, Józefik E, Rydzewska G. Rifaximin in gut microbiota modification in acute pancreatitis: 15 years of retrospective clinical study. Adv Clin Exp Med. 2022;31(4):399–405.

33. Tiong L, Jalleh R, Barreto SG. Selective digestive decontamination in severe acute pancreatitis—A review of literature. Astrocyte. 2014;1:93–9.

34. Mofidi R, Suttie SA, Patil PV, Ogston S, Parks RW. The value of procalcitonin at predicting the severity of acute pancreatitis and development of infected pancreatic necrosis: systematic review. Surgery. 2009;146(1):72–81.

35. Thandassery RB, Yadav TD, Dutta U, Appasani S, Singh K, Kochhar R. Hypotension in the first week of acute pancreatitis and APACHE II score predict development of infected pancreatic necrosis. Dig Dis Sci. 2015;60(2):537–42.

36. Talukdar R, Nechutova H, Clemens M, Vege SS. Could rising BUN predict the future development of infected pancreatic necrosis? Pancreatology. 2013;13(4):355–9.

37. Shen X, Sun J, Ke L, Zou L, Li B, Tong Z, et al. Reduced lymphocyte count as an early marker for predicting infected pancreatic necrosis. BMC Gastroenterol. 2015;15:147.

38. Sharma D, Jakkampudi A, Reddy R, Reddy PB, Patil A, Murthy HVV, et al. Association of systemic inflammatory and anti-inflammatory responses with adverse

outcomes in acute pancreatitis: preliminary results of an ongoing study. Dig Dis Sci. 2017;62(12):3468–78.

39. Jakkampudi A, Sarkar P, Chandrakanth K, Patil A, Unnisa M, Prasanna A, et al. Alteration of inflammatory modulators and plasma metabolites in patients having acute pancreatitis with infected pancreatic necrosis. Pancreas. 2021;50(7):1068.

40. Mole DJ, Webster SP, Uings I, Zheng X, Binnie M, Wilson K, et al. Kynurenine-3-monooxygenase inhibition prevents multiple organ failure in rodent models of acute pancreatitis. Nat Med. 2016;22(2):202–9.

41. Siriwardena AK, Jegatheeswaran S, Mason JM, PROCAP investigators. A procalcitonin-based algorithm to guide antibiotic use in patients with acute pancreatitis (PROCAP): a single-centre, patient-blinded, randomised controlled trial. Lancet Gastroenterol Hepatol. 2022;7(10):913–21.

42. Bassi C, Pederzoli P, Vesentini S, Falconi M, Bonora A, Abbas H, et al. Behavior of antibiotics during human necrotizing pancreatitis. Antimicrob Agents Chemother. 1994;38(4):830–6.

43. Jiang L, Peng Q, Yao Y. Penetration of ciprofloxacin and cefoperazone into human pancreas. Hua Xi Yi Ke Da Xue Xue Bao. 1997;28(4):365–8.

44. Besselink MG, van Santvoort HC, Buskens E, Boermeester MA, van Goor H, Timmerman HM, et al. Probiotic prophylaxis in predicted severe acute pancreatitis: a randomised, double-blind, placebo-controlled trial. Lancet. 2008;371(9613):651–9.

45. Besselink MG, van Santvoort HC, Renooij W, de Smet MB, Boermeester MA, Fischer K, et al. Intestinal barrier dysfunction in a randomized trial of a specific probiotic composition in acute pancreatitis. Ann Surg. 2009;250(5):712–9.

46. Bongaerts GPA, Severijnen RSVM. A reassessment of the PROPATRIA study and its implications for probiotic therapy. Nat Biotechnol. 2016;34(1):55–63.

47. Zhang MM, Cheng JQ, Lu YR, Yi ZH, Yang P, Wu XT. Use of pre-, pro- and synbiotics in patients with acute pancreatitis: a meta-analysis. World J Gastroenterol. 2010;16(31):3970–8.

48. Banks PA, Bollen TL, Dervenis C, Gooszen HG, Johnson CD, Sarr MG, et al. Classification of acute pancreatitis—2012: revision of the Atlanta classification and definitions by international consensus. Gut. 2013;62(1):102–11.

49. Marshall JC, Cook DJ, Christou NV, Bernard GR, Sprung CL, Sibbald WJ. Multiple organ dysfunction score: a reliable descriptor of a complex clinical outcome. Crit Care Med. 1995;23:1638–52.

Managing Biliary Pancreatitis

Marco J. Bruno

Key Points

1. Urgent endoscopic retrograde cholangiography (ERC) is indicated in patients with biliary pancreatitis and concomitant cholangitis.
2. In patients with predicted mild biliary pancreatitis, urgent ERC is not indicated.
3. In patients with predicted severe biliary pancreatitis, a recent study shows that urgent ERC is not indicated, even when stones or sludge is proven by imaging.
4. Cholecystectomy during index admission for mild biliary pancreatitis is safe and prevents recurrent biliary and pancreatitis events.
5. The timing of cholecystectomy in clinically severe pancreatitis with local complications such as pancreatic necrosis and organ failure should be delayed and scheduled as early as considered safe when local complications (e.g. necrosis) have resolved.

1 Introduction

1.1 Epidemiology

Acute pancreatitis (AP) is the most common gastrointestinal cause for acute hospital admissions in the United States [1]. Its global incidence has been rising steadily through the years [2]. In Europe, its incidence has been increasing at a median rate of 3.4% per year [3]. Although acute pancreatitis has multiple etiologies, biliary stone disease is the most frequent cause in Europe accounting for 45% of cases, followed by alcohol abuse (20%) [3]. Most patients with AP, including those with a biliary cause, recover quickly without major clinical sequelae. About 20% of cases, however, run a severe disease course with local (necrosis) and systemic (systemic inflammatory response syndrome, infected necrosis, multi-organ failure) complications with the need for care from a multidisciplinary team in an intensive care unit. In these patients, despite aggressive management, mortality ranges between 20 and 40% [4]. In view of the rising incidence of acute biliary pancreatitis and its associated morbidity and mortality, utilization of health care resources and costs are substantial [5].

1.2 Definitions

A biliary cause for an episode of acute pancreatitis is considered when stones in the common bile duct (CBD) are visualized on imaging, or in case of dilation of the CBD or an abnormal liver panel. The former can be regarded as a definite diagnosis of biliary pancreatitis, the latter two as circumstantial evidence of the possibility of having a biliary pancreatitis with varying degrees of

M. J. Bruno (✉)
Department of Gastroenterology and Hepatology,
Erasmus University Medical Center,
Rotterdam, The Netherlands
e-mail: m.bruno@erasmusmc.nl

© The Author(s), under exclusive license to Springer Nature Singapore Pte Ltd. 2024
J. A. Windsor et al. (eds.), *Acute Pancreatitis*, https://doi.org/10.1007/978-981-97-3132-9_13

probability depending on which criteria are used (see next section).

Disease severity is classified into three grades according to the presence or absence of organ failure and morphological features of the pancreas [7]. In 'mild' pancreatitis there is no organ failure and complications such as extra-pancreatic or pancreatic parenchymal necrosis are lacking. Organ failure lasting less than 48 h or the occurrence of pancreatic (necrosis) or systemic (e.g. exacerbation of previous illness such as chronic heart or lung disease) complications is classified as 'moderately severe'. Organ failure persisting beyond 48 h is classified as 'severe' pancreatitis and is frequently accompanied by pancreatic necrosis or fluid collections.

2 Diagnosis of a Biliary Cause of an Acute Pancreatitis Episode

Diagnosing AP is not usually difficult but demonstrating a biliary cause may prove challenging. Clinical predictors including symptoms and blood tests are unreliable, particularly early in the course of the disease [6]. A biliary cause may be suspected based on increased concentrations of bilirubin, alkaline phosphatase, gamma-glutamyl transferase, alanine aminotransferase (ALT) and aspartate aminotransferase (AST). Multiple studies show that ALT two times the upper limit of normal within 48 h of hospital admission [8] or three times the upper limit of normal regardless of timing [7, 8] are associated with a positive predictive value exceeding 80% in determining a biliary origin.

Abdominal ultrasound has a high sensitivity for cholecystolithiasis, but a sensitivity of only 20% for choledocholithiasis in AP, mainly due to the inability to visualize the CBD in its entirety due to overlying bowel loops [9, 11]. Computed tomography for the detection of CBD stones reaches a sensitivity of only 40% [7]. The sensitivity of magnetic resonance cholangiopancreatography (MRCP) to detect choledocholithiasis

in biliary pancreatitis is high at 90%. Stones smaller than 5 mm however are easily missed by MRCP [10]. This is of clinical significance because small stones, per se, are thought to be more often associated with biliary pancreatitis [11]. The most sensitive modality for diagnosing CBD stones or sludge is endoscopic ultrasonography (EUS) with a reported sensitivity between 89 and 96% [7, 12, 13]. The availability of EUS has improved considerably, but it widely available globally. It is also important to acknowledge that EUS is an operator-dependent technique. Endoscopic retrograde cholangiopancreatography (ERCP) has no place as a solely diagnostic tool to detect biliary stones because of associated complications including (aggravating) pancreatitis, perforation and bleeding [7, 14].

In summary, MRCP and EUS are the most valuable diagnostic tools to detect a biliary origin in patients presenting with AP.

3 Management

3.1 Indication for ERC and Management of Bile Duct Stones

Acute biliary pancreatitis is the result of a transient impediment of the flow of secretion from the pancreatic duct caused by gallstones and sludge obstructing the ampulla of Vater [15, 16]. The duration of the pancreatic duct obstruction appears related to the severity of inflammation of the pancreas [17]. Based on these observations, it has been postulated that the disease course could potentially be ameliorated by (early) decompression of the pancreatic duct by removing bile duct stones or sludge with endoscopic retrograde cholangiography (ERC) and endoscopic sphincterotomy (ES).

Existing guidelines state that urgent ERC with ES is warranted in patients with acute biliary pancreatitis and concomitant cholangitis, and is not recommended in patients with a predicted mild disease course. The evidence is more regarding the indication of urgent ERC with ES in patients with a predicted severe disease course [18–20]. Previously published randomized trials on this subject have substantial shortcomings. First, patients with concomitant cholangitis, patients with a predicted mild disease course and even patients with a non-gallstone aetiology were included [21–25]. Second, in most trials, ERC was performed up to 3 days after hospital admission. Presumably, for biliary decompression to be effective in preventing complications, ERC needs to be done as early as possible after the onset of symptoms [24, 26]. Third, only a small proportion of patients underwent a biliary sphincterotomy [25–27, 29]. Because microlithiasis can easily be missed on cholangiogram during ERC, and as small gallstones in particular are known to cause pancreatitis, this limitation is particularly relevant [13, 28]. Performing ES routinely during ERC for biliary pancreatitis is also supported by a previous study showing that sphincterotomy reduced complications irrespective of the presence of gallstones on cholangiogram [29]. Furthermore, biliary sphincterotomy decompresses the biliary tract, which potentially ameliorates the disease course [17, 18, 30–32]. Conversely, ERC with ES is an invasive procedure that is associated with complications in up to 10% of patients [33, 34]. Finally, the study populations of individual trials and of subsequent meta-analyses were too small to detect an effect of ERC in the group of patients with gallstone pancreatitis with a predicted severe disease course. It therefore remained unclear whether urgent ERC with ES is beneficial in patients with predicted severe acute gallstone pancreatitis, with and without cholestasis, but without cholangitis.

The recently published APEC trial investigated whether urgent biliary decompression using ERC with ES is beneficial in patients with predicted severe acute biliary pancreatitis without cholangitis [35]. In this trial, 232 patients were randomized between conservative treatment and urgent ERC with ES. 'Urgent' was defined as within 24 h after hospital presentation and within 72 h after symptom onset. Urgent biliary decompression with ERC with ES did not reduce the composite endpoint of major complications, or mortality, as compared to conservative treatment.

In the APEC trial, however, the probability for a biliary origin and the indication for ERC was based on CBD dilation, an increase in ALT or sludge or stones on imaging (located in the gallbladder or CBD). Studies have shown that elevated liver enzymes and radiological signs of CBD stones are poorly correlated to the actual presence of CBD stones or sludge during ERC [8, 36]. This was confirmed in the APEC trial, where 55% of the patients in the urgent ERC group did not show CBD stones or sludge during ERC. After spontaneous stone passage into the duodenum, biliary decompression is no longer indicated, and ERC with ES may even be harmful (e.g. haemorrhage and aggravation of pancreatitis) [35, 36]. As discussed previously, the most sensitive modality for diagnosing CBD stones or sludge is EUS [15, 37]. Although not published in a peer-reviewed journal yet (review is pending), the prospective multicentre APEC-2 cohort study found that urgent EUS-guided ERC with ES did not reduce the composite endpoint of major complications or mortality as compared to the conservative arm of the APEC randomized trial [38]. In 58% of patients, CBD stones or sludge was found with urgent EUS within 24 h after presentation at the emergency department and within 72 h of start of symptoms. Immediate ERC with ES was performed successfully in 90% of patients with a low complication rate (2%). Early EUS-guided ERC showed a more favourable outcome with regard to the readmission rate for biliary events, specifically recurrent biliary pancreatitis and symptomatic choledocholithiasis, but not for the composite primary endpoint of major complications and death.

Based on the current literature, meta-analyses and the results of the APEC and the APEC 2 study (see above), there is no indication to perform an urgent ERC in patients with acute biliary pancreatitis, regardless of predicted severity. An urgent ERC is only indicated in the case of (suspected) cholangitis. The majority of biliary stones

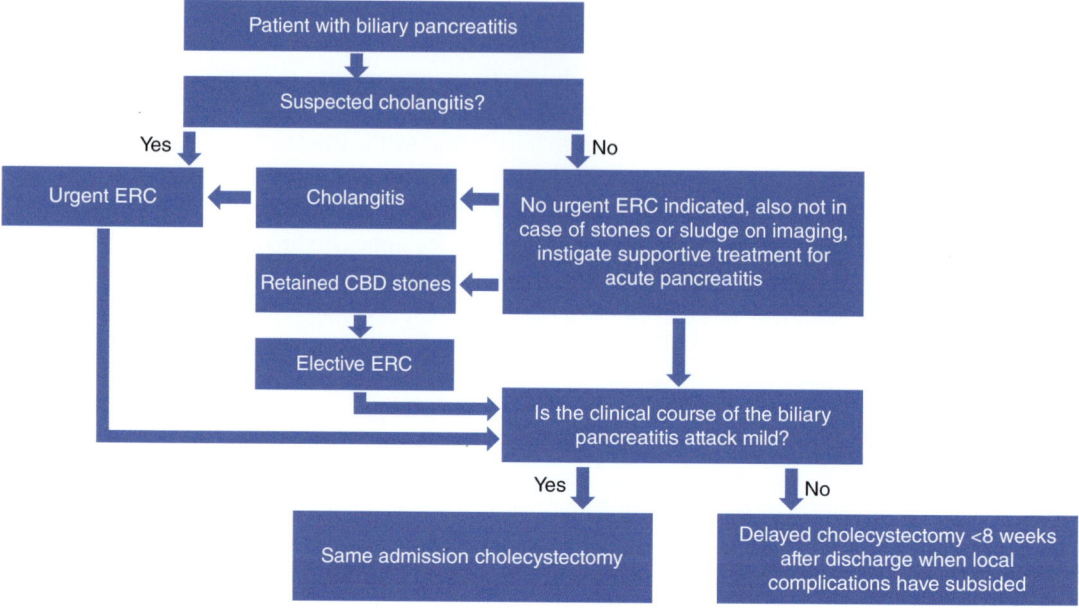

Fig. 1 Management of biliary pancreatitis. Abbreviations: *ERC* endoscopic retrograde cholangiography, *CBD* common bile duct

pass spontaneously, but when there are signs of persistent CBD stones based on symptoms and laboratory investigations, ERC with ES for stone removal should be scheduled, when the acute attack has subsided. In such cases it is our routine practice to (re)confirm the indication for ERC with EUS in the same session. Figure 1 provides a flowchart pertaining the management of biliary pancreatitis.

4 Timing of Cholecystectomy in Biliary Pancreatitis

After an initial attack of biliary pancreatitis, patients may suffer a recurrent episode of biliary pancreatitis or other biliary events, including acute cholecystitis, CBD obstruction due to stones or pancreatitis and cholangitis [39, 40]. Interval cholecystectomy after mild biliary pancreatitis is associated with a substantial risk of readmission for recurrent biliary events, especially recurrent biliary pancreatitis. To prevent such recurrent events, international guidelines advise performing a cholecystectomy after biliary pancreatitis with a secondary

role for endoscopic sphincterotomy (ES) in patients unfit for surgery [40, 41]. In patients with mild pancreatitis, international guidelines advise cholecystectomy directly after recovery or in the first 2–4 weeks after discharge for mild biliary pancreatitis [20, 21, 40]. Audits and surveys, however, show that in the majority of cases, a cholecystectomy is done 6–12 weeks after discharge, due to persistent uncertainty amongst caregivers about the efficacy and safety of an early cholecystectomy and for logistical reasons [42–44]. Meanwhile the results of the PONCHO trial, a randomized controlled study, were published. Compared with interval cholecystectomy 25–30 days after recovery, same-admission cholecystectomy within 72 h after recovery of a first episode of mild biliary pancreatitis reduced the rate of recurrent gallstone-related complications in patients with mild gallstone pancreatitis, with a very low risk of cholecystectomy-related complications [45].

The timing of cholecystectomy in patients with clinically severe pancreatitis, with local complications such as pancreatic necrosis and organ failure, is deliberately delayed until local complications have resolved [9]. There is limited scientific evidence to guide optimal timing in terms of preventing recurrent biliary events and pancreatitis from occurring and safely performing a cholecystectomy in patients with necrotizing biliary pancreatitis. In a post hoc analysis of a multicentre prospective cohort, the optimal timing of cholecystectomy after necrotizing biliary pancreatitis, in the absence of peripancreatic collections, was found to be within 8 weeks after discharge [46].

In conclusion, the only indication for urgent ERC in biliary pancreatitis is concomitant cholangitis. In the absence of cholangitis, urgent ERC is not indicated in biliary pancreatitis, as well as not in patients with a predicted severe outcome, as it does not ameliorate the disease course but potentially could induce complications. In the case of retained stones, ERC should be performed when the acute pancreatitis attack has subsided. In case of mild biliary pancreatitis, cholecystectomy during index admission is safe and prevents recurrent biliary and pancreatitis events. Cholecystectomy in clinically severe pancreatitis, with local complications such as organ failure pancreatic necrosis, should be delayed and scheduled when local complications (e.g. necrosis) have resolved, preferably within 6–8 weeks after discharge.

References

1. Yadav D, Lowenfels AB. The epidemiology of pancreatitis and pancreatic cancer. Gastroenterology. 2013;144:1252–61.
2. Iannuzzi JP, King JA, Leong JH, et al. Global incidence of acute pancreatitis is increasing over time: a systematic review and meta-analysis. Gastroenterology. 2022;162:122–34.
3. Roberts SE, Morrison-Rees S, John A, Williams JG, Brown TH, Samuel DG. The incidence and aetiology of acute pancreatitis across Europe. Pancreatology. 2017;17:155–65.
4. Schepers NJ, Bakker OJ, Besselink MG, et al. Impact of characteristics of organ failure and infected necrosis on mortality in necrotising pancreatitis. Gut. 2019;68:1044–51.
5. Fagenholz PJ, Fernandez-del Castillo C, Harris NS, Pelletier AJ, Camargo CA. Direct medical costs of acute pancreatitis hospitalizations in the United States. Pancreas. 2007;35:302–7.
6. van Santvoort HC, Bakker OJ, Besselink MG, Bollen TL, Fischer K, Nieuwenhuijs VB, Gooszen HG, Erpecum KJ, Dutch Pancreatitis Study Group. Prediction of common bile duct stones in the earliest stages of acute biliary pancreatitis. Endoscopy. 2011;43:8–13.
7. Liu CL, Fan ST, Lo CM, Tso WK, Wong Y, Poon RT, Lam CM, Wong BC, Wong J. Clinico-biochemical prediction of biliary cause of acute pancreatitis in the era of endoscopic ultrasonography. Aliment Pharmacol Ther. 2005;22:423–31.
8. Tenner S, Dubner H, Steinberg W. Predicting gallstone pancreatitis with laboratory parameters: a meta-analysis. Am J Gastroenterol. 1994;89:1863–6.
9. Moon JH, Cho YD, Cha SW, Cheon YK, Ahn HC, Kim YS, Kim YS, Lee JS, Lee MS, Lee HK, Shim CS, Kim BS. The detection of bile duct stones in suspected biliary pancreatitis: comparison of MRCP, ERCP, and intraductal US. Am J Gastroenterol. 2005;100:1051–7.
10. Kondo S, Isayama H, Akahane M, Toda N, Sasahira N, Nakai Y, Yamamoto N, Hirano K, Komatsu Y, Tada M, Yoshida H, Kawabe T, Ohtomo K, Omata M. Detection of common bile duct stones: comparison between endoscopic ultrasonography, magnetic resonance cholangiography, and helical-computed-tomographic cholangiography. Eur J Radiol. 2005;54:271–5.
11. Venneman NG, Buskens E, Besselink MG, Stads S, Go PM, Bosscha K, van Berge-Henegouwen GP, van Erpecum KJ. Small gallstones are associated with increased risk of acute pancreatitis: potential benefits of prophylactic cholecystectomy? Am J Gastroenterol. 2005;100:2540–50.
12. Stabuc B, Drobne D, Ferkolj I, Gruden A, Jereb J, Kolar G, Mlinaric V, Mervic M, Repse A, Stepec S, Markovic S. Acute biliary pancreatitis: detection of common bile duct stones with endoscopic ultrasound. Eur J Gastroenterol Hepatol. 2008;20:1171–5.
13. De Lisi S, Leandro G, Buscarini E. Endoscopic ultrasonography versus endoscopic retrograde cholangiopancreatography in acute biliary pancreatitis: a systematic review. Eur J Gastroenterol Hepatol. 2011;23:367–74.
14. Cotton PB, Garrow DA, Gallagher J, Romagnuolo J. Risk factors for complications after ERCP: a multivariate analysis of 11,497 procedures over 12 years. Gastrointest Endosc. 2009;70:80–8.
15. Lerch MM, Saluja AK, Runzi M, Dawra R, Saluja M, Steer ML. Pancreatic duct obstruction triggers acute necrotizing pancreatitis in the opossum. Gastroenterology. 1993;104:853–61.
16. Opie EL. The aetiology of acute haemorrhagic pancreatitis. Bull Johns Hop Hosp. 1901;xii:182–8.
17. Acosta JM, Rubio Galli OM, Rossi R, Chinellato AV, Pellegrini CA. Effect of duration of ampullary gallstone obstruction on severity of lesions of acute pancreatitis. J Am Coll Surg. 1997;184:499–505.
18. Tenner S, Baillie J, DeWitt J, Vege SS, American College of G. American College of Gastroenterology

guideline: management of acute pancreatitis. Am J Gastroenterol. 2013;108:1400–15.

19. Working Group IAP/APA Acute Pancreatitis Guideline. IAP/APA evidence-based guidelines for the management of acute pancreatitis. Pancreatology. 2013;13:e1–15.

20. Crockett SD, Wani S, Gardner TB, Falck-Ytter Y, Barkun AN, American Gastroenterological Association Institute Clinical Guidelines C. American gastroenterological association institute guideline on initial management of acute pancreatitis. Gastroenterology. 2018;154:1096–101.

21. Chen P, Hu B, Wang C, Kang Y, Jin X, Tang C. Pilot study of urgent endoscopic intervention without fluoroscopy on patients with severe acute biliary pancreatitis in the intensive care unit. Pancreas. 2010;39:398–402.

22. Fan ST, Lai EC, Mok FP, Lo CM, Zheng SS, Wong J. Early treatment of acute biliary pancreatitis by endoscopic papillotomy. N Engl J Med. 1993;328:228–32.

23. Neoptolemos JP, Carr-Locke DL, London NJ, Bailey IA, James D, Fossard DP. Controlled trial of urgent endoscopic retrograde cholangiopancreatography and endoscopic sphincterotomy versus conservative treatment for acute pancreatitis due to gallstones. Lancet. 1988;2:979–83.

24. Zhou MQ, Li NP, Lu RD. Duodenoscopy in treatment of acute gallstone pancreatitis. Hepatobiliary Pancreat Dis Int. 2002;1:608–10.

25. Folsch UR, Nitsche R, Ludtke R, Hilgers RA, Creutzfeldt W. Early ERCP and papillotomy compared with conservative treatment for acute biliary pancreatitis. The German study group on acute biliary pancreatitis. N Engl J Med. 1997;336:237–42.

26. Oria A, Cimmino D, Ocampo C, Sliva W, Kohan G, Szelagowski C, Chiapetta L. Early endoscopic intervention versus early conservative management in patients with acute gallstone pancreatitis and biliopancreatic obstruction: a randomized clinical trial. Ann Surg. 2007;245:10–7.

27. Acosta JM, Katkhouda N, Debian KA, Groshen SG, Tsao-Wei DD, Berne TV. Early ductal decompression versus conservative management for gallstone pancreatitis with ampullary obstruction: a prospective randomized clinical trial. Ann Surg. 2006;243:33–40.

28. Kim HS, Moon JH, Choi HJ, Lee JC, Han SH, Hong SJ, Lee TH, Cheon YK, Cho YD, Park SH, Lee MS. The role of intraductal US in the management of idiopathic recurrent pancreatitis without a definite cause on ERCP. Gastrointest Endosc. 2011;73:1148–54.

29. Lee HS, Chung MJ, Park JY, Bang S, Park SW, Song SY, Chung JB. Urgent endoscopic retrograde cholangiopancreatography is not superior to early ERCP in acute biliary pancreatitis with biliary obstruction without cholangitis. PLoS One. 2018;13:e0190835.

30. Runzi M, Saluja A, Lerch MM, Dawra R, Nishino H, Steer ML. Early ductal decompression prevents the progression of biliary pancreatitis: an experi-

mental study in the opossum. Gastroenterology. 1993;105:157–64.

31. Senninger N, Moody FG, Coelho JC, Van Buren DH. The role of biliary obstruction in the pathogenesis of acute pancreatitis in the opossum. Surgery. 1986;99:688–93.

32. Stone HH, Fabian TC, Dunlop WE. Gallstone pancreatitis: biliary tract pathology in relation to time of operation. Ann Surg. 1981;194:305–12.

33. Andriulli A, Loperfido S, Napolitano G, et al. Incidence rates of post-ERCP complications: a systematic survey of prospective studies. Am J Gastroenterol. 2007;102:1781–8.

34. Freeman ML, Nelson DB, Sherman S, et al. Complications of endoscopic biliary sphincterotomy. N Engl J Med. 1996;335:909–18.

35. *Schepers NJ, Hallensleben NDL, Besselink MG, Anten MGF, Bollen TL, da Costa DW, van Delft F, van Dijk SM, van Dullemen HM, Dijkgraaf MGW, van Eijck CHJ, Erkelens GW, Erler NS, Fockens P, van Geenen EJM, van Grinsven J, Hollemans RA, van Hooft JE, van der Hulst RWM, Jansen JM, Kubben FJGM, Kuiken SD, Laheij RJF, Quispel R, de Ridder RJJ, Rijk MCM, Römkens TEH, Ruigrok CHM, Schoon EJ, Schwartz MP, Smeets XJNM, Spanier BWM, Tan ACITL, Thijs WJ, Timmer R, Venneman NG, Verdonk RC, Vleggaar FP, van de Vrie W, Witteman BJ, van Santvoort HC, Bakker OJ, Bruno MJ; Dutch Pancreatitis Study Group. Urgent endoscopic retrograde cholangiopancreatography with sphincterotomy versus conservative treatment in predicted severe acute gallstone pancreatitis (APEC): a multicentre randomised controlled trial. Lancet 2020; 396: 167–176. *RCT showing that urgent ERCP is not indicated in patients with predicted severe biliary pancreatitis.

36. Anderloni A, Galeazzi M, Ballare M, Pagliarulo M, Orsello M, Del Piano M, Repici A. Early endoscopic ultrasonography in acute biliary pancreatitis: a prospective pilot study. World J Gastroenterol. 2015;21:10427–34.

37. Giljaca V, Gurusamy KS, Takwoingi Y, et al. Endoscopic ultrasound versus magnetic resonance cholangiopancreatography for common bile duct stones. Cochrane Database Syst Rev. 2015;2:CD011549.

38. Hallensleben ND, for the Dutch Pancreatitis Study Group. Urgent endoscopic ultrasound-guided ERC in predicted severe acute biliary pancreatitis (APEC-2): a multicenter prospective study. United Eur Gastroenterol. 2021;9(S8, OP131):101–2.

39. Forsmark CE, Baillie J. AGA institute technical review on acute pancreatitis. Gastroenterology. 2007;132:2022–44.

40. Banks PA, Freeman ML. Practice guidelines in acute pancreatitis. Am J Gastroenterol. 2006;101:2379–400.

41. Uhl W, Warshaw A, Imrie C, Bassi C, McKay CJ, Lankisch PG, Carter R, Di Magno E, Banks PA, Whitcomb DC, Dervenis C, Ulrich CD, Satake K, Ghaneh P, Hartwig W, Werner J, McEntee G,

Neoptolemos JP, Büchler MW. International association of pancreatology: IAP guidelines for the surgical management of acute pancreatitis. Pancreatology. 2002;2:565–73.

42. Nguyen GC, Boudreau H, Jagannath SB. Hospital volume as a predictor for undergoing cholecystectomy after admission for acute biliary pancreatitis. Pancreas. 2010;39:e42–7.

43. Pezzilli R, Uomo G, Gabbrielli A, Zerbi A, Frulloni L, De Rai P, Castoldi L, Cavallini G, Di Carlo V. A prospective multicentre survey on the treatment of acute pancreatitis in Italy. Dig Liver Dis. 2007;39:838–46.

44. Green R, Charman SC, Palser T. Early definitive treatment rate as a quality indicator of care in acute gallstone pancreatitis. Br J Surg. 2017;104:1686–94.

45. *da Costa DW, Bouwense SA, Schepers NJ, Besselink MG, van Santvoort HC, van Brunschot S, Bakker OJ, Bollen TL, Dejong CH, van Goor H, Boermeester MA, Bruno MJ, van Eijck CH, Timmer R, Weusten BL, Consten EC, Brink MA, Spanier BWM, Spillenaar Bilgen EJ, Nieuwenhuijs VB, Hofker HS, Rosman C, Voorburg AM, Bosscha K, van Duijvendijk P, Gerritsen JJ, Heisterkamp J, de Hingh IH, Witteman BJ, Kruyt PM, Scheepers JJ, Molenaar IQ, Schaapherder AF, Manusama ER, van der Waaij LA, van Unen J, Dijkgraaf MG, van Ramshorst B, Gooszen HG, Boerma D, Dutch Pancreatitis Study Group. Same-admission versus interval cholecystectomy for mild gallstone pancreatitis (PONCHO): a multicentre randomised controlled trial. Lancet 2015;386(10000):1261–1268. *RCT showing that same-admission cholecystectomy is safe in patients with mild gallstone pancreatitis.

46. *Hallensleben ND, Timmerhuis HC, Hollemans RA, Pocornie S, van Grinsven J, van Brunschot S, Bakker OJ, van der Sluijs R, Schwartz MP, van Duijvendijk P, Römkens T, Stommel MWJ, Verdonk RC, Besselink MG, Bouwense SAW, Bollen TL, van Santvoort HC, Bruno MJ, Dutch Pancreatitis Study Group. Optimal timing of cholecystectomy after necrotising biliary pancreatitis. Gut 2022; 71: 974–982. *Study showing that the optimal interval for cholecystectomy after necrotising biliary pancreatitis is within 8 weeks after discharge when local complications (e.g. necrosis) have resolved.

Managing Hypertriglyceridaemia-Associated Acute Pancreatitis

Wei Huang and Qing Xia

Key Points

1. Obesity, uncontrolled diabetes, and alcohol misuse together with genetic variants of lipoprotein lipase pathway are substantial contributors to hypertriglyceridaemia and hypertriglyceridaemia-associated acute pancreatitis (HTG-AP).
2. HTG-AP can be diagnosed on admission by measuring serum triglyceride levels ≥ 11.2 mmol/L, or ≥ 5.6 mmol/L with past hypertriglyceridaemia history or milky plasma, after ruling out other aetiologies.
3. Compound (two or more) aetiology with admission serum triglyceride levels ≥ 11.2 mmol/L should be recognised as a more severe phenotype of HTG-AP.
4. Fat emulsion should be avoided in HTG-AP patients requiring total parental nutrition but can be administered with caution in those with a serum triglyceride level <5.6 mmol/L.
5. Insulin (normally 0.1–0.3 units/kg/h) with or without heparin (depending on the contradictory conditions) should be considered as the first-line therapy approach for early management of HTG-AP.
6. The role of extracorporeal therapies in early management of HTG-AP patients remain uncertain, but can serve as a last resort for individuals.
7. Risk factor screening programmes are important for preventing recurrence of HTG-AP and its sequelae.
8. Lipid-lowering drugs with concomitant control of secondary causes are important for prevention of HTG-AP and its sequelae.
9. Genetic testing should be performed for individuals with persistently severe hypertriglyceridaemia and/or cholesterol despite optimal lipid-lowing drug treatment.

W. Huang (✉) · Q. Xia
West China Centre of Excellence for Pancreatitis,
Institute of Integrated Traditional Chinese and
Western Medicine, West China-Liverpool Biomedical
Research Centre, West China Hospital, Sichuan
University, Chengdu, China
e-mail: dr_wei_huang@scu.edu.cn;
xiaqing@medmail.com.cn

1 Introduction

1.1 Epidemiology and Clinical Characteristics

Hypertriglyceridaemia is a component of metabolic syndrome that is often associated with the

© The Author(s), under exclusive license to Springer Nature Singapore Pte Ltd. 2024
J. A. Windsor et al. (eds.), *Acute Pancreatitis*, https://doi.org/10.1007/978-981-97-3132-9_14

development of atherosclerosis, fatty liver disease, and acute pancreatitis, resulting in a major health concern and economic burden [1]. Acute pancreatitis is one of the most common digestive disorders [2, 3] with an increasing global incidence [2, 4, 5]. With the high prevalence of obesity [6], diabetes [7, 8], and metabolic syndrome [9], all known factors that contribute to hypertriglyceridaemia, the incidence of hypertriglyceridaemia-associated acute pancreatitis (HTG-AP) has dramatically increased to being the third most common type following that of biliary origin and excessive alcohol consumption worldwide [10–16]. This phenomenon is more profound in China as per reports from recent large cohorts ($n > 500$) of acute pancreatitis in which the proportion of HTG-AP accounted for around one-third of all cases, similar to, or more than, that of contemporaneous biliary aetiology [17–21]. Moreover, in most recent randomised controlled trials conducted in China, HTG-AP accounted for around 50% of all cases, making it an important ethology for acute pancreatitis [22, 23].

Population-based studies have demonstrated a stepwise relationship between elevated serum triglyceride (TG) levels and the increased incidence [24–26] of HTG-AP. Intriguingly, high TG variability also increased the risk of first-attack acute pancreatitis [27]. High body mass index or central obesity [28], diabetes mellitus [29], alcoholism and diabetes in combination [30], third trimester of pregnancy [31, 32], and genetic variants [33] and metabolic traits [34] related to TG-rich lipoprotein (TGRL) metabolism pathway are common situations often associated with elevated serum TG levels. They are in themselves known independent risk factors for AP.

Compared to other aetiologies, patients with HTG-AP are often younger, are more likely to be male, have heavier alcohol use, and have a higher rate of comorbid metabolic disorders (obesity, fatty liver disease, diabetes, and metabolic syndrome) as well as pre-existing kidney disease [18, 35]. Patients with HTG-AP are more likely to develop multiple organ dysfunction syndrome (MODS) with higher mortality [36], recurrent AP [37], and long-term diabetes mellitus [17],

exocrine pancreatic insufficiency [38], and chronic pancreatitis [26, 39, 40]. The severity of HTG-AP has been reported to proportionally correlate with escalating admission serum TG levels [41–43].

2 Clinically Relevant Science

Triglycerides are an essential energy source for mammals and are absorbed in the intestine, stored in adipose tissue, resynthesised in liver, and utilised in muscle, all processes that are finely orchestrated by TGRL metabolism to maximise resource use [44]. Factors affecting the metabolism of TGRLs are the determinants for dyslipidaemias including severe (11.2–22.4 mmol/L) or very severe (>22.4 mmol/L; Endocrine Society Guidelines (2012) [45]) classify hypertriglyceridaemia as primary (genetic) and secondary. The latter include life-style factors (excess alcohol consumption, smoking, diet, and decreased physical activity), comorbid metabolic disorders (obesity, uncontrolled diabetes mellitus, and other medical conditions) or pregnancy, and use of certain drugs (oral oestrogen, tamoxifen, isotretinoin, ciclosporin, L-asparaginase, etc.) [46]. The role of TGRLs and their cholesterol-enriched remnants in the pathogenesis of atherosclerosis [46] and AP [47] is well established.

The enzymes involved in TGRL metabolism include lipoprotein lipase (LPL), hormone sensitive lipase, and hepatic lipase [46, 47]. LPL is an indispensable rate-limiting enzyme that catalyses TGRL into free fatty acids (FFAs), monoacylglycerols, and remnant lipoproteins [48]. Dysfunction of LPL would result in impaired utility of available FFAs and monoacylglycerols for peripheral tissue cells and development of hypertriglyceridaemia [48]. The maturation, transportation, stabilisation, and activation are achieved by a co-ordinated network composed of lipase maturation factor 1 (LMF1), glycosylphosphatidylinositol-anchored high-density lipoprotein-binding protein 1 (GPIHBP1), apolipoprotein A-V, and apolipoprotein C-II (activator). Apolipoprotein C-I, apolipoprotein C-III, apolipoprotein E, as well as angiopoietin-like protein 3 and 4 (ANGPTL3/4) inhibit activity of LPL [46]. Hormone-sensitive lipase hydrolyses adipose tissue triglyceride to release FFAs, while hepatic lipase hydrolyses intermediate-density lipoproteins to generate low-density lipoproteins [46, 47]. So far, genomic research of blood lipids from large cohorts has identified more than 300 genetic loci that are associated with TG levels, and these genome-wide association studies have been recently reviewed [49]. Loss-of-function mutations in genes *LPL*, *APOC2*, *APOA5*, *LMF1*, *GPIHBP1*, or *GPD1* result in increased serum TG levels, while loss-of-function mutations in genes *APOC3*, *ANGPTL3*, or *ANGPTL4* result in decreased serum TG levels.

The pathogenesis of HTG-AP is incompletely understood, but the proposed mechanisms are summarised as follows:

1. Elevated levels of chylomicrons in pancreatic capillaryes lead to ischaemia and acidosis [50].
2. Excessive free fatty acids released from lipolysis cause acinar cell calcium overload, mitochondrial injury, and cell death [51–53].
3. Endoplasmic reticulum, oxidative stress, and post-translational modification play important roles in the pathobiology of HTG-AP [54, 55].

4. Large triglyceride-rich lipoproteins in hypertriglyceridaemia are associated with the onset and severity of HTG-AP [56].
5. Genetic variants of TGRL metabolism pathway together with secondary causes are substantial contributors to the development of HTG-AP [33, 57].
6. High TG variability-associated subclinical inflammation may partially predispose to onset of HTG-AP [27].

3 General Management in the Acute Presentation

On admission, patients with AP should be diagnosed and triaged in a timely manner. Clinicians should note that elevated TG levels affect routine detection of amylase, sodium, and low-density lipoproteins. Therefore, the diagnosis of HTG-AP is generally based on serum lipase and imaging. For patients admitted within 48 h of symptom onset, the diagnosis of HTG-AP is made if patients have serum triglyceride levels ≥11.2 mmol/L, or ≥5.6 mmol/L with past hypertriglyceridaemia history or lactescent blood (Fig. 1), and after ruling out other aetiologies [58]. The TG levels after initial 48 h of symptoms

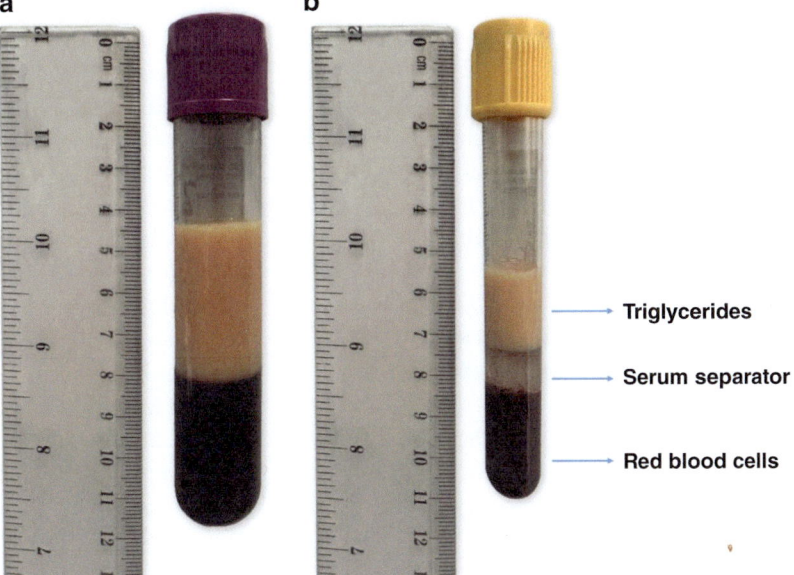

Fig. 1 Lactescent blood samples from a patient with hypertriglyceridaemia-associated acute pancreatitis. Blood samples obtained from a 50-year-old male patient after 26 hours from abdominal pain onset (serum triglyceride levels = 31.3 mmol/L). (**a**) 10 mL EDTA tube and (**b**) 5 mL serum separator tube containing lactescent blood samples after centrifugation at 1500 g × 15 min at room temperature

makes it more difficult to diagnose and assess HTG-AP [59].

Severity assessment should be completed on admission, within 24 h, and after every 24 h for the first week using appropriate biochemical markers and clinical scoring systems [60]. Comorbid metabolic disorders (i.e. fatty liver diseases) [61, 62], body composition [63], admission glucose levels [64–66], and detailed lipid profile (i.e. apolipoprotein A-I [63], TG/high-density lipoprotein ratio [20, 67]) may have additional value for severity prediction. Compound (two or more) aetiologies in association with HTG-AP are associated with an increased severity of disease that clinicians should be mindful of [17, 68–70]. There is an increased risk of developing any organ failure, persistent organ failure, and pancreatic necrosis for single aetiology, dual aetiology (hypertriglyceridaemia-biliary or hypertriglyceridaemia-alcohol), and triple aetiology (hypertriglyceridaemia-biliary-alcohol) [70]. Therefore, HTG-AP patients with compound aetiology warrant timely and prioritised triage, monitoring, and treatment.

The initial management of AP should follow the 2018 American Gastroenterological Association (AGA) Institute Guideline on Initial Management of Acute Pancreatitis [71]. Some specific aspects of care include moderate (not aggressive) fluid resuscitation [72], nonsteroidal anti-inflammatory drugs are equivalent to opiates for managing predicted mild patients [73, 74], and epidural analgesia is safe and effective in improving clinical outcomes in moderately severe and severe acute pancreatitis (persistent organ failure of respiratory, circulatory, and/or renal system with Sequential Organ Failure Assessment [SOFA] score $\geq$ 2 for 48 h) [71] and should be implemented if possible [74].

4 Specific Management of HTG-AP in the Acute Stage

For patients with HTG-AP in the primary admission, they should be kept fasted for the first 48 h and then followed with an oral low-fat soft diet. When this is not well tolerated, enteral nutrition via nasogastric or nasojejunal tubes should be implemented. In patients requiring total parenteral nutrition, fat emulsion needs to be avoided but can be considered with caution when serum TG levels are <5.6 mmol/L.

Besides control of confounding factors, intravenous infusion of insulin and/or heparin to enhance LPL activity should be considered, the use of extracorporeal therapies for TG reduction in HTG-AP patients is not recommended. No clear indications exist for the use of oral lipid-lowering drugs during the acute stage of HTG-AP. However, they can be administered once patients are commenced on and tolerate (to ingest >50% of each meal) [75] an oral diet. The primary goal is to maintain serum TG levels <5.65 mmol/L.

5 Insulin

In addition to its glucose-lowering effect, recent experimental findings have revealed that insulin reduces pancreatitis associated acinar cell injury by reducing cytotoxic ionic calcium overload [76–78]. Furthermore, insulin has been found to stimulate LPL activity while reducing the activity of hormone-sensitive lipase, thus decreasing the release of FFAs from adipocytes and subsequent hepatic TG synthesis and very low-density lipoprotein generation. These functions of insulin eventually accelerate TG degradation to FFAs and glycerol, thereby catalysing the breakdown of chylomicrons.

No randomised controlled trials (RCTs) have been conducted to compare insulin-based therapy with conventional treatment in HTG-AP. So far, the largest case series ($n = 23$) appraised the effect of insulin-based treatment in the management of severe hypertriglyceridaemia (median baseline TG levels 42.5 mmol/L). Weight-based intravenous infusion at 0.1 units/kg/h was safe and resulted in reduction of triglyceride levels to less than 11.2 mmol/L in approximately 2 days and less than 5.6 mmol/L in approximately 3 days [79]. The most recent meta-analysis [80] comparing insulin-based treatment with blood purification in HTG-AP patients included 15 ($n = 909$; 1 randomised, 2 prospective case-control, and 12 retrospective cohort) studies. Pooled results demonstrated that insulin-based treatments were significantly less efficient than blood purification in reducing serum TG levels (Δ-TG) in the first 24 h (weighted mean difference [WMD], -666; 95% confidence interval [CI], -1130 to -202), at 48 h (WMD, -673; 95% CI, -1233 to -112) and overall Δ-TG by day 7 (WMD, -386; 95% CI, -711 to -61). However, insulin-based treatments were associated with significantly less adverse events (odds ratio [OR], 0.09; 95% CI, 0.03 to 0.27) and costs (WMD, -2.5; 95% CI, -3.61 to -1.39). The reduction in serum C-reactive protein levels and Acute Physiology and Chronic Health Evaluation II (APACHE II) scores and major clinical outcomes (including organ failure, local complication, mortality, length of hospital stay, and recurrence of AP) were not significantly different between insulin-based treatment and blood purification. Of particular note, only one retrospective study [81] in this meta-analysis included consecutive patients admitted with very high levels of serum TGs (>45.6 mmol/L). The authors inferred that in HTG-AP patients without MODS, no significant benefit to either mortality or length of hospital stay was observed when superimposing therapeutic plasma exchange even when patients presented with severely elevated levels of TGs. More recently, a randomised, open-label, parallel group, single-centre interventional trial ($n = 22$) [82] compared insulin-based treatment and therapeutic plasma exchange (admission TG levels in mmol/L: 26 ± 8 vs. 31 ± 9, $P = 0.21$) in managing HTG-AP patients. The authors found that despite a trend towards slower reduction of serum TGs with insulin, the clinical outcomes were comparable between the two regimens.

On a separate note, admission stress hyperglycaemia (≥ 7 mmol/L for non-diabetes and ≥ 10 mmol/L for diabetes) [65] and persistent elevation of glucose levels [64, 83] correlate with worsening clinical outcomes in AP, and more so for HTG-AP patients [64]. For critically ill patients, it is advisable to use intravenous insulin

to control blood glucose levels at 7.8–10 mmol/L with monitoring of fingertip blood glucose levels every 4–6 h.

Since HTG-AP patients are prone to develop concomitant hyperglycaemia, current available evidence is in support of using insulin as the first-line therapy for the management of these patients.

6 Heparin

Heparin increases the release of endothelial LPL into circulation. When administered intravenously, heparin's intrinsic affinity for LPL is markedly increased and may thus help catabolise TGRLs resulting in lowered serum TG levels. However, heparin's TG-lowering effect is transient, and chylomicrons will accumulate when LPL is exhausted due to its easy absorption and degradation in the circulation.

A RCT [84] compared insulin with low-molecular-weight heparin (LMWH; $n = 32$, admission TG, 22 ± 8.8 mmol/L) versus early high-volume haemofiltration ($n = 34$, admission TG, 22.4 ± 9.4 mmol/L) in treating HTG-AP patients who were admitted within 72 h after abdominal pain onset. High-volume haemofiltration starting from admission was not found to be superior to the comparable insulin and LMWH regimen in terms of major clinical outcomes, but was more expensive. These findings were supported by a retrospective study [85] in which the authors found that insulin with an unfractionated heparin regimen ($n = 34$, admission TG, 39.4 ± 23.8 mmol/L) had similar effects to therapeutic plasma exchange ($n = 30$, admission TG, 41.4 ± 37.7 mmol/L) in terms of TG reduction rate and clinical outcomes. However, the costs were significantly lower using the unfractionated heparin and insulin regimen and without adverse events. A recent meta-analysis [86] included 4 studies comparing LMWH + conventional treatment ($n = 289$) with conventional treatment alone ($n = 283$) in patients with moderately severe and severe AP. It was found that LMWH was associated with a reduced incidence of MODS, vascular thrombosis, and mortality with a reasonable safety profile.

Taken together, it can be inferred that the insulin and heparin regimens are safe and effective in reducing TG levels in HTG-AP patients. In the absence of contra-indications (e.g. persistent single organ failure, MODS, disseminated intravascular coagulation or severe active bleeding, etc.) an insulin + heparin regimen for up to 3 days is a plausible option.

7 Extracorporeal Therapies

Extracorporeal therapies used in patients with AP principally include continuous veno-venous haemofiltration, high-volume haemofiltration, haemoperfusion, and therapeutic plasma exchange [87, 88]. The applications of these modalities in HTG-AP are rarely indicated.

7.1 Continuous Veno-Venous Haemofiltration

A Cochrane systematic review [89] and meta-analysis of two RCTs comparing continuous veno-venous haemofiltration ($n = 97$) with conventional treatment ($n = 92$) in AP patients found very low-certainty evidence that continuous veno-venous haemofiltration reduces length of stay in the intensive care unit or hospital, as well as total hospital costs. Results were ambiguous when comparing high-volume with standard continuous veno-venous haemofiltration procedures. There are no RCTs addressing continuous veno-venous haemofiltration in HTG-AP patients.

7.2 High-Volume Haemofiltration

A single-centre prospective pilot study [90] showed that early high-volume haemofiltration ($n = 32$) reduced local and systemic complications as well as mortality in patients with predicted severe acute pancreatitis with APACHE II score > 15 when compared to conventional treatment ($n = 29$). Similarly, a prospective controlled pilot study [91] demonstrated that high-volume

haemofiltration with haemoperfusion ($n = 10$) significantly reduced serum TG and multiple cytokine levels, APACHE II scores, and SOFA scores as well as duration of ICU stay in HTG-AP patients when compared to conventional treatment ($n = 10$).

7.3 Therapeutic Plasma Exchange

The guidelines of American Society for Apheresis (ASFA) [92] recommend therapeutic plasma exchange to be used for management of severe HTG-AP, or prevention of HTG-AP relapse. However, this recommendation was based on retrospective case-control studies which have not been validated. A meta-analysis [93] of 15 ($n = 1080$; 13 historical cohort) studies compared the effect of therapeutic plasma exchange with conventional treatment in HTG-AP patients. The authors found that therapeutic plasma exchange achieved faster serum TG reduction in the first 24 h after hospital admission (standardised mean difference [SMD], 0.58; 95% CI, 0.17 to 0.99; $P = 0.005$) but was associated with increased costs of hospitalisation (WMD, 24.32; 95% CI, 12.96 to 35.68; $P < 0.001$). Additionally, no significant differences were found in systemic and local complications, need for surgery, mortality, and length of hospital stay. These findings were confirmed by another meta-analysis [94] on the same topic which included 16 ($n = 1476$; 14 retrospective) studies. Further, a meta-analysis [88] of 13 studies comparing blood purification modalities ($n = 263$; 152 received therapeutic plasma exchange) with conventional treatment (together $n = 671$) arrived at similar conclusions to the aforementioned meta-analyses on plasmapheresis [93, 94]. A multicentre, prospective cohort study (the PERFORM) [95], aiming to enrol 300 HTG-AP patients, is underway, which may provide better evidence on this topic.

In summary, the above evidence does not support general use of any extracorporeal therapies for TG reduction in HTG-AP patients. However, haemofiltration, plasmapheresis, or therapeutic plasma exchange are a last resort therapy and should be tailored to selected HTG-AP patients after treatment with insulin and/or heparin over 48 h. These patients include, but are not restricted to, those who experience a severe clinical course (e.g. admission APACHE II > 15, acute kidney injury, MODS, or severe acidosis) and/or have very high admission TG levels (i.e. TG ≥ 33.9 mmol/L). The treatment window and the technical aspects of extracorporeal therapies in stratified HTG-AP patients remain largely unexplored.

8 Prevention of Recurrent Acute Pancreatitis and Long-Term Complications

Appropriate screening programmes need to be established for high-risk individuals. The American College of Obstetricians and Gynecologists (ACOG) advises lipid assessment of females before pregnancy at their annual doctor's visits [96]. Furthermore, lipid assessment should be conducted at each trimester [31]. The American Academy of Pediatrics (AAP) also recommends lipid screening for all children between 9–11 and 17–21 years old with additional screening procedure performed when any secondary causes for hypertriglyceridaemia are present [97]. Genetic testing is recommended to identify variants in genes of TGRL metabolism and stratify patients with refractory severe hypertriglyceridemia who can potentially benefit maximally from novel TG-lowering therapies [98].

The primary goal of treatment after screening is to reduce serum TG concentration to below 5.65 mmol/L by traditional lipid-lowering drugs (fibrates, omega-3 fatty acids, and niacin) [47]. In a large cohort of 41,210 patients with severe hypertriglyceridemia, it has been reported that patients whose serum TG levels were maintained <5.6 mmol/L (compared to those ≥5.6 mmol/L) had a significantly reduced hazard ratio for AP, cardiovascular events, diabetes-related events, and kidney diseases. In a population-based study [26], the use of statins, fibrates, or any lipid-lowering drugs was associated with a reduced risk of developing new-onset diabetes mellitus

and myocardial infarction. However, a similar trend in terms of reducing acute and chronic pancreatitis was not observed. In severe elevations of serum TGs and/or cholesterols despite optimal use of lipid-lowering drugs and management, genetic testing must be considered to rule out rare dyslipidaemias associated with monogenic and polygenetic hypertriglyceridaemia [98]. A recent phase 2 RCT has demonstrated that evinacumab, a novel ANGPTL3 inhibitor, significantly reduced fasting serum TG levels of patients with severe HTG and a past history of AP, except for those who had familial chylomicronemia syndrome lacking functional LPL [99]. Of note, serum apolipoprotein C-III levels were substantially reduced for patients in all groups, indicating improved TGRL metabolism. Results from multi-centre RCTs are awaited regarding the potential benefit of apolipoprotein C-III and ANGPTL3 antagonists as preventative strategies for HTG-AP. Until such time, in general, the use of lipid-lowering drugs and controlling secondary causes by achieving weight loss through dietary changes and exercise and abstinence from alcohol confer some protection [47].

9 Concluding Remarks and Perspectives

The incidence of HTG-AP has risen in recent years. Its management during the acute stage is not substantially different from the current practice guidelines for AP. However, specific areas that warrant attention include the avoidance of fat emulsion infusions (should the patient require total parenteral nutrition) and the need to lower the serum TG levels. Insulin with, or without, heparin remains the first-line therapy to lower serum TG levels in HTG-AP patients during the acute stage. The safety and efficacy of extracorporeal therapies need to be compared with insulin-based treatment in individuals who may benefit from any of the extracorporeal therapies (e.g. haemofiltration, plasmapheresis, and therapeutic plasma exchange) in well-designed RCTs. However, haemofiltration, plasmapheresis, or therapeutic plasma exchange are a last resort therapy and should be tailored to selected HTG-AP patients after treatment with insulin and/or heparin over 48 h. Screening, use of lipid-lowering drugs, and the control of associated factors related to metabolic syndrome are important strategies for targeting hypertriglyceridaemia and its sequelae including the prevention of HTG-AP. The role of genetic testing and novel lipid-lowering drugs need to be considered in individuals with severe hypertriglyceridaemia refractory to current management modalities.

References

1. Pirillo A, Casula M, Olmastroni E, et al. Global epidemiology of dyslipidaemias. Nat Rev Cardiol. 2021;18:689–700.
2. Mederos MA, Reber HA, Girgis MD. Acute pancreatitis: a review. JAMA. 2021;325:382–90.
3. Szatmary P, Grammatikopoulos T, Cai W, et al. Acute pancreatitis: diagnosis and treatment. Drugs. 2022;82:1251–76.
4. Cho J, Petrov MS. Pancreatitis, pancreatic cancer, and their metabolic sequelae: projected burden to 2050. Clin Transl Gastroenterol. 2020;11:e00251.
5. Iannuzzi JP, King JA, Leong JH, et al. Global incidence of acute pancreatitis is increasing over time: a systematic review and meta-analysis. Gastroenterology. 2022;162:122–34.
6. Bluher M. Obesity: global epidemiology and pathogenesis. Nat Rev Endocrinol. 2019;15:288–98.
7. Zheng Y, Ley SH, Hu FB. Global aetiology and epidemiology of type 2 diabetes mellitus and its complications. Nat Rev Endocrinol. 2018;14:88–98.
8. Ke C, Narayan KMV, Chan JCN, et al. Pathophysiology, phenotypes and management of type 2 diabetes mellitus in Indian and Chinese populations. Nat Rev Endocrinol. 2022;18:413–32.
9. Saklayen MG. The global epidemic of the metabolic syndrome. Curr Hypertens Rep. 2018;20:12.
10. Adiamah A, Psaltis E, Crook M, et al. A systematic review of the epidemiology, pathophysiology and current management of hyperlipidaemic pancreatitis. Clin Nutr. 2018;37:1810–22.
11. Mukherjee R, Nunes Q, Huang W, et al. Precision medicine for acute pancreatitis: current status and future opportunities. Precis Clin Med. 2019;2:81–6.
12. Pothoulakis I, Paragomi P, Archibugi L, et al. Clinical features of hypertriglyceridemia-induced acute pancreatitis in an international, multicenter, prospective cohort (APPRENTICE consortium). Pancreatology. 2020;20:325–30.
13. Tan HLE, McDonald G, Payne A, et al. Incidence and management of hypertriglyceridemia-associated acute pancreatitis: a prospective case series in a single Australian tertiary centre. J Clin Med. 2020;9:9.
14. Mosztbacher D, Hanak L, Farkas N, et al. Hypertriglyceridemia-induced acute pancreatitis: a prospective, multicenter, international cohort analysis of 716 acute pancreatitis cases. Pancreatology. 2020;20:608–16.
15. Dancu G, Bende F, Danila M, et al. Hypertriglyceridaemia-induced acute pancreatitis: a different disease phenotype. Diagnostics (Basel). 2022;12:12.
16. Olesen SS, Harakow A, Krogh K, et al. Hypertriglyceridemia is often under recognized as an aetiologic risk factor for acute pancreatitis: a population-based cohort study. Pancreatology. 2021;21:334–41.
17. Zhang R, Deng L, Jin T, et al. Hypertriglyceridaemia-associated acute pancreatitis: diagnosis and impact on severity. HPB (Oxford). 2019;21:1240–9.
18. Shi N, Liu T, de la Iglesia-Garcia D, et al. Duration of organ failure impacts mortality in acute pancreatitis. Gut. 2020;69:604–5.
19. He W, Wang G, Yu B, et al. Elevated hypertriglyceridemia and decreased gallstones in the etiological composition ratio of acute pancreatitis as affected by seasons and festivals: a two-center real-world study from China. Front Cell Infect Microbiol. 2022;12:976816.
20. Huang Y, Zhu Y, Peng Y, et al. Triglycerides to high-density lipoprotein cholesterol (TG/HDL-C) ratio is an independent predictor of the severity of hyperlipidaemic acute pancreatitis. J Hepatobiliary Pancreat Sci. 2022;30:784–91.
21. Lin XY, Zeng Y, Zhang ZC, et al. Incidence and clinical characteristics of hypertriglyceridemic acute pancreatitis: a retrospective single-center study. World J Gastroenterol. 2022;28:3946–59.
22. Ke L, Zhou J, Mao W, et al. Immune enhancement in patients with predicted severe acute necrotising pancreatitis: a multicentre double-blind randomised controlled trial. Intensive Care Med. 2022;48:899–909.
23. He W, Chen P, Lei Y, et al. Randomized controlled trial: neostigmine for intra-abdominal hypertension in acute pancreatitis. Crit Care. 2022;26:52.
24. Murphy MJ, Sheng X, MacDonald TM, et al. Hypertriglyceridemia and acute pancreatitis. JAMA Intern Med. 2013;173:162–4.
25. Pedersen SB, Langsted A, Nordestgaard BG. Nonfasting mild-to-moderate hypertriglyceridemia and risk of acute pancreatitis. JAMA Intern Med. 2016;176:1834–42.
26. Patel RS, Pasea L, Soran H, et al. Elevated plasma triglyceride concentration and risk of adverse clinical outcomes in 1.5 million people: a CALIBER linked electronic health record study. Cardiovasc Diabetol. 2022;21:102.
27. Tung YC, Hsiao FC, Lin CP, et al. Triglyceride variability and risk of first acute pancreatitis: a retrospective multi-institutional cohort study. Am J Gastroenterol. 2023;118:1080.

28. Aune D, Mahamat-Saleh Y, Norat T, et al. High body mass index and central adiposity is associated with increased risk of acute pancreatitis: a meta-analysis. Dig Dis Sci. 2021;66:1249–67.

29. Aune D, Mahamat-Saleh Y, Norat T, et al. Diabetes mellitus and the risk of pancreatitis: a systematic review and meta-analysis of cohort studies. Pancreatology. 2020;20:602–7.

30. Lai SW, Muo CH, Liao KF, et al. Risk of acute pancreatitis in type 2 diabetes and risk reduction on antidiabetic drugs: a population-based cohort study in Taiwan. Am J Gastroenterol. 2011;106:1697–704.

31. Gupta M, Liti B, Barrett C, et al. Prevention and management of hypertriglyceridemia-induced acute pancreatitis during pregnancy: a systematic review. Am J Med. 2022;135:709–14.

32. Madro A. Pancreatitis in pregnancy-comprehensive review. Int J Environ Res Public Health. 2022;19:16179.

33. Hansen SEJ, Madsen CM, Varbo A, et al. Genetic variants associated with increased plasma levels of triglycerides, via effects on the lipoprotein lipase pathway, increase risk of acute pancreatitis. Clin Gastroenterol Hepatol. 2021;19:1652–1660 e6.

34. Mi J, Liu Z, Jiang L, et al. Mendelian randomization in blood metabolites identifies triglycerides and fatty acids saturation level as associated traits linked to pancreatitis risk. Front Nutr. 2022;9:1021942.

35. Qureshi TM, Khan A, Javaid H, et al. Secondary causes of hypertriglyceridemia are prevalent among patients presenting with hypertriglyceridemia induced acute pancreatitis. Am J Med Sci. 2021;361:616–23.

36. Wang Q, Wang G, Qiu Z, et al. Elevated serum triglycerides in the prognostic assessment of acute pancreatitis: a systematic review and meta-analysis of observational studies. J Clin Gastroenterol. 2017;51:586–93.

37. Balint ER, Fur G, Kiss L, et al. Assessment of the course of acute pancreatitis in the light of aetiology: a systematic review and meta-analysis. Sci Rep. 2020;10:17936.

38. Yang N, Li B, Pan Y, et al. Hypertriglyceridaemia delays pancreatic regeneration after acute pancreatitis in mice and patients. Gut. 2019;68:378–80.

39. Vipperla K, Somerville C, Furlan A, et al. Clinical profile and natural course in a large cohort of patients with hypertriglyceridemia and pancreatitis. J Clin Gastroenterol. 2017;51:77–85.

40. Yuan S, Giovannucci EL, Larsson SC. Gallstone disease, diabetes, calcium, triglycerides, smoking and alcohol consumption and pancreatitis risk: Mendelian randomization study. NPJ Genom Med. 2021;6:27.

41. Pascual I, Sanahuja A, Garcia N, et al. Association of elevated serum triglyceride levels with a more severe course of acute pancreatitis: cohort analysis of 1457 patients. Pancreatology. 2019;19:623–9.

42. Pothoulakis I, Paragomi P, Tuft M, et al. Association of Serum Triglyceride Levels with severity in acute pancreatitis: results from an international, multicenter cohort study. Digestion. 2021;102:809–13.

43. Sanchez RJ, Ge W, Wei W, et al. The association of triglyceride levels with the incidence of initial and recurrent acute pancreatitis. Lipids Health Dis. 2021;20:72.

44. Cham BE. Importance of apolipoproteins in lipid metabolism. Chem Biol Interact. 1978;20:263–77.

45. Expert Panel on Detection E, Treatment of High Blood Cholesterol in A. Executive summary of the third report of the national cholesterol education program (NCEP) expert panel on detection, evaluation, and treatment of high blood cholesterol in adults (adult treatment panel III). JAMA. 2001;285:2486–97.

46. Boren J, Taskinen MR, Bjornson E, et al. Metabolism of triglyceride-rich lipoproteins in health and dyslipidaemia. Nat Rev Cardiol. 2022;19:577–92.

47. *Simha V. Management of hypertriglyceridemia. BMJ 2020;371:m3109. *A comprehensive review on the clinical management of hypertriglyceridaemia.

48. Olivecrona G. Role of lipoprotein lipase in lipid metabolism. Curr Opin Lipidol. 2016;27:233–41.

49. Carrasquilla GD, Christiansen MR, Kilpelainen TO. The genetic basis of hypertriglyceridemia. Curr Atheroscler Rep. 2021;23:39.

50. Havel RJ. Pathogenesis, differentiation and management of hypertriglyceridemia. Adv Intern Med. 1969;15:117–54.

51. Yang F, Wang Y, Sternfeld L, et al. The role of free fatty acids, pancreatic lipase and ca+ signalling in injury of isolated acinar cells and pancreatitis model in lipoprotein lipase-deficient mice. Acta Physiol (Oxf). 2009;195:13–28.

52. Navina S, Acharya C, DeLany JP, et al. Lipotoxicity causes multisystem organ failure and exacerbates acute pancreatitis in obesity. Sci Transl Med. 2011;3:107ra110.

53. de Oliveira C, Khatua B, Bag A, et al. Multimodal transgastric local pancreatic hypothermia reduces severity of acute pancreatitis in rats and increases survival. Gastroenterology. 2019;156(735–747):e10.

54. Chen W, Wang Y, Xia W, et al. Neddylation-mediated degradation of hnRNPA2B1 contributes to hypertriglyceridemia pancreatitis. Cell Death Dis. 2022;13:863.

55. Kiss L, Fur G, Pisipati S, et al. Mechanisms linking hypertriglyceridemia to acute pancreatitis. Acta Physiol (Oxf). 2023;237:e13916.

56. Zhang Y, He W, He C, et al. Large triglyceride-rich lipoproteins in hypertriglyceridemia are associated with the severity of acute pancreatitis in experimental mice. Cell Death Dis. 2019;10:728.

57. Hegele RA, Ginsberg HN, Chapman MJ, et al. The polygenic nature of hypertriglyceridaemia: implications for definition, diagnosis, and management. Lancet Diabetes Endocrinol. 2014;2:655–66.

58. Scherer J, Singh VP, Pitchumoni CS, et al. Issues in hypertriglyceridemic pancreatitis: an update. J Clin Gastroenterol. 2014;48:195–203.

59. Dong X, Pan S, Zhang D, et al. Hyperlipemia pancreatitis onset time affects the association between elevated serum triglyceride levels and disease severity. Lipids Health Dis. 2022;21:49.

60. Mounzer R, Langmead CJ, Wu BU, et al. Comparison of existing clinical scoring systems to predict persistent organ failure in patients with acute pancreatitis. Gastroenterology. 2012;142:1476–82; quiz e15–6

61. Hou S, Tang X, Cui H, et al. Fatty liver disease is associated with the severity of acute pancreatitis: a systematic review and meta-analysis. Int J Surg. 2019;65:147–53.

62. Vancsa S, Nemeth D, Hegyi P, et al. Fatty liver disease and non-alcoholic fatty liver disease worsen the outcome in acute pancreatitis: a systematic review and meta-analysis. J Clin Med. 2020;9:9.

63. Chen L, Huang Y, Yu H, et al. The association of parameters of body composition and laboratory markers with the severity of hypertriglyceridemia-induced pancreatitis. Lipids Health Dis. 2021;20:9.

64. Yang X, Shi N, Yao L, et al. Impact of admission and early persistent stress hyperglycaemia on clinical outcomes in acute pancreatitis. Front Endocrinol (Lausanne). 2022;13:998499.

65. Yang X, Zhang R, Jin T, et al. Stress hyperglycemia is independently associated with persistent organ failure in acute pancreatitis. Dig Dis Sci. 2022;67:1879–89.

66. Jin Y, Tao S, Yu G, et al. Predictive value of hyperglycemia on infection in critically ill patients with acute pancreatitis. Sci Rep. 2023;13:4106.

67. Cho SK, Kim JW, Huh JH, et al. Atherogenic index of plasma is a potential biomarker for severe acute pancreatitis: a prospective observational study. J Clin Med. 2020;9:9.

68. Wang YH, Xu ZH, Zhou YH, et al. The clinical characteristic of biliary-hyperlipidemic etiologically complex type of acute pancreatitis: a retrospective study from a tertiary center in China. Eur Rev Med Pharmacol Sci. 2021;25:1462–71.

69. Chen EX, Tu Ya SQ, She ZF, et al. The clinical characteristic of alcohol-hyperlipidemia etiologically complex type of acute pancreatitis. Eur Rev Med Pharmacol Sci. 2022;26:7212–8.

70. Yang DD, Gao J, Liu J, et al. Patients-associated compound etiology may have more severe acute pancreatitis: a retrospective cohort study. Quant Imaging Med Surg. 2022;12:4109–19.

71. Crockett SD, Wani S, Gardner TB, et al. American Gastroenterological Association Institute guideline on initial management of acute pancreatitis. Gastroenterology. 2018;154:1096–101.

72. de Madaria E, Buxbaum JL, Maisonneuve P, et al. Aggressive or moderate fluid resuscitation in acute pancreatitis. N Engl J Med. 2022;387:989–1000.

73. Cai W, Liu F, Wen Y, et al. Pain Management in Acute Pancreatitis: a systematic review and meta-analysis of randomised controlled trials. Front Med (Lausanne). 2021;8:782151.

74. Thavanesan N, White S, Lee S, et al. Analgesia in the initial Management of Acute Pancreatitis: a systematic review and meta-analysis of randomised controlled trials. World J Surg. 2022;46:878–90.

75. Ramirez-Maldonado E, Lopez Gordo S, Pueyo EM, et al. Immediate Oral refeeding in patients with mild and moderate acute pancreatitis: a multicenter, randomized controlled trial (PADI trial). Ann Surg. 2021;274:255–63.

76. Mankad P, James A, Siriwardena AK, et al. Insulin protects pancreatic acinar cells from cytosolic calcium overload and inhibition of plasma membrane calcium pump. J Biol Chem. 2012;287:1823–36.

77. Samad A, James A, Wong J, et al. Insulin protects pancreatic acinar cells from palmitoleic acid-induced cellular injury. J Biol Chem. 2014;289:23582–95.

78. Bruce JIE, Sanchez-Alvarez R, Sans MD, et al. Insulin protects acinar cells during pancreatitis by preserving glycolytic ATP supply to calcium pumps. Nat Commun. 2021;12:4386.

79. Hoff A, Piechowski K. Treatment of hypertriglyceridemia with aggressive continuous intravenous insulin. J Pharm Pharm Sci. 2021;24:336–42.

80. He W, Cai W, Yang X, et al. Insulin or blood purification treatment for hypertriglyceridaemia-associated acute pancreatitis: a systematic review and meta-analysis. Pancreatology. 2022;22:846–57.

81. Webb CB, Leveno M, Quinn AM, et al. Effect of TPE vs medical management on patient outcomes in the setting of hypertriglyceridemia-induced acute pancreatitis with severely elevated triglycerides. J Clin Apher. 2021;36:719–26.

82. Gubensek J, Andonova M, Jerman A, et al. Comparable triglyceride Reduction with plasma exchange and insulin in acute pancreatitis—a randomized trial. Front Med (Lausanne). 2022;9:870067.

83. Nagy A, Juhasz MF, Gorbe A, et al. Glucose levels show independent and dose-dependent association with worsening acute pancreatitis outcomes: post-hoc analysis of a prospective, international cohort of 2250 acute pancreatitis cases. Pancreatology. 2021;21:1237–46.

84. *He WH, Yu M, Zhu Y, et al. Emergent triglyceride-lowering therapy with early high-volume hemofiltration against low-molecular-weight heparin combined with insulin in hypertriglyceridemic pancreatitis: a prospective randomized controlled trial. J Clin Gastroenterol 2016;50:772–778. *A single-centre randomised controlled trial demonstrated that early high-volume haemofiltration was not superior to low-molecular-weight heparin + insulin in terms of clinical outcomes and costs, despite faster triglyceride-lowering effect.

85. Jin M, Peng JM, Zhu HD, et al. Continuous intravenous infusion of insulin and heparin vs plasma exchange in hypertriglyceridemia-induced acute pancreatitis. J Dig Dis. 2018;19:766–72.

86. He K, Zhang Y, Song K, et al. Randomized controlled trials of low molecular weight heparin in non-mild acute pancreatitis: a systemic review and meta-analysis. Thromb Res. 2023;221:26–9.

87. Villa G, Neri M, Bellomo R, et al. Nomenclature for renal replacement therapy and blood purification techniques in critically ill patients: practical applications. Crit Care. 2016;20:283.

88. Zhang Y, Lin J, Wu L, et al. Blood purification for hypertriglyceridemia-induced acute pancreatitis: a meta-analysis. Pancreas. 2022;51:531–9.

89. Lin Y, He S, Gong J, et al. Continuous veno-venous hemofiltration for severe acute pancreatitis. Cochrane Database Syst Rev. 2019;10:CD012959.

90. Guo J, Huang W, Yang XN, et al. Short-term continuous high-volume hemofiltration on clinical outcomes of severe acute pancreatitis. Pancreas. 2014;43:250–4.

91. Sun S, He L, Bai M, et al. High-volume hemofiltration plus hemoperfusion for hyperlipidemic severe acute pancreatitis: a controlled pilot study. Ann Saudi Med. 2015;35:352–8.

92. Padmanabhan A, Connelly-Smith L, Aqui N, et al. Guidelines on the use of therapeutic apheresis in clinical practice—evidence-based approach from the writing Committee of the American Society for apheresis: the eighth special issue. J Clin Apher. 2019;34:171–354.

93. Yan LH, Hu XH, Chen RX, et al. Plasmapheresis compared with conventional treatment for hypertriglyceridemia-induced acute pancreatitis: a systematic review and meta-analysis. J Clin Apher. 2022;38:4.

94. Lin YF, Yao Y, Xu Y, et al. Apheresis technique for acute hyperlipidemic pancreatitis: a systemic review and meta-analysis. Dig Dis Sci. 2023;68(3):948–56.

95. Cao L, Zhou J, Chen M, et al. The effect of plasma triglyceride-lowering therapy on the evolution of organ function in early hypertriglyceridemia-induced acute pancreatitis patients with worrisome features (PERFORM study): rationale and Design of a Multicenter, prospective, observational, cohort study. Front Med (Lausanne). 2021;8:756337.

96. Christopher BA, Pagidipati NJ. Clinical updates in women's health care summary: evaluation and management of lipid disorders: primary and preventive care review. Obstet Gynecol. 2019;133:609.

97. Expert Panel on Integrated Guidelines for Cardiovascular H, Risk Reduction in C, Adolescents, et al. Expert panel on integrated guidelines for cardiovascular health and risk reduction in children and adolescents: summary report. Pediatrics. 2011;128(Suppl 5):S213–56.

98. *Deshotels MR, Hadley TD, Roth M, et al. Genetic testing for hypertriglyceridemia in academic lipid clinics: implications for precision medicine-brief report. Arterioscler Thromb Vasc Biol 2022;42:1461–1467. *This study demonstrated that patients with both pathogenic variants and high polygenic risk score of triglyceride-rich lipoprotein metabolism had significantly increased risk for very severe hypertriglyceridemia and acute pancreatitis, highlighting an important role for genetic testing to identify individuals who can maximally benefit from novel triglyceride-lowering therapies.

99. *Rosenson RS, Gaudet D, Ballantyne CM, et al. Evinacumab in severe hypertriglyceridemia with or without lipoprotein lipase pathway mutations: a phase 2 randomized trial. Nat Med 2023;29:729–737. *A phase 2 clinical trial which demonstrated that evinacumab, a novel angiopoietin-like 3 inhibitor, reduced serum triglyceride levels of patients with severe hypertriglyceridaemia and a past history of acute pancreatitis except for those who had familial chylomicronemia syndrome without functional lipoprotein lipase.

Managing Idiopathic Pancreatitis

Rowan W. Parks and Elizabeth Gleeson

Key Points

1. "Idiopathic" pancreatitis is a diagnosis of exclusion, and true idiopathic cases should account for ≤20% of all acute pancreatitis etiologies after meticulous investigation.
2. Initial management of idiopathic acute pancreatitis is similar to management of other etiologies of pancreatitis.
3. Extensive workup should be performed to identify the cause of pancreatitis in order to provide adequate and appropriate treatment which will, in turn, reduce recurrence. These studies include serum IgG4 testing, genetic testing in appropriate patient populations, EUS, ERCP with biliary analysis, contrast-enhanced CT, and MRCP.
4. Laparoscopic cholecystectomy should be performed if microlithiasis is found.
5. Further studies should be conducted to investigate multiple, or interacting, factors leading to idiopathic acute pancreatitis.

R. W. Parks (✉)
Royal Infirmary of Edinburgh, University of Edinburgh, Edinburgh, UK
e-mail: r.w.parks@ed.ac.uk

E. Gleeson
University of North Carolina, Chapel Hill, NC, USA
e-mail: elizabeth_gleeson@med.edu.edu

1 Introduction

The term "idiopathic pancreatitis" has long been defined as pancreatitis when the etiology cannot be explained by thorough history, physical examination, laboratory studies, and imaging including transabdominal ultrasound and computed tomography (CT). Previously, the prevalence of idiopathic pancreatitis was reported to be as high as 40% [1–3]. However, with advances in genetic testing, computed tomography (CT), magnetic resonance cholangiopancreatography (MRCP), endoscopic retrograde cholangiopancreatography (ERCP), and endoscopic ultrasound (EUS), 79–80% of cases previously defined as idiopathic now have a defined etiology [4–6]. Overall, the mortality rate of acute pancreatitis is 2–11% but is reportedly higher (14%) when the etiology is idiopathic, or miscellaneous [2, 7]. Likewise, recurrence of acute pancreatitis is also higher when the etiology is idiopathic [3].

Patients for whom a diagnosis cannot be determined using conventional workup often undergo multiple, expensive, and invasive procedures, as early diagnosis and etiology-based therapy are critical to achieve best outcomes and prevention of recurrence [8]. Patients with true idiopathic pancreatitis generally have had a comprehensive assessment and the most common causes (Fig. 1) have been eliminated [6]. Table 1 shows an exhaustive list of possible etiologies for idiopathic pancreatitis. After exclusion of other diagnoses, generally only 10% of cases persist as

© The Author(s), under exclusive license to Springer Nature Singapore Pte Ltd. 2024
J. A. Windsor et al. (eds.), *Acute Pancreatitis*, https://doi.org/10.1007/978-981-97-3132-9_15

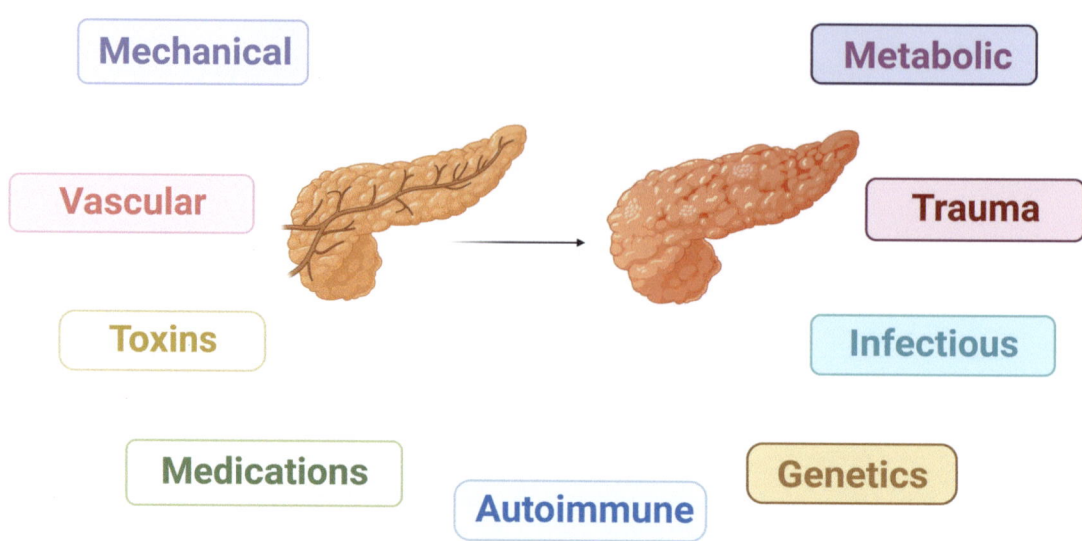

Fig. 1 Causes of idiopathic pancreatitis

Table 1 Possible etiologies of idiopathic pancreatitis

Category	Etiology
Toxin	Alcohol-related (>5 drinks daily)
	Scorpion venom
	Organophosphorus insecticides
	Cannabis
	Cocaine
	Opiates
Mechanical	Gallstones
	Microlithiasis/biliary sludge
	Sphincter of Oddi dysfunction
	Pancreas divisum
	Autoimmune pancreatitis
	Annular pancreas
	Pancreatobiliary tumors
	Choledochocele
	Duodenal stricture or obstruction
	Ascariasis
Metabolic	Hypertriglyceridemia
	Hypercalcemia
	Hyperparathyroidism
Trauma	Blunt or penetrating abdominal injury
	Post-ERCP pancreatitis
	ERCP sphincterotomy
	Sphincter of Oddi manometry
	Iatrogenic surgical complication
Viral	Mumps
	Coxsackievirus type B

Table 1   (continued)

Category	Etiology
	Hepatitis B
	Cytomegalovirus
	Herpes simplex
	Varicella zoster
	HIV
	Rubella
	SARS-CoV-2
Bacterial	Legionella
	Leptospira
	Salmonella
	Mycoplasma
	Brucella
	Salmonella typhi
Fungal	Aspergillus
Parasites	Toxoplasma
	Cryptosporidium
	Ascaris lumbricoides
Antimicrobial medications	Metronidazole
	Stibogluconate
	Sulfonamides
	Tetracycline
	Nitrofurantoin
	Erythromycin
	Isoniazid
HIV medications	Didanosine
	Pentamidine
Diuretics	Furosemide
	Thiazides
GI medications	5-ASA

Table 1 (continued)

Category	Etiology
	Sulfasalazine
	Cimetidine
	Ranitidine
	Mercaptopurine
	Proton pump inhibitors
Cardiac medications	Procainamide
Immunosuppressives	L-asparaginase
	Azathioprine
	Cytosine
	Arabinoside
	Dexamethasone
Neuropsychiatric medications	Valproic acid
	Alpha-methyl dopa
Other medications	Acetaminophen
	Salicylates
	Sulindac
	Calcium
	Ethinylestradiol
	Norethindrone
Autoimmune	Sjogren's syndrome
	Primary biliary cirrhosis
	Renal tubular acidosis
	Hyper IgG4 disease
	Celiac disease
Genetic	CFTR
	Serine protease inhibitor Kazal type 1
	Cationic trypsinogen gene PRSS1
Vascular	Atheroembolism
	Intraoperative hypotension
	Hemorrhagic shock
	Vasculitis (lupus and polyarteritis nodosa)
Miscellaneous	Renal transplant

Refs. [6, 40, 41, 58]

truly idiopathic, and multiple guidelines state that no more than 20% should be classified as idiopathic [9–11].

2 Initial Management

Initial management of idiopathic pancreatitis is similar to acute pancreatitis due to other causes. As discussed previously in this book, management should include fluid resuscitation, analge-sia, nutritional support, antibiotics (if indicated), additional procedures (if indicated), workup for causes, and treatment of any identified cause. Patients should be asked about previous gall-stones, alcohol intake, family history of pancre-atitis, pancreatic cancer, recurrent undiagnosed abdominal pain or type 1 diabetes, drug intake, exposure to known viral causes, or whether they have prodromal symptoms. Laboratory tests including plasma pancreatic enzymes and liver function tests should be performed. As the vast majority of patients with idiopathic pancreatitis are due to undiagnosed stones or microlithiasis [12], high-quality transabdominal ultrasound should be conducted at least twice prior to deter-mination of idiopathic pancreatitis [10].

Serum triglyceride and calcium levels should be drawn at admission since these will need to be corrected at the outset. In the recovery phase fol-lowing an episode of pancreatitis, investigations should include viral antibody titers (mumps, Coxsackie B4, and others), repeat biliary ultra-sound, MRCP, and contrast-enhanced CT (helical or multi-slice with pancreas protocol). If these investigations do not yield a diagnosis, then fur-ther investigations are necessary and include an additional transabdominal ultrasound, endo-scopic ultrasound (EUS), immunoglobulin gamma-4 (IgG4), antinuclear antibodies (ANA), MRCP with secretin stimulation (MRCP-S), ERCP—bile for cytology, ERCP—bile and pan-creatic cytology, and sphincter of Oddi manome-try. Pancreatic function tests, including breath tests, may also be performed to exclude chronic pancreatitis. These tests include noninvasive fecal fat measurements, fecal elastase or invasive tests that require endoscopy, injection of secretin, and analysis of pancreatic fluid production.

3 Subsequent Management

If the cause of acute pancreatitis cannot be treated because it is not identified, patients can develop idiopathic recurrent acute pancreatitis (IRAP). IRAP has a much higher risk for chronic pancre-atitis than a single episode of acute pancreatitis.

Furthermore, chronic pancreatitis puts patients at risk for the development of pancreas cancer [9]. Thus, clinicians must determine whether the patient has true idiopathic pancreatitis or if this has an identifiable and potentially treatable cause.

3.1 Hereditary Pancreatitis and Genetic Testing

If there is any family history of pancreatitis, patients should be referred for, as a minimum, genetic counseling [10]. Hereditary pancreatitis (HP) is defined as two, or more, individuals in a family developing pancreatitis in two, or more, generations, or pancreatitis associated with mutation of the serine protease 1 gene, PRSS1, p.N29I, and p.R122H variants [13]. The PRSS1 gene encodes cationic trypsinogen, and mutation in this gene leads to premature activation of trypsin in the acinar cell leading to pancreatic parenchymal destruction [9]. Interestingly, loss of function of anionic trypsinogen, coded by PRSS2 gene, affords a protective effect against pancreatitis [14]. Loss of function variants in two trypsinogen inhibitor genes, serine protease inhibitor Kazal type 1 (SPINK1) [15] and chymotrypsin C (CTRC) [16], are also associated with acute pancreatitis. Lastly, a variant of the cystic fibrosis transmembrane conductance regulator gene (CFTR) leads to impaired bicarbonate secretion and, thus, impaired flushing out of trypsinogen from the pancreatic duct [17, 18].

The median age of patients with HP is 10 years [19, 20]. Genetic testing should be offered to all young patients with RAP who have undergone a cholecystectomy or sphincterotomy (thus ruling out a biliary etiology) and who do not binge drink alcohol (<5 drinks per day) [9]. The rationale for genetic testing is to (1) ascertain the etiology and limit the need for further investigation; (2) define an etiologic-based pathway; (3) foresee any potential complications; (4) develop management plans; and (5) enable counseling of patients about the cause and prognosis of their disease [9]. Patients should be advised to cease smoking and avoid alcohol, as both substances increase the risk of pancreatitis and smoking increases the risk of pancreatic cancer. Pancreatic cancer risk increases with increasing age in these patients and is 40% by age 70 years in these patients [21].

A total pancreatectomy with islet autotransplantation (TPIAT) is and option to be considered in patients with unremitting chronic pain who have failed medical and/or endoscopic treatments with ongoing recurrent pancreatitis. However, it is advisable to consider TPAIT before the onset of central sensitization. However, postoperative glucose control is dependent on the islet cell yield, and the majority of patients ultimately develop diabetes. TPIAT should not be offered if the only concern is of developing pancreatic cancer [9, 22].

3.2 Autoimmune Pancreatitis

Autoimmune pancreatitis (AIP) is primarily a histologic diagnosis although it can be diagnosed using clinical (obstructive jaundice, abdominal pain), radiologic (diffusely enlarged pancreas or "sausage-shaped" pancreas), and serologic (elevated serum immunoglobulin gamma-4 [IgG4]) markers. Diagnosis of AIP also requires the exclusion of pancreatic cancer. International consensus guidelines categorize AIP into type 1, type 2, and not otherwise specified (NOS) [23]. Type 2 AIP is often referred to as idiopathic duct-centric pancreatitis [9]. Both types are found in adults with a median age between 40 and 50 years. However, patients with type 1 AIP are diagnosed at a mean age of about 10–15 years older than those with type 2 AIP [24]. AIP has a sex predilection for males at a ratio of 2.94:1 [25].

The basis of treatment of AIP is corticosteroids followed by immunomodulators, or, if patients are unable to tolerate corticosteroids, they can be started on rituximab as a single agent [23]. In a randomized controlled trial of prednisolone taper followed by long-term maintenance therapy (3 years) vs. short-term maintenance therapy (26 weeks), patients who underwent long-term maintenance therapy experienced almost 50%

fewer recurrent pancreatitis episodes (3-year follow-up period) [26]. The combination of corticosteroids and immunomodulators has not been well studied, and guidelines lack detail regarding dosing and duration of treatment. When imaging suggests a mass, the patient should be presented at a multidisciplinary tumor board for discussion. In certain cases, when the mass is concerning for cancer, surgery may be recommended.

3.3 Sphincter of Oddi Dysfunction (SOD)

Sphincter of Oddi dysfunction (SOD) is defined as the presence of biliary pain, elevation of liver enzymes or dilated bile duct (but not both), and absence of biliary stones or other structural abnormalities [27]. SOD is thought to cause pancreatitis by obstructing outflow of pancreatic juices or by causing reflux of bile into the pancreatic duct. Sphincter of Oddi manometry (SOM) is the gold standard for diagnosing SOD. SOM is performed via ERCP and cannulation of the biliary and pancreatic ducts with a water-perfused catheter system to measure the pressure [28]. SOD is identified as the cause of idiopathic pancreatitis in up to 31% of cases [4].

In a randomized controlled trial of ERCP+SOM for patients with recurrent acute pancreatitis, 69 patients with pancreatic SOD were assigned biliary endoscopic sphincterotomy (BES) or dual (biliary and pancreatic) endoscopic sphincterotomy (DES). There was no difference in incidence of recurrent episodes of acute pancreatitis after a median follow-up of 78 months. Those with normal SOM were randomized to BES or sham surgery with no difference in recurrent episodes of acute pancreatitis. However, the analysis of normal SOM patients was underpowered as the authors did not meet their target sample size. Overall, patients with pancreatic SOD were more likely to develop recurrent acute pancreatitis than patients with normal SOM (HR 3.5, 95% 1.07–11.4, $p < 0.04$) [29].

SOM is not performed as a standard of care as outcomes are dependent on the technical skill of the proceduralist and there is still a risk for post-ERCP pancreatitis. To avoid post-ERCP complications, a secretin stimulated MRCP (MRCP-S) can be performed. It shows the anatomy and function of the pancreatic ducts at the same time [30, 31]. The pancreatic duct size is measured at baseline and at 15 min after secretin stimulation. The difference in the pancreatic duct size serves as a marker for sphincter of Oddi function [32–34], with dilation of the main pancreatic duct reflecting a functional obstruction at the ampulla.

In a study by Testoni and colleagues, 37 consecutive patients with unexplained recurrent acute pancreatitis, who also had a nondiagnostic EUS, underwent MRCP-S to identify the cause of pancreatitis. In patients in whom this MRCP-S did not identify a cause or in those for whom an ERCP was required for treatment, an ERCP was performed. The positive and negative predictive values of the MRCP-S for diagnosing pancreatic outflow obstruction were 100% and 64%, respectively. The positive and negative predictive values of the test for SOD were 92% and 64%, respectively [30].

3.4 Pancreatic Divisum (PD)

Pancreatic divisum (PD) comprises 25–50% of idiopathic pancreatitis cases [35, 36]. PD is the absence of fusion of the dorsal and ventral pancreatic ducts that develop as pancreatic buds during embryology. Thus, two separate ducts drain the pancreas through two papillae: the dorsal duct into the minor and the ventral duct with the main bile duct into the major papilla [35]. Patients with PD are considered to be more at risk for acute pancreatitis. In the presence of risk factors (i.e., sludge, alcohol use, minor elevations in serum triglycerides) that would not ordinarily trigger an episode of pancreatitis in patients with normal anatomy, it is felt that the minor papilla may be "too small" in patients with PD to accommodate adequate flow of pancreatic juice and this may predispose to an episode of pancreatitis [35, 37]. Treatment is case specific and may consist of cholecystectomy for biliary sludge, abstinence from alcohol if alcohol is the trigger, control of serum triglycerides in cases of hypertriglyceridemia, and, sometimes, improving drainage through the minor papilla using endoscopic techniques (papillotomy ± stenting).

In a trial by Lans et al., 19 patients with PD and at least 2 episodes of pancreatitis were randomized to prophylactic dorsal stent placement, or no intervention. One of the ten patients (10%) in the intervention group developed pancreatitis compared to seven of nine (78%) in the control group ($p < 0.05$, mean follow-up 28.6 and 31.5 months, respectively). Based on the results of this study, the authors recommended dorsal pancreatic duct stent placement for patients with PD to prevent recurrent pancreatitis and improve quality of life [37]. However, these numbers are exceptionally small and the context with which the patient with PD developed pancreatitis must be taken into account. Counseling should be directed toward prevention of pancreatitis based on the triggering events.

3.5 Microlithiasis

Biliary stones <3 mm are unlikely to be detected by transabdominal ultrasound, or CT, and are termed "microlithiasis." Although technically incorrect, microlithiasis has also been used to describe sludge, biliary sediment, biliary "sand," microcrystalline disease, and pseudolithiasis [38]. Given that many patients with biliary sludge eventually develop gallstones, many clinicians believe that sludge is a precursor to microlithiasis, and thus the terms are used interchangeably [12]. Microlithiasis is responsible for about half of all idiopathic pancreatitis cases.

Identification of microlithiasis is done by either EUS or ERCP with bile sampling (Fig. 2). EUS has the advantage over transabdominal ultrasound in that it minimizes interference of bowel gas and peripheral fat on image quality, leading to a high diagnostic yield [38]. EUS has a sensitivity of 95% for microliths, whereas biliary fluid analysis via ERCP detects with a sensitivity of 65–95% [38]. If microlithiasis is diagnosed, the patient should undergo cholecystectomy as

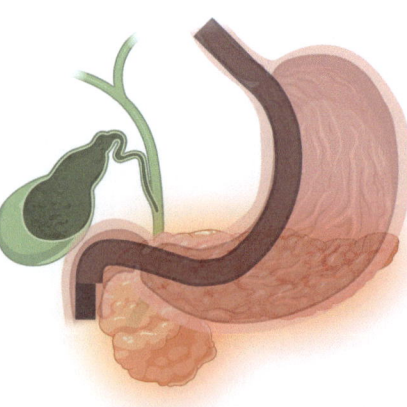

EUS

Can identify:

- Microlithiasis
- Sludge
- Gallstones
- Pancreatic masses/cysts
- Pancreatic divisum
- Choledochocele

ERCP

Can perform:

- Bile aspirate for fluid analysis
- SOM
- Sphincterotomy for SOD
- Stent insertion
- Cholangiogram for pancreatic divisum

Fig. 2 Endoscopic techniques. *EUS* endoscopic ultrasound, *ERCP* endoscopic retrograde cholangiopancreatography, *SOM* sphincter of Oddi manometry, *SOD* sphincter of Oddi dysfunction

the mechanism of microlithiasis in causing pancreatitis is thought to be obstruction of the pancreatic duct.

3.6 Combination of Etiologies

In a study that compared the frequency of PD in a cohort of patients with idiopathic pancreatitis and a control cohort, no differences in rates of PD were observed. These results suggest that another etiology may be at play. Potentially, the combination of PD and microlithiasis led to pancreatitis [39]. Future research should focus on the combination of etiologies in identifying and treating idiopathic pancreatitis.

3.7 SARS-CoV-2

With the recent COVID−19 pandemic (caused by SARS-CoV-2), authors from the United Kingdom have reported a high percentage of COVID-19-positive patients with idiopathic pancreatitis (25%) [40]. Furthermore, those with pancreatitis and COVID-19 have worse outcomes than those with acute pancreatitis alone [41]. These patients were more likely to require ICU admission, develop local complications, have persistent organ failure, and have a prolonged length of stay and increased 30-day mortality [41].

3.8 EUS

There are multiple reasons why EUS is critical in the workup of patients with idiopathic pancreatitis. The diagnosis of microlithiasis can be detected with greater sensitivity on EUS when compared to transabdominal ultrasound. Additionally, EUS can identify masses within the pancreas causing obstruction where MRCP and CT cannot. In a systematic review and meta-analysis of EUS compared to MRI/MRCP, EUS had a diagnostic yield of >60% in patients with idiopathic acute pancreatitis and was statistically better at detecting biliary sludge or microlithiasis [42, 43]. It is technically feasible to perform sphincterotomy in addition to stone extraction using EUS. As the technology improves, EUS will become the primary tool for therapy and should minimize or eliminate post-ERCP pancreatitis risks [44].

While rare, pancreatitis is the presenting symptom in 5–11% of patients with pancreatic ductal adenocarcinoma (PDAC) [45, 46]. Although PDAC generally occurs in only 1–5% of patients with acute pancreatitis, this rate is higher than the rate of PDAC in the general population [47, 48]. The possibility of an unidentified pancreatic ductal adenocarcinoma (PDAC) causes great distress among patients who present with idiopathic pancreatitis. In a retrospective study of 565 patients who had no discrete mass identified on imaging (CT, MRI, and/or US) performed after an episode of acute pancreatitis, EUS with biopsy identified a pancreatic cancer in 30 (5.3%) patients [48]. More than 50% of patients with a pancreatic mass were stage I–II, consistent with previous studies showing that EUS is particularly accurate in identifying tumors <2 cm in size [49]. EUS should be performed at ≥6 weeks following the episode of pancreatitis [50].

Because EUS has increased the diagnostic yield so greatly in patients with idiopathic pancreatitis, many believe that EUS should be utilized routinely [51]. However, all invasive procedures come with risk. In order to avoid patients undergoing an unnecessary procedure, Cortés and colleagues have created a risk score for identifying patients who are most likely to have a positive EUS. They identified the criteria of delayed EUS, obesity, repeat transabdominal ultrasound, male sex, and age over 65 years as risk factors and have named this score DORM65 (Table 2). This risk score has a positive predictive value of 86% (sensitivity 35% and specificity 92%) with an AUC of 0.77 [52]. While further validation is needed, this score may be used to rule out patients who would unlikely benefit from an EUS.

Table 2 DORM65 risk score and point assignment for likelihood of positive EUS

Factor	Points
Delayed EUS	+0.5
Obesity	+1.5
Repeat transabdominal ultrasound	−1
Male sex	+1
Age ≥ 65	+1.5

3.9 Laparoscopic Cholecystectomy

In a prospective trial in Finland, 85 patients with a first episode of idiopathic acute pancreatitis were randomized to either laparoscopic cholecystectomy (LC) or observation. During the 24-month follow-up, 30% (14/46) of the patients in the control group developed recurrent pancreatitis compared to 10% (4/39) of the patients in the LC group ($p = 0.016$). Examination of the gallbladders during surgery revealed that 59% (23/39) contained biliary stones or sludge [53].

In general, utilization of LC during admission for idiopathic pancreatitis has been low. In a study from the US National Inpatient Sample, of all patients with idiopathic pancreatitis between 2015 and 2018 (62,305 patients), only 1% had LC performed during the index admission. Hispanics, those on total parenteral nutrition (TPN), and those with private insurance were more likely to undergo LC during the index admission [54].

4 Medical Therapies

Since microlithiasis is one of the most common causes of idiopathic pancreatitis, use of ursodeoxycholic acid (UDCA) has the potential to reduce recurrence. Multiple small, non-randomized studies of patients with idiopathic pancreatitis have reported success with UDCA [55, 56]. However, in a randomized, controlled trial of UDCA vs. placebo for patients with highly symptomatic gallstones awaiting cholecystectomy, no reduction in biliary symptoms, including pancreatitis, was seen in the UDCA group compared to controls [57]. This study was not powered to focus on pancreatitis events but suggests that UDCA may not be as effective as previously thought.

Pancreatic enzyme therapy has long been used to treat symptoms from pancreatitis, namely, abdominal pain and steatosis. However, there is limited research on whether it treats the underlying cause of idiopathic pancreatitis. Likewise, octreotide has been prescribed in order to reduce the severity of acute pancreatitis, and the same principles would be applied in the acute setting of idiopathic pancreatitis. Octreotide has also been used to reduce output of postoperative pancreatic fistulas, but no data exist on its use for treating underlying causes of idiopathic pancreatitis. In summary, the role of medical therapy in idiopathic pancreatitis lacks a significant evidence base.

5 Management Algorithm

Based on evidence from several studies, a proposed algorithm for working up patients with idiopathic pancreatitis is presented (Fig. 3) [58, 59]. Additional diagnostic testing in a modern retrospective study from the Netherlands revealed the etiology of idiopathic pancreatitis in 36% (64/176) of patients. These authors recommend, as a minimum, a repeat ultrasound followed by either EUS or MRCP in all patients with a first episode of idiopathic pancreatitis [59].

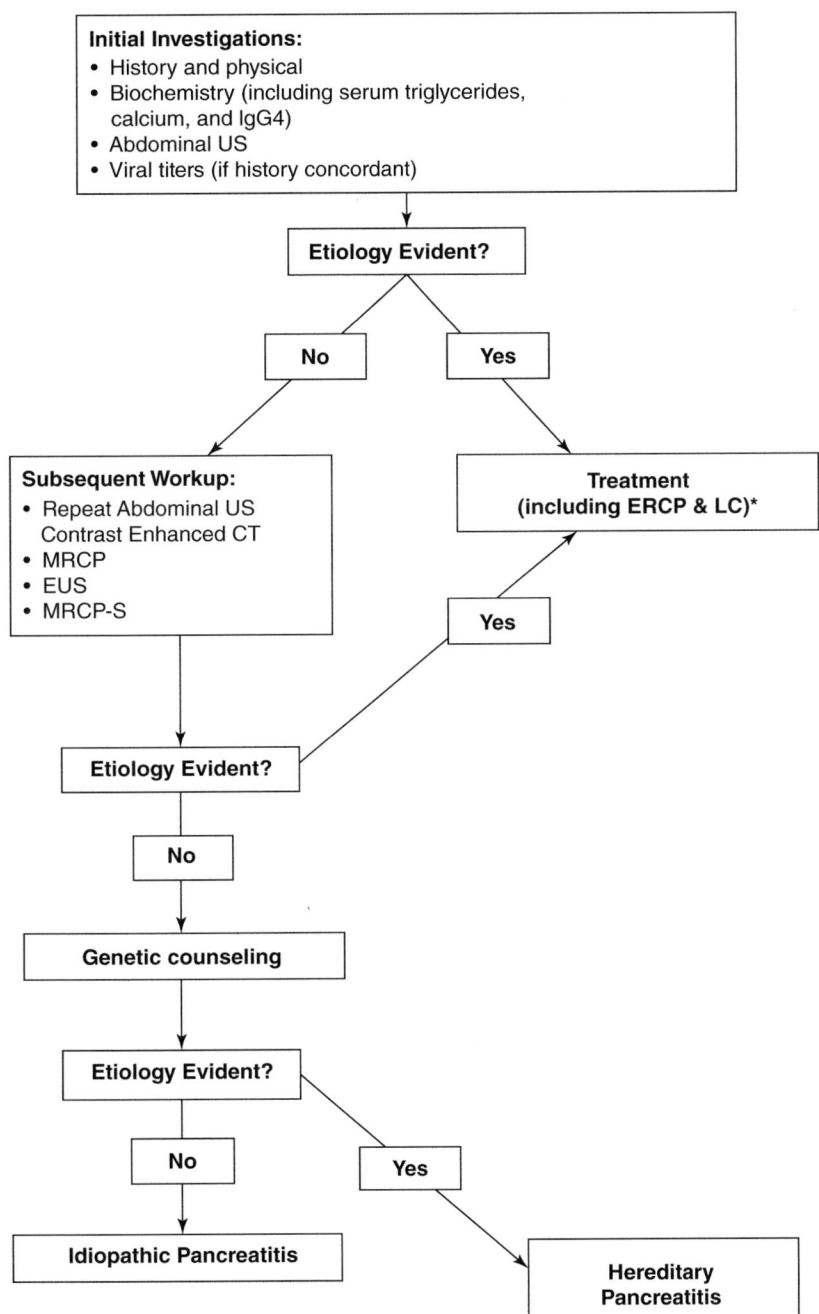

Fig. 3 Recommended algorithm for the diagnosis of idiopathic pancreatitis. *If clinically indicated. *IgG4* immunoglobulin G4, *US* ultrasound, *CT* computed tomography, *MRCP* magnetic resonance cholangiopancreatography, *EUS* endoscopic ultrasound, *ERCP* endoscopic retrograde cholangiopancreatography, *MRCP-S* magnetic resonance cholangiopancreatography with secretin stimulation, *LC* laparoscopic cholecystectomy

6 Ongoing Trials and Future Directions

Several trials are ongoing that may reveal best practices for managing idiopathic pancreatitis. The SpHincterotomy for Acute Recurrent Pancreatitis (SHARP) trial is currently recruiting patients with recurrent acute pancreatitis in the setting of pancreatic divisum to be randomized to either minor papilla endoscopic sphincterotomy (miES) or sham surgery. The primary outcome measure will be risk reduction of subsequent acute pancreatitis episodes by 33% [60].

The Pancreatitis of Idiopathic origin: Clinical added value of endoscopic UltraSonography (PICUS) Study is enrolling patients who have had their first episode of presumed idiopathic acute pancreatitis. All patients will undergo routine EUS. If the diagnostic yield is >10%, the authors will recommend routine EUS for all patients with idiopathic acute pancreatitis [61].

In the EFFORT study, patients who have had at least two episodes of idiopathic acute pancreatitis in the preceding 2 years will be randomized to either a "reduced fat diet" (15% fat, 65% carbohydrate, 20% protein) or a "standard healthy diet" (30% fat, 50% carbohydrate, 20% protein according to the World Health Organization [WHO]). Patients will be followed for 2 years to see if diet can prevent recurrence of pancreatitis [62].

Future research studies should focus on identifying ways to prevent idiopathic pancreatitis, calculating the prevalence of occult intraductal papillary mucinous neoplasm (IPMN) in patients with idiopathic pancreatitis, determine disparities in care after diagnosis of idiopathic pancreatitis, and define the role of combination etiologies in the diagnosis of idiopathic pancreatitis [11, 54].

7 Conclusion

In summary, true idiopathic pancreatitis is a diagnosis of exclusion and should account for no more than 20% of all pancreatitis etiologies. Initial management of idiopathic acute pancreatitis is similar to other acute pancreatitis episodes. Acute pancreatitis may incorrectly be diagnosed as idiopathic when workup is incompletely performed. Thorough diagnostic studies should be conducted to identify the cause in order to provide quality care and prevent recurrence. These studies include serum IgG4 testing, genetic testing in appropriate patient populations, EUS, ERCP with biliary analysis, contrast-enhanced CT, and MRCP (see Fig. 1).

In patients in whom microlithiasis is the etiology, LC should be performed. Future studies should be conducted to investigate multiple or interacting factors contributing to idiopathic acute pancreatitis and to investigate reasons for incomplete workup, or disparities in care.

Acknowledgments Images 1 and 2 were created with BioRender.com.

Conflicts of Interest The authors have no conflicts of interest.

References

1. Trapnell JE, Duncan EH. Patterns of incidence in acute pancreatitis. BMJ. 1975;2(5964):179–83.
2. Thomson SR, Hendry WS, McFarlane GA, Davidson AI. Epidemiology and outcome of acute pancreatitis. Br J Surg. 1987;74(5):398–401.
3. Venu RP, Geenen JE, Hogan W, Stone J, Johnson GK, Soergel K. Idiopathic recurrent pancreatitis: an approach to diagnosis and treatment. Dig Dis Sci. 1989;34(1):56–60.
4. Coyle WJ, Pineau BC, Tarnasky PR, Knapple WL, Aabakken L, Hoffman BJ, et al. Evaluation of unexplained acute and acute recurrent pancreatitis using endoscopic retrograde cholangiopancreatography, sphincter of Oddi manometry and endoscopic ultrasound. Endoscopy. 2002;34(08):617–23.
5. Kaw M, Brodmerkel GJ. ERCP, biliary crystal analysis, and sphincter of Oddi manometry in idiopathic recurrent pancreatitis. Gastrointest Endosc. 2002;55(2):157–62.
6. Lee JK, Enns R. Review of idiopathic pancreatitis. World J Gastroenterol. 2007;13(47):6296–313.
7. Birgisson H, Möller PH, Birgisson S, Thoroddsen Á, Ásgeirsson KS, Sigurjónsson SV, et al. Acute pancreatitis: a prospective study of its incidence, aetiology, severity, and mortality in Iceland. Eur J Surg. 2002;168(5):278–82.

8. Sajith KG, Chacko A, Dutta AK. Recurrent acute pancreatitis: clinical profile and an approach to diagnosis. Dig Dis Sci. 2010;55(12):3610–6.

9. Guda NM, Muddana V, Whitcomb DC, Levy P, Garg P, Cote G, et al. Recurrent acute pancreatitis: international state-of-the-science conference with recommendations. Pancreas. 2018;47(6):653–66.

10. UK Working Party on Acute Pancreatitis. UK guidelines for the management of acute pancreatitis. Gut. 2005;54(suppl_3):iii1–9:iii1.

11. Tenner S, Baillie J, DeWitt J, Vege SS. American College of Gastroenterology guideline: management of acute pancreatitis. Am J Gastroenterol. 2013;108(9):1400–15.

12. Biliary sludge: more than a curiosity. Lancet. 1992;339(8801):1087:1087.

13. Suzuki M, Minowa K, Nakano S, Isayama H, Shimizu T. Genetic abnormalities in pancreatitis: an update on diagnosis, clinical features, and treatment. Diagnostics. 2020;11(1):31.

14. Witt H, Sahin-Tóth M, Landt O, Chen JM, Kähne T, Drenth JP, et al. A degradation-sensitive anionic trypsinogen (PRSS2) variant protects against chronic pancreatitis. Nat Genet. 2006;38(6):668–73.

15. Pfützer RH, Barmada MM, Brunskill APJ, Finch R, Hart PS, Neoptolemos J, et al. SPINK1/PSTI polymorphisms act as disease modifiers in familial and idiopathic chronic pancreatitis. Gastroenterology. 2000;119(3):615–23.

16. Rosendahl J, Witt H, Szmola R, Bhatia E, Ózsvári B, Landt O, et al. Chymotrypsin C (CTRC) variants that diminish activity or secretion are associated with chronic pancreatitis. Nat Genet. 2008;40(1):78–82.

17. Sharer N, Schwarz M, Malone G, Howarth A, Painter J, Super M, et al. Mutations of the cystic fibrosis gene in patients with chronic pancreatitis. N Engl J Med. 1998;8:645.

18. Cohn JA, Friedman KJ, Noone PG, Knowles MR, Silverman LM, Jowell PS. Relation between mutations of the cystic fibrosis gene and Idiopathic pancreatitis. N Engl J Med. 1998;339(10):653–8.

19. Rebours V, Lévy P, Ruszniewski P. An overview of hereditary pancreatitis. Dig Liver Dis. 2012;44(1):8–15.

20. Howes N, Lerch MM, Greenhalf W, Stocken DD, Ellis I, Simon P, et al. Clinical and genetic characteristics of hereditary pancreatitis in Europe. Clin Gastroenterol Hepatol. 2004;2(3):252–61.

21. Lowenfels AB, Maisonneuve P, DiMagno EP, Elitsur Y, Gates LK, Perrault J, et al. Hereditary pancreatitis and the risk of pancreatic cancer. JNCI J Natl Cancer Inst. 1997;89(6):442–6.

22. Chinnakotla S, Bellin MD, Schwarzenberg SJ, Radosevich DM, Cook M, Dunn TB, et al. Total pancreatectomy and islet autotransplantation in children for chronic pancreatitis: indication, surgical techniques, postoperative management, and long-term outcomes. Ann Surg. 2014;260(1):56–64.

23. Madhani K, Farrell JJ. Management of Autoimmune Pancreatitis. Gastrointest Endosc Clin N Am. 2018;28(4):493–519.

24. Poddighe D. Autoimmune pancreatitis and pancreatic cancer: epidemiological aspects and immunological considerations. World J Gastroenterol. 2021;27(25):3825–36.

25. Drake M, Dodwad SJM, Davis J, Kao LS, Cao Y, Ko TC. Sex-related differences of acute and chronic pancreatitis in adults. JCM. 2021;10(2):300.

26. Masamune A, Nishimori I, Kikuta K, Tsuji I, Mizuno N, Iiyama T, et al. Randomised controlled trial of long-term maintenance corticosteroid therapy in patients with autoimmune pancreatitis. Gut. 2017;66(3):487–94.

27. Cotton PB, Elta GH, Carter CR, Pasricha PJ, Corazziari ES. Gallbladder and sphincter of Oddi disorders. Gastroenterology. 2016;150(6):1420–1429.e2.

28. Kim HJ, Kim MH, Bae JS, Lee SS, Seo DW, Lee SK. Idiopathic acute pancreatitis. J Clin Gastroenterol. 2003;37(3):13.

29. Coté GA, Imperiale TF, Schmidt SE, Fogel E, Lehman G, McHenry L, et al. Similar efficacies of biliary, with or without pancreatic, Sphincterotomy in treatment of idiopathic recurrent acute pancreatitis. Gastroenterology. 2012;143(6):1502–1509.e1.

30. Testoni PA, Mariani A, Curioni S, Zanello A, Masci E. MRCP-secretin test–guided management of idiopathic recurrent pancreatitis: long-term outcomes. Gastrointest Endosc. 2008;67(7):1028–34.

31. Nicaise N, Pellet O, Metens T, Devière J, Braudé P, Struyven J, et al. Magnetic resonance cholangiopancreatography: interest of IV secretin administration in the evaluation of pancreatic ducts. Eur Radiol. 1998;8(1):16–22.

32. Soto J, Barish M, Yucel E, Siegenberg D, Ferrucci J, Chuttani R. Magnetic resonance cholangiography: comparison with endoscopic retrograde cholangiopancreatography. Gastroenterology. 1996;110(2):589–97.

33. Francesco VD, Brunori MP, Rigo L, Uli JT, Angelini G, Frulloni L, et al. Comparison of ultrasound-secretin test and sphincter of Oddi manometry in patients with recurrent acute pancreatitis. Dig Dis Sci. 1999;44(2):5.

34. Khalid A, Peterson M, Slivka A. Secretin-stimulated magnetic resonance pancreaticogram to assess pancreatic duct outflow obstruction in evaluation of idiopathic acute recurrent pancreatitis: a pilot study. Dig Dis Sci. 2003;48(8):1475–81.

35. Bernard JP, Sahel J, Giovannini M, Sarles H. Pancreas divisum is a probable cause of acute pancreatitis: a report of 137 cases. Pancreas. 1990;5(3):248–54.

36. Cruz LM, Kwon JY, Oman SP, Zaver H, Bolaños GA, Kröner PT, et al. Comparison of idiopathic recurrent acute pancreatitis [IRAP] and recurrent acute

pancreatitis with genetic mutations. Dig Liver Dis. 2021;53(10):1294–300.

37. Lans JI, Geenen JE, Johanson JF, Hogan WJ. Endoscopic therapy in patients with pancreas divisum and acute pancreatitis: a prospective, randomized, controlled clinical trial. Gastrointest Endosc. 1992;38(4):430–4.

38. Levy MJ. The hunt for microlithiasis in idiopathic acute recurrent pancreatitis: Should we abandon the search or intensify our efforts? Gastroint Endosc. 2002;55(2):286–93.

39. Matos C, Metens T, Devière J, Delhaye M, Le Moine O, Cremer M. Pancreas divisum: evaluation with secretin-enhanced magnetic resonance cholangiopancreatography. Gastrointest Endosc. 2001;53(7):728–33.

40. Nayar M, Varghese C, Kanwar A, Siriwardena AK, Haque AR, Awan A, et al. SARS-CoV-2 infection is associated with an increased risk of idiopathic acute pancreatitis but not pancreatic exocrine insufficiency or diabetes: long-term results of the COVIDPAN study. Gut. 2022;71(7):1444–7.

41. Pandanaboyana S, Moir J, Leeds JS, Oppong K, Kanwar A, Marzouk A, et al. SARS-CoV-2 infection in acute pancreatitis increases disease severity and 30-day mortality: COVID PAN collaborative study. Gut. 2021;70(6):1061–9.

42. Wan J, Ouyang Y, Yu C, Yang X, Xia L, Lu N. Comparison of EUS with MRCP in idiopathic acute pancreatitis: a systematic review and meta-analysis. Gastrointest Endosc. 2018;87(5):1180–1188.e9.

43. Tepox-Padrón A, Bernal-Mendez RA, Duarte-Medrano G, Romano-Munive AF, Mairena-Valle M, Ramírez-Luna MÁ, et al. Utility of endoscopic ultrasound in idiopathic acute recurrent pancreatitis. BMJ Open Gastroenterol. 2021;8(1):e000538.

44. Artifon ELA, Kumar A, Eloubeidi MA, Chu A, Halwan B, Sakai P, et al. Prospective randomized trial of EUS versus ERCP-guided common bile duct stone removal: an interim report (with video). Gastrointest Endosc. 2009;69(2):238–43.

45. Coté GA, Xu H, Easler JJ, Imler TD, Teal E, Sherman S, et al. Informative patterns of health-care utilization prior to the diagnosis of pancreatic ductal adenocarcinoma. Am J Epidemiol. 2017;186(8):944–51.

46. Singhi AD, Koay EJ, Chari ST, Maitra A. Early detection of pancreatic cancer: opportunities and challenges. Gastroenterology. 2019;156(7):2024–40.

47. Easler JJ. Detecting pancreatic carcinoma in the setting of idiopathic pancreatitis and negative cross-sectional imaging: why EUS is useful. Dig Dis Sci. 2019;64(12):3372–4.

48. Bartell N, Bittner K, Vetter MS, Kothari T, Kaul V, Kothari S. Role of endoscopic ultrasound in detecting pancreatic cancer missed on cross-sectional imaging in patients presenting with pancreatitis: a retrospective review. Dig Dis Sci. 2019;64(12):3623–9.

49. Wang W, Shpaner A, Krishna SG, Ross WA, Bhutani MS, Tamm EP, et al. Use of EUS-FNA in diagnosing pancreatic neoplasm without a definitive mass on CT. Gastrointest Endosc. 2013;78(1):73–80.

50. Khoury T, Shahin A, Sbeit W. Exploring the optimal timing of endoscopic ultrasound performance post-acute idiopathic pancreatitis. Diagnostics. 2022;12(8):1808.

51. Pereira R, Eslick G, Cox M. Endoscopic ultrasound for routine assessment in idiopathic acute pancreatitis. J Gastrointest Surg. 2019;23(8):1694–700.

52. Cortés P, Kumbhari V, Antwi SO, Wallace MB, Raimondo M, Ji B, et al. A simple risk score to predict the likelihood of a positive endoscopic ultrasound in idiopathic acute pancreatitis. Gastrointest Endosc. 2022;S0016510722018284:993.

53. Räty S, Pulkkinen J, Nordback I, Sand J, Victorzon M, Grönroos J, et al. Can laparoscopic cholecystectomy prevent recurrent idiopathic acute pancreatitis?: a prospective randomized multicenter trial. Ann Surg. 2015;262(5):736–41.

54. Etheridge JC, Cooke RM, Castillo-Angeles M, Jarman MP, Havens JM. Disparities in uptake of cholecystectomy for idiopathic pancreatitis: a nationwide retrospective cohort study. Surgery. 2022;172(2):612–6.

55. Saraswat VA, Sharma BC, Agarwal DK, Kumar R, Negi TS, Tandon RK. Biliary microlithiasis in patients with idiopathic acute pancreatitis and unexplained biliary pain: response to therapy. J Gastroenterol Hepatol. 2004;19(10):1206–11.

56. Ros E, Navarro S, Bru C, Garcia-Pugés A, Valderrama R. Occult microlithiasis in "idiopathic" acute pancreatitis: prevention of relapses by cholecystectomy or ursodeoxycholic acid therapy. Gastroenterology. 1991;101(6):1701–9.

57. Venneman NG, Besselink MGH, Keulemans YCA, vanBerge-Henegouwen GP, Boermeester MA, Broeders IAMJ, et al. Ursodeoxycholic acid exerts no beneficial effect in patients with symptomatic gallstones awaiting cholecystectomy. Hepatology. 2006;43(6):1276–83.

58. Del Vecchio BG, Gesuale C, Varanese M, Monteleone G, Paoluzi OA. Idiopathic acute pancreatitis: a review on etiology and diagnostic work-up. Clin J Gastroenterol. 2019;12(6):511–24.

59. Hallensleben ND, Umans DS, Bouwense SA, Verdonk RC, Romkens TE, Witteman BJ, et al. The diagnostic work-up and outcomes of 'presumed' idiopathic acute pancreatitis: a post-hoc analysis of a multicentre observational cohort. United European Gastroenterol J. 2020;8(3):340–50.

60. Coté GA, Durkalski-Mauldin VL, Serrano J, Klintworth E, Williams AW, Cruz-Monserrate Z, et al. SpHincterotomy for acute recurrent pancreatitis randomized trial: rationale, methodology, and potential implications. Pancreas. 2019;48(8):1061–7.

61. Umans DS, Timmerhuis HC, Hallensleben ND, Bouwense SA, Anten MPG, Bhalla A, et al. Role of endoscopic ultrasonography in the diagnostic work-up of idiopathic acute pancreatitis (PICUS): study protocol for a nationwide prospective cohort study. BMJ Open. 2020;10(8):e035504.

62. Juhász MF, Vereczkei Z, Ocskay K, Szakó L, Farkas N, Szakács Z, et al. The EFFect of dietary fat content on the recurrence of pancreaTitis (EFFORT): protocol of a multicenter randomized controlled trial. Pancreatology. 2022;22(1):51–7.

Managing Local Complications

Hannah S. Pauw and Hjalmar C. van Santvoort

Key Points

1. Local peripancreatic fluid complications are categorized based on symptom duration (±4 weeks), the nature of the content (solid, liquid, or gas), and whether it is infected.
2. Most sterile peripancreatic fluid collections resolve spontaneously over time and can therefore be treated conservatively.
3. Infected peripancreatic fluid collections, once walled off by 4 weeks, are treated by the step-up approach for necrotizing pancreatitis. According to the step-up approach, invasive intervention is most effective and associated with a lower risk of complications when performed after 4 weeks, when necrosis has become walled off.

1   Introduction

In the majority of patients with acute pancreatitis, the disease course is mild and self-limiting requiring supportive care only. However, a wide

H. S. Pauw
Department of Surgery, St. Antonius Hospital, Nieuwegein, The Netherlands
e-mail: ha.pauw@antoniusziekenhuis.nl

H. C. van Santvoort (✉)
Department of Surgery, St. Antonius Hospital, Nieuwegein, The Netherlands

Department of Surgery, University Medical Center Utrecht, Utrecht, The Netherlands
e-mail: H.C.vanSantvoort-2@umcutrecht.nl

variety of complications can occur in patients with acute pancreatitis and these can be classified as local or systemic. Early detection of complications following acute pancreatitis is essential for accurate treatment. For this chapter we will only address the local complications and its management. Chapter "Managing Organ Dysfunction/Failure" will further address (the management of) the systemic complications.

Over the past decades, the strategies and techniques for invasive treatment of local complications have greatly evolved. The historical treatment of acute and infected necrotizing pancreatitis was open surgical debridement in all patients. For example, Beger et al. promoted early debridement of sterile necrosis [1]. The mortality rate for these open surgery strategies was above the 50%; still it was considered standard treatment till around the 1930s [2]. In the 1980s, a series of prospective studies demonstrated the superior efficacy of conservative treatment over surgical treatment in patients with sterile necrosis, causing a shift in therapeutic approach [3–5]. In 1979, the value of abdominal abscess drainage under ultrasound or CT was discovered, while in 1987, the possibility of using ultrasound or CT-guided aspiration for early diagnosis of infected necrosis was realized [6, 7]. At the beginning of this century, the first study was published on laparoscopic necrosectomy followed by a study involving endoscopic necrosectomy in 2009 [8, 9]. At the end of the 1990s and early 2000s, the necessity of surgical debride-

© The Author(s), under exclusive license to Springer Nature Singapore Pte Ltd. 2024

J. A. Windsor et al. (eds.), *Acute Pancreatitis*, https://doi.org/10.1007/978-981-97-3132-9_16

ment was being questioned when it was shown that initial conservative therapy, including antibiotic treatment, can be successful in a subgroup of patients [10]. Mortality in patients managed with surgery was identical to those managed conservatively [11]. Surgical therapy, when required, was often delayed to a later stage of disease when the systemic inflammatory response has stabilized and the necrotic pancreas had become demarcated. In 2010, the randomized PANTER trial confirmed that a minimally invasive step-up approach (percutaneous catheter drainage ± minimally invasive debridement) prevents the need for open surgical debridement in around 30% of patients [12]. It also demonstrated that drainage alone was sufficient in 35% of patients. Since then, the step-up approach has become the standard of care and is recommended in all guidelines [13–17]. The choice of which intervention strategy is most suitable depends on the location of the walled-off necrosis, whether there is evidence of encapsulation, and if there is apparent adherence to adjacent organs. Endoscopic transgastric necrosectomy has gained widespread popularity and has the advantage of internal drainage with prevention of external pancreatic fistula, which is often seen after percutaneous drainage of surgical intervention [14, 18]. Invasive intervention can be altogether avoided in some cases, as shown in the randomized POINTER trial in 2022 [19]. In this study, 39% of patients with infected necrosis did not require intervention at all and were successfully treated with antibiotics alone. Over the years, significant progress has been made regarding the optimal timing and type of treatment to manage the local complications of acute pancreatitis. With this chapter we aim to provide the best clinical guidance on how and

when to treat the local complications of acute pancreatitis.

2   Definitions of Local Complications

The most frequent local complications associated with acute pancreatitis are pancreatic and/or peripancreatic fluid collections. These can arise with either interstitial or necrotizing pancreatitis. The collections were defined by the Revised Atlanta Classification (RAC) based on chronicity, content, and whether they are infected or not (see Table 1) [20]. The content is not well determined by CT scanning, and ultrasound or MR scanning is preferred to determine whether the collection contains solid material (i.e., necrosis). The morphology of the local complications is also important in deciding treatment and is not covered by this classification. Central collections in the region of the lesser sac are most common, but extensions can occur into the small bowel mesentery, and down both paracolic gutters, into the pelvis, scrotum, and pleura.

2.1   Interstitial Pancreatitis

Interstitial pancreatitis consists of edema and inflammation of the pancreas. CT demonstrates a localized or diffuse enlargement of the pancreas with homogeneous or slightly heterogeneous enhancement of the pancreatitis parenchyma. There are no signs of (peri)pancreatic necrosis (hypoperfusion or Hounsfield unit (HU) is <30). Normal pancreatic parenchyma should display a homogeneous increase

Table 1 Morphological classification of local complications (adapted from the Revised Atlanta Classification)

Content	Acute (<4 weeks, no defined wall)		Chronic (>4 weeks, defined wall)	
	No infection	Infection	No infection	Infection
Fluid	Acute pancreatic fluid collection	Infected APFC	Pseudocyst	Infected pseudocyst
Solid ± fluid	Acute necrotic collection	Infected ANC	Walled-off necrosis	Infected WON

APFC acute pancreatic fluid collection, *ANC* acute necrotic collection, *WON* walled-off necrosis

in attenuation with intravenous contrast agent of 100–150 HU. Parenchymal necrosis is seen as focal or diffuse zones of non-enhanced or minimally enhanced (<30 HU) pancreatic parenchyma on contrast-enhanced CT [21–24].

2.1.1 Acute Pancreatic Fluid Collection (APFC)

APFC is defined as a nonencapsulated homogeneous peripancreatic collection that develops within the first 4 weeks of the disease, and only contains fluid APFCs are caused by (peri)pancreatic inflammation or as a consequence of rupture of small peripheral pancreatic side duct branches. Generally, these collections remain sterile and will resolve spontaneously over time without the need for invasive intervention. Infection is rare. When these collections persist beyond 4 weeks, they are referred to as pseudocysts.

2.1.2 Pseudocysts

Pseudocysts are filled with fluid which consists of fluid debris, blood, and inflammatory cells, no solid necrotic material, and they are walled off by a thick fibrous wall. They can be either asymptomatic or symptomatic: causing biliary or gastric outlet obstruction, bleeding, or secondary infection. It is a complication most often seen in chronic pancreatitis patients, but it also occurs in a small proportion (approximately 10–20%) of patients with acute pancreatitis. The majority of the pseudocysts will spontaneously resolve over time. Indication for intervention depends on symptoms and less on the size. Interventions are only needed in a small subset of patients with pseudocysts.

2.2 Necrotizing Pancreatitis

Approximately 5–10% of the patients will develop necrotizing pancreatitis (NP). This is characterized by necrosis of the pancreatic or peripancreatic tissue, as seen on contrast-enhanced CT scanning. There are three different subgroups of NP as defined by the Revised Atlanta Classification depending on the involvement of the pancreas: pancreatic parenchymal necrosis alone, peripancreatic necrosis alone, and acute pancreatic parenchymal necrosis with peripancreatic necrosis. In most patients with necrotizing pancreatitis (approximately 75–80%), the combined type is seen. Necrosis of the pancreatic or peripancreatic tissue is sterile at first but may become secondarily infected. The risk of secondary infection is around 30% [25, 26].

2.2.1 Acute Necrotic Collection (ANC)

In necrotizing pancreatitis, collections that develop during the first 4 weeks from the onset of disease are referred to as acute necrotic collections. These collections contain variable amounts of fluid and solid necrotic debris which distinguish them from APFCs. Necrosis usually involves both the pancreas and peripancreatic tissue, and in approximately 50% of necrotic collections, it is located outside of the pancreas without apparent direct involvement of the pancreatic parenchyma [27]. The process of encapsulation (formation of inflammatory fibrotic capsule) starts to develop during the arbitrary 4 week period that is used for the definition.

2.2.2 Walled-off Necrosis (WON)

When ANC matures and encapsulates, they are referred to as walled-off necrosis (WON). Usually this happens after 4 weeks in the disease. In contrast to ANC, WON is surrounded by a fibrotic capsule. These collections can vary in size and may or may not become secondarily infected.

2.2.3 Infected Walled-off Necrosis

Infected necrosis is suspected when a patient clinically deteriorates despite maximal conservative support and other sources of infection are ruled out. CT imaging may show gas in the necrotic collections in around 40% of patients [28], as shown in Fig. 1d. Infected necrosis usually takes up to 2–4 weeks to develop, but it can also occur in the first week of pancreatitis or much later [14].

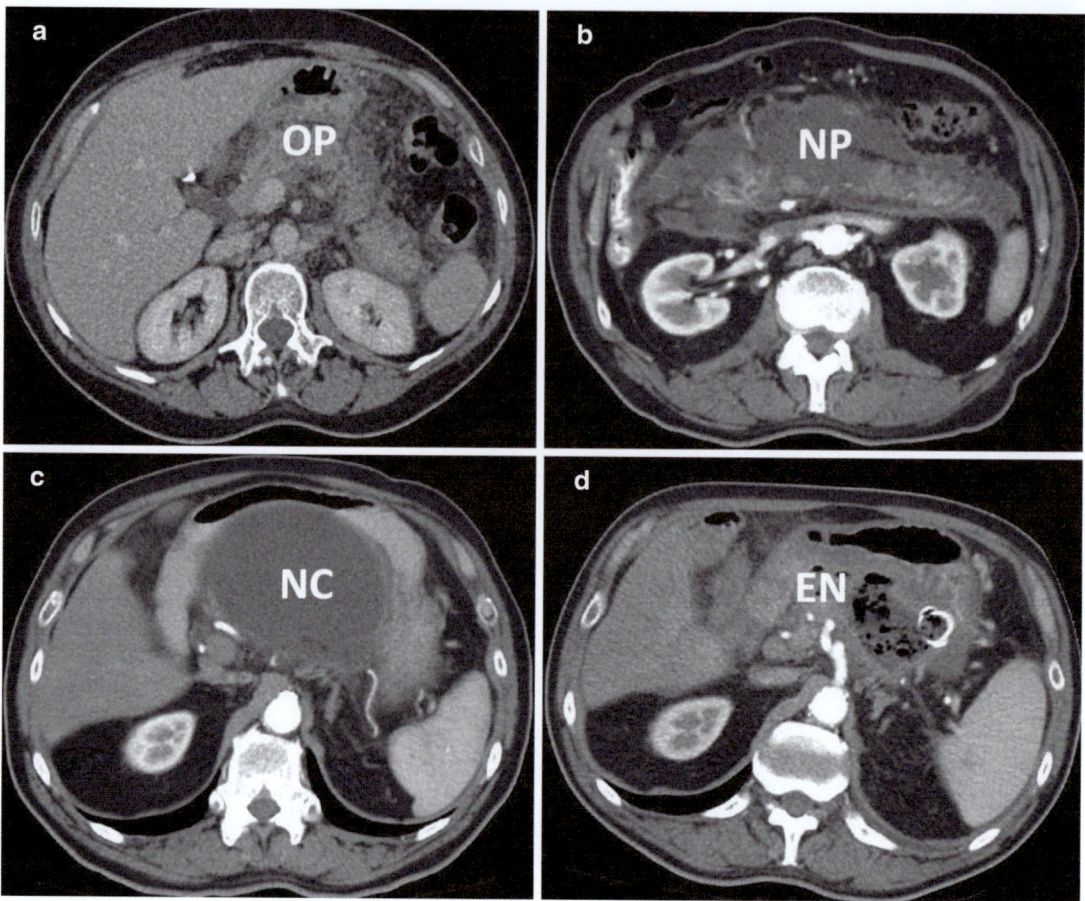

Fig. 1 Contrast-enhanced computerized tomography scans of patients with acute pancreatitis, with application of specialist interventions for pancreatic necrosis. (**a**) Uncomplicated acute edematous pancreatitis (OP) is seen with perfusion of the pancreatic parenchyma, surrounded by inflammation. (**b**) Acute necrotizing pancreatitis (NP) with loss of most of the parenchyma, excepting a small portion in the head and separate small portion of the tail of the gland. This scan was taken 2 weeks into the attack and the necrosis with associated inflammation is diffuse and poorly localized. (**c**) More than 4 weeks after the onset of acute pancreatitis in the same patient as in b, the walled-off necrosis (WON) (designated NC in Figure) has become localized and walled off close to the posterior wall of the stomach, making it suitable for endoscopic drainage. (**d**) In the same patient as in **b**, infection has supervened, identified by the presence of radiolucent black gas bubbles within the collection, which was treated by endoscopic necrosectomy (EN). The endoscopically inserted self-expanding metal stent between the stomach and necrotic cavity is visible as a radiopaque white ring; flushing the cavity endoscopically every 7–10 days was necessary to empty and allow collapse of the cavity, following which the stent was removed. (Reprinted from Szatmary et al. [76])

3 Management of Local Complications: Interstitial Edematous Pancreatitis

3.1 Acute Peripancreatic Fluid Collection (APFC)

In general, the vast majority of acute pancreatic or peripancreatic fluid collections resolve spontaneously in the first few weeks after onset. They do not require invasive intervention. Drainage of sterile collections can do harm by introducing iatrogenic infection [29].

3.2 Pseudocysts

In general, the indication for intervention of pancreatic pseudocysts is determined by the presence of symptoms (e.g., persistent abdominal pain, anorexia, a new abdominal mass after an episode of pancreatitis) and/or the presence of complications (e.g., gastric and/or biliary outlet obstruction, bleeding, or secondary infection) [30]. Current guidelines do not recommend intervention based on the diameter of pseudocysts. When drainage is indicated, it should preferably be performed 4–6 weeks after onset of disease because the collection is usually fully encapsulated by then which reduces the risk of procedure related complications [20, 31]. The first choice of treatment is endoscopic transluminal drainage. If there is communication with the main pancreatic duct, additional transpapillary drainage or stenting should be considered. An alternative would be laparoscopic cystogastrostomy or Roux-en-Y cystojejunostomy, which may required depending on the location and morphology of the pseudocyst.

4 Management of Local Complications: Necrotizing Pancreatitis

The majority of patients with sterile pancreatic or peripancreatic necrosis can be successfully treated conservatively, regardless of the size and extension of the collections. Most acute necrotic collections will resolve spontaneously over time. In some cases (e.g., ongoing organ failure for several weeks, or ongoing [arbitrarily >4–8 weeks after onset of pancreatitis] gastric outlet, intestinal, or biliary obstruction due to mass effect from large walled-off necrosis), intervention is indicated without the suspicion or documented infection of the necrotizing pancreatitis [14]. Invasive intervention is generally only indicated in patients who are deteriorating despite the best conservative management and in whom infected necrosis is suspected (Fig. 2). Clinical decision-making on timing and type of invasive intervention can be complex and requires a multidisciplinary team approach. The different strategies and techniques, as part of a step-up approach, are discussed below and summarized in a treatment algorithm.

4.1 Investigation for Suspected Infected Pancreatic Necrosis

Infected pancreatic necrosis can be suspected based on clinical deterioration (persisting sepsis, new/prolonged organ failure, increased need for cardiovascular and/or respiratory and/or renal support, leukocytosis, elevated or increasing C-reactive protein [CRP], and fever) despite adequate support, in the absence of an alternative source of infection [32]. In case of clinical deterioration, we recommend to perform a CT scan to further investigate the possibility of infection of the pancreatic necrosis and to evaluate other possible local complications (such as extrapancreatic necrosis, arterial pseudoaneurysms, venous thrombosis). On CT, presence of extraluminal gas in the pancreatic and/or peripancreatic tissues can be seen as a sign of infection [33]. To formally diagnose infection of the pancreatic necrosis, tissue obtained from percutaneous, endoscopic, or surgical drainage should test positive for bacteria and/or fungi on Gram stain or culture.

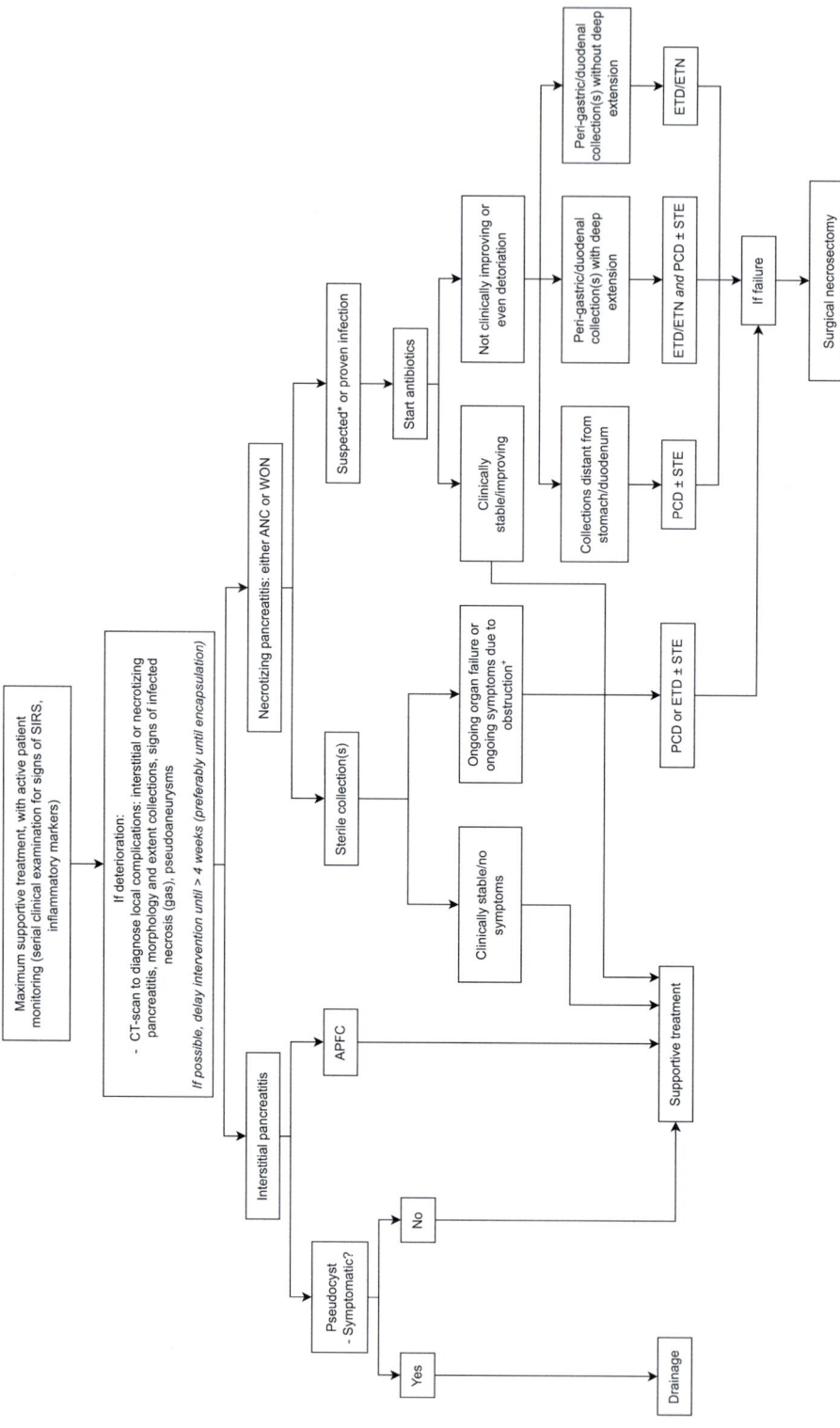

Fig. 2 Algorithm for managing suspected infected pancreatic necrosis. Definitions and further explanation: * Infected pancreatic necrosis can be suspected based on clinical deterioration (persisting sepsis, new/prolonged organ failure, increased need for cardiovascular and/or respiratory and/or renal support, leukocytosis, elevated or increasing C-reactive protein [CRP], and fever) despite adequate support, in the absence of an alternative source of infection. + Ongoing organ failure for several weeks, or ongoing [arbitrarily >4–8 weeks after onset of pancreatitis] gastric outlet, intestinal, or biliary obstruction due to mass effect from large walled-off necrosis. Abbreviations: *ANC* acute necrotic collection, *WON* walled-off necrosis, *APFC* acute peripancreatic fluid collection, *PCD* percutaneous catheter drainage, *ETD* endoscopic transluminal drainage, *STE* step-up approach; endoscopic

4.2 Antibiotic Management

There is no established role for prophylactic antibiotics as proven by various meta-analysis [34, 35]. Also, no reduction in the risk of IPN or associated mortality was found with or without probiotic prophylaxis. Intravenous antibiotics are indicated in patients with strong suspicion of infected pancreatic necrosis. The choice of which type of antibiotics relies on the studies that demonstrate that the majority of infections are due to bacteria derived from the intestine, but not all. Initial antibiotics should therefore be effective against gut-derived bacteria that are known to penetrate pancreatic tissue well, such as carbapenems, quinolones, metronidazole, third-generation cephalosporins [14, 15, 36]. Note that the penetration data may not applicable in the presence of necrotic tissue. After starting empirical treatment, the antibiotics should be adjusted once pancreatic bacterial culture results have been obtained. In current guidelines it is recommended that antibiotics are discontinued once the last percutaneous catheter drain has been removed for more than 48 h and/or pancreatic cultures remain negative [14]. In addition, improvement of clinical, biochemical, and radiological signs aids in the decision to stop antibiotics [18, 37, 38]. A recent RCT implemented a procalcitonin-based algorithm to guide antibiotic use in patients with acute pancreatitis. If patients were randomized for the intervention, they used the cutoff value of procalcitonin level <1.0 µg/L to not start or stop antibiotics and >1.0 µg/L to start or continue antibiotics. The other arm was treated according to the IAP/APA guidelines. The result was a lower percentage of prescribed antibiotics in the intervention group (45 vs. 63% in the usual care group) without increasing infection or harm [39].

4.2.1 Timing of Invasive Intervention

When possible, invasive interventions should be postponed until infected necrotic collections have become walled off, typically after 4 weeks. In the recent multicenter randomized POINTER trial, no difference in the rate of complications or mortality was found between patients randomly assigned to immediate drainage (<24 h after suspected or proven infected necrosis, 55 patients) or postponed drainage (when the collections were walled off, 49 patients). The mean number of pancreatic interventions was higher in the group of patients who underwent immediate drainage [19].

When considering mortality, it is important to note that a meta-analysis showed that late surgery resulted in a significant better survival compared to early surgery (e.g., 72 h and 12 days). This improvement seems to be related to lower bleeding risk and a more effective necrosectomy [40]. However, it remains unknown how long surgery can be postponed and if patients do tolerate the delay of intervention with the risk of sepsis syndrome and organ failure. If possible, delaying surgical intervention for more than 4 weeks is recommended in order to minimize mortality and bleeding risk and to optimize the efficiency of the necrosectomy.

4.3 Invasive Intervention: A Minimally Invasive Step-Up Approach

4.3.1 Step 1: Percutaneous or Endoscopic Drainage

In general, the first step of the step-up approach in patients with (suspected) infected necrosis after failure of antibiotic treatment is image-guided percutaneous or endoscopic ultrasound-guided drainage.

The choice of one approach (percutaneous vs. endoscopic) over another is based on multiple factors, including characteristics of the collection (i.e., location, extent, integrity of the pancreatic duct) and clinical (i.e., hemodynamic) status of the patient. For example, percutaneous catheter drainage can be the first choice in patients with extended collections to the flank or pelvic region. In the PANTER trial, percutaneous catheter drainage was technically feasible in more than 95% of the patients [12]. The preferred route is through the retroperitoneum, as this route can be used for navigation in a later phase or, if needed, for minimally invasive retroperitoneal debridement or necrosectomy. Percutaneous catheter drainage can be performed with either ultrasound guidance or CT guidance. Drain diameter may vary, but large-bore catheter of more than 14 French obstruct less frequently [41]. In about half of the patients, upsizing or replacing the initial drains is required. The success of initial percutaneous drainage can be predicted when the collection shows a decrease of at least 75% of its original size within the first 10–14 days after drainage [42, 43]. In about 50–70% of the patients, drainage is inadequate and debridement or necrosectomy is required [41, 44].

The randomized TENSION trial assigned 98 patients to either the endoscopic step-up approach (51 patients) or the surgical step-up approach (47 patients). No difference was found in major complications or death during a 6-month follow-up between the two groups. However, the endoscopic approach demonstrated a lower rate of pancreatic fistula and shorter length of hospital stay, making it the preferred approach to drainage, unless the collections are far removed from the stomach or duodenum, necessitating a percutaneous approach to drainage [18].

Several endoscopic techniques are used to treat infected walled-off necrosis. All of these techniques are performed via the transmural access route, through the stomach or duodenal wall. During endoscopic drainage, a transmural drain is inserted into the cavity through one or several access sites. The multiple transluminal gateway technique with several access sites showed a higher clinical success rate compared to single-access drainage [45, 46]. After accessing the cavity, balloon dilation is performed to create a wider fistula between the gastrointestinal tract and the collection. This is done by inserting either multiple plastic double-pigtail stents or a self-expandable metal stent (e.g., lumen-apposing metal stents [LAMS]). In a recently published study by the Dutch Pancreatitis Study Group, two patient groups from two multicenter prospective studies with a similar design were compared, and the results suggest that LAMS does not reduce the need for endoscopic transluminal necrosectomy when compared with plastic double-pigtail stents. The rate of bleeding complications and

mortality was comparable. There is a tendency for all drains to become obstructed with solid necrosum, including LAMS. Sometimes it is necessary to use pigtail stents through the LAMS to prevent the solid necrosum from plugging the LAMS.

Attempts to improve the efficiency and efficacy of drainage have included the use of saline irrigation through a nasocystic catheter during the access phase of the WON and between each necrosectomy session, and irrigation use during a session of necrosectomy, sometimes with a large volume of warmed antibiotic or with a smaller volume of hydrogen peroxide [15, 45]. No prospective randomized trials have assessed the duration, type, and volume of irrigation. One large multicenter study reported no significant difference in clinical success with or without nasocystic tube placement [47]. Also, high clinical success was reported by two studies without any irrigation protocol or with only irrigation performed during the debridement phase [48, 49].

Regarding the removal of endoscopic drains, plastic double-pigtail stents can be left in situ indefinitely, unlike LAMS. LAMS are advised to be removed within 6 weeks after initial placement to prevent long-term adverse events [15, 50]. When there is a disruption of the pancreatic duct present, the LAMS should be replaced by plastic double-pigtail stents because long-term indwelling of transluminal plastic stents is indicated to create an internal fistula, preventing recurrence of peripancreatic collections [15]. The recurrence rate of fluid collections when there was a disruption of the pancreatic duct after drainage with LAMS is 13% [51].

4.3.2 Step 2: Endoscopic or Surgical Debridement of Infected Necrosis

When there are no signs of clinical improvement of when patients show clinical deterioration after percutaneous or endoscopic drainage, and attempts have been made to improve the efficacy of drainage (upsizing, irrigating, replacing, and/or additional drains), debridement of pancreatic necrosis is indicated. If clinically possible, the debridement should be performed after the collection has become walled off, as early necrosectomy is associated with poor outcomes [52]. The choice between endoscopic and surgical necrosectomy should be based on patient's characteristics, availability of expertise, experience and equipment, and location of the necrosis. It should preferably be performed in a minimally invasive fashion (see Figs. 3 and 4) [12, 14, 18]. In critically ill patients, minimally invasive surgery and endoscopic necrosectomy have been shown to be associated with lower death rates and fewer cases of new-onset organ failure as compared with open surgical necrosectomy [53].

Both surgical and endoscopic transluminal necrosectomy are time-consuming interventions and typically require more than one procedure. Endoscopic necrosectomy is performed by combining the suctioning of necrotic debris through the working channel of the endoscopic device, which is directly inserted into the necrotic collection, with the removal of necrotic tissue with a removal device, and applying irrigation. A variety of auxiliary instruments have been used for endoscopic necrosectomy, including polypectomy snares, Dormia and other stone removal baskets, balloons, nets, tripod retrieval forceps, or grasping/rat-tooth/pelican forceps [15]. Until recently, there were no specifically designed endoscopic tools for debridement, but an ongoing international trial is investigating a new device called the EndoRotor. This automated mechanical endoscopic resection system is designed for tissue debridement with a single device. This device can be advanced through the working channel of a large caliber endoscope, and once in the necrotic collection, necrotic tissue can be dabraded using a rotation mechanism with a protective sheath and

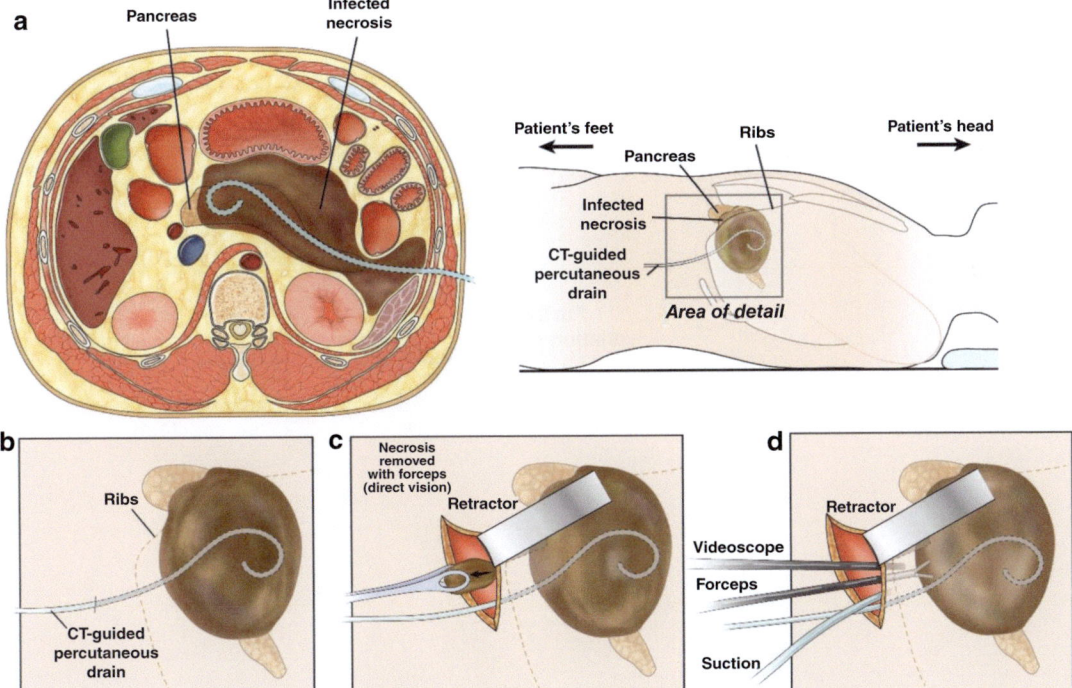

Fig. 3 Surgical step-up approach consisting of percutaneous catheter drainage and VARD. (**a**) Cross-sectional image and torso depicting a peripancreatic collection. The preferred route is through the left retroperitoneal space between the kidney, spleen, and descending colon. A percutaneous catheter drain is inserted in the collection to mitigate sepsis and postpone or even obviate necrosectomy. The area of detail is shown in **b**. (**c**) A 5 cm subcostal incision is made and the percutaneous drain is followed into the collection. The first necrosis is removed under direct vision with a long grasping forceps, followed by further debridement under videoscopic assistance (**d**). (Reprinted from van Brunschot et al. [77])

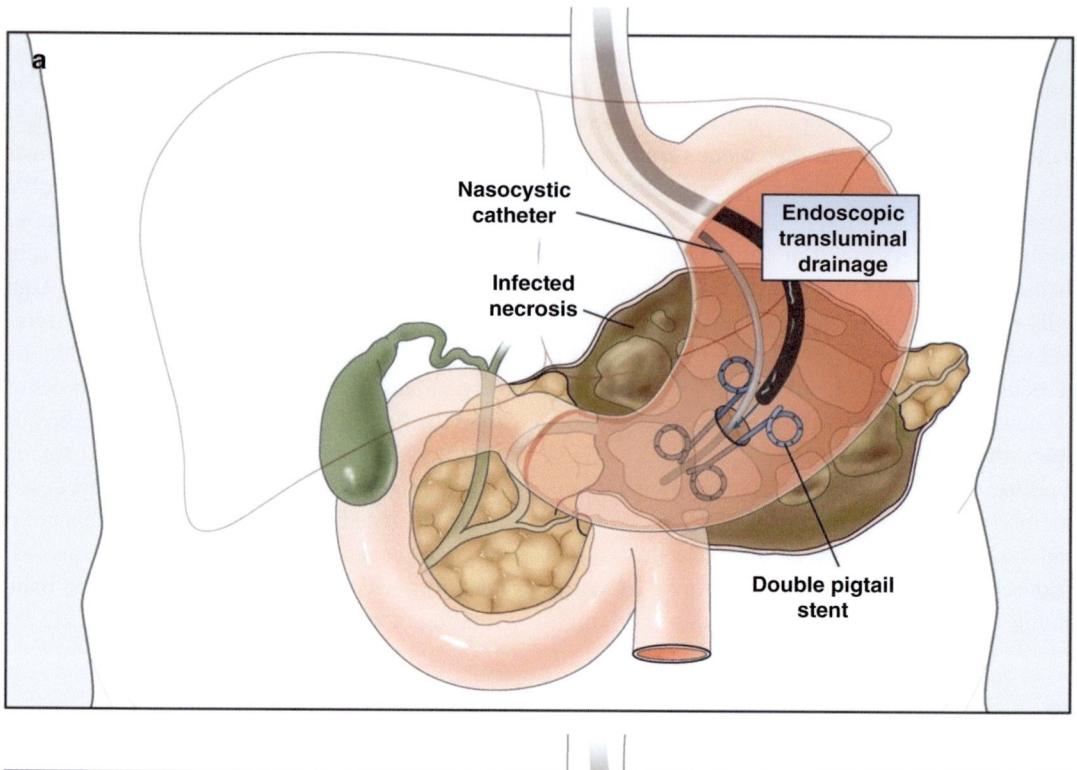

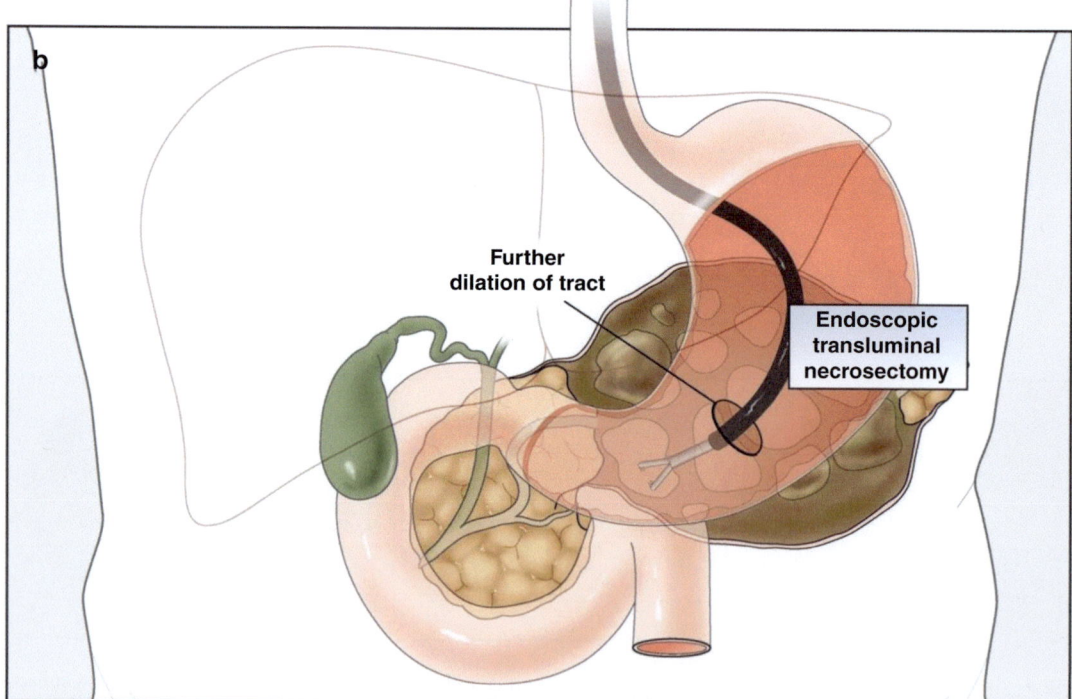

Fig. 4 Endoscopic step-up approach consisting of endoscopic transluminal drainage (ETD) and endoscopic transluminal necrosectomy (ETN). A large peripancreatic collection containing fluid and necrosis is shown. (**a**) ETD: The collection is punctured through the gastric wall, followed by balloon dilatation of the tract. Two double-pigtail stents and a nasocystic catheter for continuous postoperative irrigation are placed. (**b**) ETN: The cystostomy tract is dilated, the collection is entered with an endoscope, and necrosectomy is performed (Reprinted from van Brunschot et al. [77])

aspirated at the same time. Preliminary results suggest that the EndoRotor can safely, rapidly, and effectively be used to remove necrotic tissue from within an (infected) walled-off necrosis [54].

In surgical necrosectomy, a range of minimally invasive techniques have been developed. Minimally invasive necrosectomy is indicated as a continuum in the step-up approach after percutaneous and/or endoscopic drainage has failed, and endoscopic interventions are not available or feasible. There are various minimal invasive approaches, including percutaneous necrosectomy, video-assisted retroperitoneal debridement (VARD), laparoscopic transgastric necrosectomy, laparoscopic cystogastrostomy, and other variations [55–59]. These techniques generally involve a laparoscope, nephroscope, or percutaneous flexible endoscope. The limitation of all of these methods is that the removal of necrotic tissue is inefficient and multiple procedures are often required. There has been a shift away from trying to achieve a complete necrosectomy to ensuring effective drainage. The VARD procedure can be highly effective in removing large portions of necrotic debris with the use of larger forceps and a flank incision.

Open surgical necrosectomy is generally indicated in patients where a minimally invasive approach is technically not feasible or has failed. Open debridement with external drainage is performed through a laparotomy followed by entry into the retroperitoneum to remove necrotic tissue and leaving two to four closed suction drains to facilitate drainage of the cavity. There are other indications for open surgery in necrotizing pancreatitis, including treatment of abdominal compartment syndrome by laparostomy, resection of ischemic bowel, and when angiographic embolization has failed to control bleeding [60].

4.4 Follow-Up Imaging After Invasive Interventions

Although there is no specific evidence regarding the appropriate timing of follow-up imaging, it seems more practical to perform follow-up imaging based on relevant clinical indications or when invasive treatment is being considered, rather than providing routine follow-up [14, 17]. Relevant clinical indicators include sudden-onset or increased abdominal pain, organ dysfunction, signs of sepsis, and other indications of local complications (such as a sudden drop in hemoglobin levels). Contrast-enhanced CT is the preferred imaging method for evaluating developing local complications, providing guidance on when and how to use invasive treatment, monitoring response to treatment, and ensuring successful placement of stents and drains [15].

5 Other Local Complications and Their Management

5.1 (Splanchnic) Bleeding

Bleeding in patients with acute pancreatitis has an estimated occurrence of 1–6.2% [61]. Bleeding can occur in different locations, such as the gastrointestinal tract, peritoneal cavity, fluid collections, or the pancreatic parenchyma. Bleedings usually result from enzymatic degradation of local vessels in the peripancreatic tissues and the development of pseudoaneurysms [62]. Drains can cause erosion of vessels. Bleeding is one of reasons why it is recommended that patients with infected pancreatic necrosis should be managed in centres with immediate access to interventional radiology. Presenting symptoms often include sudden deterioration in hemodynamics with a decrease in hemoglobin levels, hemorrhagic shock, gastrointestinal blood loss (e.g., melena or hematemesis), or bloody output from drains. It is important to locate the bleeding by angiography and if possible perform immediate embolization. Surgery should only be performed when embolization fails [63]. Adequate drainage of infected peripancreatic collections is important to prevent further bleeding.

5.2 Gastric Outlet Dysfunction

Persistent vomiting or high-volume gastric aspirates from a nasogastric tube can be due to delayed gastric emptying or a gastric outlet obstruction in patients with acute pancreatitis. Mechanical obstruction of the stomach can occur as a consequence of ANCs, pancreatic pseudocysts, or WON. Treatment is indicated when patients experience persistent gastric dysfunction, which usually resolves with the treatment of these retrogastric local collections. These patients may require parenteral nutrition during this period, if nasojejunal feeding is not possible or not tolerated.

5.3 Disconnected Pancreatic Duct Syndrome

Necrosis of the pancreatic parenchyma can result in a partial disruption or a complete disconnection of the pancreatic duct. Both conditions will lead to the leaking of pancreatic fluid, resulting in disconnected pancreatic duct syndrome (DPDS). Symptoms of DPDS can range from persistent or recurrent (peri)pancreatic collections, pancreatic ascites, external pancreatic fistulas, pleural effusions to recurrent acute or chronic pancreatitis in the isolated upstream glands [64]. Several diagnostic modalities can be used in daily clinical practice to diagnose a disrupted or disconnected pancreatic duct, such as endoscopic retrograde cholangiopancreatography (ERCP), magnetic resonance cholangiopancreatography (MRCP), and measuring of amylase in external drain fluids. The treatment of DPDS ranges from conservative treatment to invasive radiological (advanced), endoscopic, or surgical interventions. A systematic review compared treatments for DPDS, presenting high pooled success rates (>80%) for all different treatment strategies [65]. There are no evidence-based standardized guidelines available for DPDS, so treatment is based on the judgment of treating clinicians and available local expertise. In cases of a partial disruption of the pancreatic duct, an endoprosthesis can bridge the disruption, whereas with a total pancreatic duct disruption, that is not feasible [66, 67].

The standard treatment for recurrent fluid collections due to DPDS is EUS-guided drainage with placement of long-term indwelling plastic double-pigtail stents [67]. This not only resolves the fluid collection but also maintains and estab-

lishes an alternative and internal drainage route for secretions from viable distal disconnected pancreas. In the absence of a large drainable fluid collection, different advanced endoscopy techniques are described, such as EUS-guided pancreaticogastrostomy techniques, or in case of a pancreaticocutaneous fistula using different rendezvous techniques to internalize the fistula tract back into the stomach or duodenum [68]. Although these advanced techniques are very interesting, they are rarely indicated and beyond the scope of this practical guide.

Despite the improvements made with the endoscopic treatment options for DPDS, some patients still require surgery. Previous endoscopic treatment fortunately does not preclude surgery. Surgery for DPDS provides a definitive option, but postprocedure morbidity is considerably higher. The different procedure options also include a distal pancreatectomy or a Roux-en-Y internal drainage of the cyst or fistula tract. There was a significantly higher risk of developing endocrine insufficiency following distal pancreatectomy, but the risk of exocrine insufficiency was comparable [65].

5.4 Gastrointestinal Perforation or Fistula

An enteric perforation (e.g., duodenal or colon) is a rare complication following acute pancreatitis. Perforation and fistula are defined as discontinuation of the gastrointestinal wall, either without or with a connection to another organ. Perforations and fistulas within the gastrointestinal tract may involve the stomach, duodenum, jejunum, ileum, and colon [69, 70]. It is more often seen in patients with necrotizing pancreatitis [69]. It can result from the action of pancreatic enzymes or, more commonly, due to iatrogenic instrumental injury or erosion caused by a drain. When there is output of any measurable volume of fluid with an increased amylase concentration from a percutaneous drain, drainage canal after removal of the drain or from a surgical site wound, it is called an external pancreatic fistula. Depending on the severity of the complication, additional antibiotics and/or interventional treatment is recommended. However, most of the gastrointestinal fistulas are described within the upper gastrointestinal tract (i.e., stomach, duodenum) and can often be treated conservatively without any form of intervention [69, 71, 72].

When an external pancreatic fistula is associated with a partial main pancreatic duct disruption and no PFC larger than 5 cm present, transpapillary stenting can be considered. However, transpapillary stenting is only successful in 27% of the patients, and no significant difference in closing time was found between the stenting group and conservative treatment group [15]. In cases of persistent or recurrent external pancreatic fistulas and/or treatment failures, surgery is indicated as a last resort treatment (e.g., distal pancreatectomy or pancreaticojejunostomy) [73].

5.5 Colonic Ischemia

Colonic ischemia is a rare complication that is potentially life-threatening. It is hypothesized that pancreatic enzymes spread through the retroperitoneum to the mesocolon and contribute to colonic ischemia. Other causes may include a "low flow state," thrombosis, or compression of one of the mesenteric arteries causing ischemia. Colonic ischemia almost always requires surgical intervention in the form of resection and colostomy.

5.6 Nonocclusive Mesenteric Ischemia

This is seen on CT scan as pneumatosis intestinalis. It is thought to occur in patient when the metabolic demand on the intestine exceeds the blood supply [74]. This can occur with aggressive enteral nutrition in hypovolemic patients with splanchnic vasoconstriction, especially with the addition of nonselective inotropes. This may precede bacterial translocation and the seeding of pancreatic necrosis. Management requires early diagnosis, addressing contributing factors (e.g.,

fluid resuscitation, stopping enteral feeding, considering alternative inotropes), and if the patient is deteriorating and there is evidence of peritonitis with possible perforation, surgical intervention will be required.

5.7 Venous Thrombosis

Patients with severe acute pancreatitis are at a high risk of developing venous thromboembolic disease. It is usually an incidental finding on radiological imaging. The thrombosis most commonly affects the splenic vein, portal vein, and superior mesenteric vein, either isolated or effecting several venous segments. The exact underlying pathophysiologic mechanism remains unclear, but it is believed to involve compression of the veins from the enlarged pancreas and inflammation causing a hypercoagulable state leading to thrombosis. It is still debated as to whether to start prophylactic anticoagulation in patients at risk and also whether therapeutic anticoagulation is indicated. It is unclear if the benefits of anticoagulation, such as preventing progression of thrombosis and recurrent venous thromboembolism, outweigh the risks of hemorrhage (related to portal hypertension and pseudoaneurysms). Since hemorrhage is a well-recognized complication of acute severe pancreatitis, the threshold for anticoagulation might be higher in patients with acute pancreatitis [26]. A recent systematic review and meta-analysis of seven retrospective cohort studies concluded that it still remains unclear if therapeutic anticoagulation provides benefit to acute pancreatitis patients with splanchnic vein thrombosis [75].

6 Conclusion

The treatment of local complications of acute (necrotizing) pancreatitis often requires a multidisciplinary team of gastroenterologists, pancreatobiliary surgeons, and radiologists. Local availability of different techniques and expertise should be taken into account when choosing the best treatment strategy.

The most common local complication of acute pancreatitis is the development of acute peripancreatic fluid collections. Most collections will resolve spontaneously over time and do not require further invasive intervention. Sterile necrotizing can usually be managed conservatively with adequate supportive treatment. When infection of the necrosis is suspected, the first step in treatment is starting antibiotics. Over time, the treatment of infected necrotizing pancreatitis has become less invasive, and in some cases, even conservative treatment was sufficient (e.g., prescribing antibiotics besides standard supportive treatment) [19]. When possible, invasive interventions should be delayed until infected necrotic collections have become walled off after around 4 weeks. The choice of which approach is best for the patient is based on multiple factors including characteristics of the infected collection (i.e., location, extent, integrity of the pancreatic duct) and clinical (i.e., hemodynamic) status of the patient. In this field further developments are expected to come from new endoscopy techniques and devices (e.g., EndoRotor), which will hopefully lead to a more efficient and successful treatment of infected necrosis. Additionally, new drainage and stenting techniques are being developed to optimize treatment strategies.

In conclusion, the optimal treatment of local complications of acute pancreatitis requires a tailored approach based on individual patient characteristics, available expertise, and the resources of the treating center.

References

1. Beger HG, Büchler M, Bittner R, Block S, Nevalainen T, Roscher R. Necrosectomy and postoperative local lavage in necrotizing pancreatitis. Br J Surg. 1988;75(3):207–12. https://doi.org/10.1002/bjs.1800750306.
2. Moynihan B. Acute pancreatitis. Ann Surg. 1925;81(1):132–42. https://doi.org/10.1097/00000658-192501010-00013.
3. McCarthy MC, Dickerman RM. Surgical management of severe acute pancreatitis. Arch Surg. 1982;117(4):476–80. https://doi.org/10.1001/archsurg.1982.01380280060012.
4. Warshaw AL, Jin GL. Improved survival in 45 patients with pancreatic abscess. Ann Surg. 1985;202(4):408–17. https://doi.org/10.1097/00000658-198510000-00002.
5. Mayer AD, McMahon MJ, Corfield AP, et al. Controlled clinical trial of peritoneal lavage for the treatment of severe acute pancreatitis. N Engl J Med. 1985;312(7):399–404. https://doi.org/10.1056/NEJM198502143120703.
6. Gerzof SG, Banks PA, Robbins AH, et al. Early diagnosis of pancreatic infection by computed tomography-guided aspiration. Gastroenterology. 1987;93(6):1315–20. https://doi.org/10.1016/0016-5085(87)90261-7.
7. Gerzof SG, Robbins AH, Birkett DH, Johnson WC, Pugatch RD, Vincent ME. Percutaneous catheter drainage of abdominal abscesses guided by ultrasound and computed tomography. AJR Am J Roentgenol. 1979;133(1):1–8. https://doi.org/10.2214/ajr.133.1.1.
8. Pamoukian VN, Gagner M. Laparoscopic necrosectomy for acute necrotizing pancreatitis. J Hepato-Biliary-Pancreat Surg. 2001;8(3):221–3. https://doi.org/10.1007/s005340170020.
9. Seifert H, Biermer M, Schmitt W, et al. Transluminal endoscopic necrosectomy after acute pancreatitis: a multicentre study with long-term follow-up (the GEPARD study). Gut. 2009;58(9):1260–6. https://doi.org/10.1136/gut.2008.163733.
10. Mier J, León EL, Castillo A, Robledo F, Blanco R. Early versus late necrosectomy in severe necrotizing pancreatitis. Am J Surg. 1997;173(2):71–5. https://doi.org/10.1016/S0002-9610(96)00425-4.
11. Runzi M, Niebel W, Goebell H, Gerken G, Layer P. Severe acute pancreatitis: nonsurgical treatment of infected necroses. Pancreas. 2005;30(3):195–9. https://doi.org/10.1097/01.mpa.0000153613.17643.b3.
12. van Santvoort HC, Besselink MG, Bakker OJ, et al. A step-up approach or open necrosectomy for necrotizing pancreatitis. N Engl J Med. 2010;362(16):1491–502. https://doi.org/10.1056/NEJMoa0908821.
13. Crockett SD, Wani S, Gardner TB, et al. American gastroenterological association institute guideline on initial management of acute pancreatitis. Gastroenterology. 2018;154(4):1096–101. https://doi.org/10.1053/j.gastro.2018.01.032.
14. IAP/APA evidence-based guidelines for the management of acute pancreatitis. Pancreatology. 2013;13(4):e1–e15. https://doi.org/10.1016/j.pan.2013.07.063.
15. Arvanitakis M, Dumonceau J-M, Albert J, et al. Endoscopic management of acute necrotizing pancreatitis: European Society of Gastrointestinal Endoscopy (ESGE) evidence-based multidisciplinary guidelines. Endoscopy. 2018;50(05):524–46. https://doi.org/10.1055/a-0588-5365.
16. Yokoe M, Takada T, Mayumi T, et al. Japanese guidelines for the management of acute pancreatitis: Japanese guidelines 2015. J Hepatobiliary Pancreat Sci. 2015;22(6):405–32. https://doi.org/10.1002/jhbp.259.

17. Leppäniemi A, Tolonen M, Tarasconi A, et al. 2019 WSES guidelines for the management of severe acute pancreatitis. World J Emerg Surg. 2019;14(1):27. https://doi.org/10.1186/s13017-019-0247-0.

18. van Brunschot S, van Grinsven J, van Santvoort HC, et al. Endoscopic or surgical step-up approach for infected necrotising pancreatitis: a multicentre randomised trial. Lancet. 2018;391(10115):51–8. https://doi.org/10.1016/S0140-6736(17)32404-2.

19. Boxhoorn L, van Dijk SM, van Grinsven J, et al. Immediate versus postponed intervention for infected necrotizing pancreatitis. N Engl J Med. 2021;385(15):1372–81. https://doi.org/10.1056/nejmoa2100826.

20. Banks PA, Bollen TL, Dervenis C, et al. Classification of acute pancreatitis—2012: revision of the Atlanta classification and definitions by international consensus. Gut. 2013;62(1):102–11. https://doi.org/10.1136/gutjnl-2012-302779.

21. Balthazar EJ. Acute pancreatitis: assessment of severity with clinical and CT evaluation. Radiology. 2002;223(3):603–13. https://doi.org/10.1148/radiol.2233010680.

22. Balthazar EJ, Freeny PC, vanSonnenberg E. Imaging and intervention in acute pancreatitis. Radiology. 1994;193(2):297–306. https://doi.org/10.1148/radiology.193.2.7972730.

23. Balthazar EJ, Robinson DL, Megibow AJ, Ranson JH. Acute pancreatitis: value of CT in establishing prognosis. Radiology. 1990;174(2):331–6. https://doi.org/10.1148/radiology.174.2.2296641.

24. Türkvatan A, Erden A, Türkoğlu MA, Seçil M, Yener Ö. Imaging of acute pancreatitis and its complications. Part 1: acute pancreatitis. Diagn Interv Imaging. 2015;96(2):151–60. https://doi.org/10.1016/j.diii.2013.12.017.

25. Wolbrink DRJ, Kolwijck E, Ten Oever J, Horvath KD, Bouwense SAW, Schouten JA. Management of infected pancreatic necrosis in the intensive care unit: a narrative review. Clin Microbiol Infect. 2020;26(1):18–25. https://doi.org/10.1016/j.cmi.2019.06.017.

26. van Santvoort HC, Bakker OJ, Bollen TL, et al. A conservative and minimally invasive approach to necrotizing pancreatitis improves outcome. Gastroenterology. 2011;141(4):1254–63. https://doi.org/10.1053/j.gastro.2011.06.073.

27. Bakker OJ, van Santvoort H, Besselink MGH, et al. Extrapancreatic necrosis without pancreatic parenchymal necrosis: a separate entity in necrotising pancreatitis? Gut. 2013;62(10):1475–80. https://doi.org/10.1136/gutjnl-2012-302870.

28. van Grinsven J, van Brunschot S, Bakker OJ, et al. Diagnostic strategy and timing of intervention in infected necrotizing pancreatitis: an international expert survey and case vignette study. HPB. 2016;18(1):49–56. https://doi.org/10.1016/j.hpb.2015.07.003.

29. Boxhoorn L, Fockens P, Besselink MG, et al. Endoscopic management of infected necrotizing pancreatitis: an evidence-based approach. Curr Treat Options Gastroenterol. 2018;16(3):333–44. https://doi.org/10.1007/s11938-018-0189-8.

30. Habashi S, Draganov PV. Pancreatic pseudocyst. World J Gastroenterol. 2009;15(1):38. https://doi.org/10.3748/wjg.15.38.

31. Varadarajulu S, Bang JY, Sutton BS, Trevino JM, Christein JD, Wilcox CM. Equal efficacy of endoscopic and surgical cystogastrostomy for pancreatic pseudocyst drainage in a randomized trial. Gastroenterology. 2013;145(3):583–590.e1. https://doi.org/10.1053/j.gastro.2013.05.046.

32. van Baal MC, Bollen TL, Bakker OJ, et al. The role of routine fine-needle aspiration in the diagnosis of infected necrotizing pancreatitis. Surgery. 2014;155(3):442–8. https://doi.org/10.1016/j.surg.2013.10.001.

33. Bollen T. Imaging assessment of etiology and severity of acute pancreatitis. The pancreapedia: exocrine pancreas knowledge base. 2016.

34. Villatoro E, Mulla M, Larvin M. Antibiotic therapy for prophylaxis against infection of pancreatic necrosis in acute pancreatitis. Cochrane Database Syst Rev. 2010;2010(5):CD002941. https://doi.org/10.1002/14651858.CD002941.pub3.

35. Wittau M, Mayer B, Scheele J, Henne-Bruns D, Dellinger EP, Isenmann R. Systematic review and meta-analysis of antibiotic prophylaxis in severe acute pancreatitis. Scand J Gastroenterol. 2011;46(3):261–70. https://doi.org/10.3109/00365521.2010.531486.

36. Baron TH, DiMaio CJ, Wang AY, Morgan KA. American gastroenterological association clinical practice update: management of pancreatic necrosis. Gastroenterology. 2020;158(1):67–75.e1. https://doi.org/10.1053/j.gastro.2019.07.064.

37. Da Costa DW, Boerma D, Van Santvoort HC, et al. Staged multidisciplinary step-up management for necrotizing pancreatitis. Br J Surg. 2014;101(1):65–79. https://doi.org/10.1002/bjs.9346.

38. De Waele JJ. Rational use of antimicrobials in patients with severe acute pancreatitis. Semin Respir Crit Care Med. 2011;32(2):174–80. https://doi.org/10.1055/s-0031-1275529.

39. Siriwardena AK, Jegatheeswaran S, Mason JM, et al. A procalcitonin-based algorithm to guide antibiotic use in patients with acute pancreatitis (PROCAP): a single-centre, patient-blinded, randomised controlled trial. Lancet Gastroenterol Hepatol. 2022;7(10):913–21. https://doi.org/10.1016/S2468-1253(22)00212-6.

40. Mowery NT, Bruns BR, MacNew HG, et al. Surgical management of pancreatic necrosis. J Trauma Acute Care Surg. 2017;83(2):316–27. https://doi.org/10.1097/TA.0000000000001510.

41. van Baal MC, van Santvoort HC, Bollen TL, Bakker OJ, Besselink MG, Gooszen HG. Systematic review of percutaneous catheter drainage as primary treatment for necrotizing pancreatitis. Br J Surg. 2010;98(1):18–27. https://doi.org/10.1002/bjs.7304.

42. Horvath K. Safety and efficacy of video-assisted retroperitoneal debridement for infected pancreatic collections. Arch Surg. 2010;145(9):817. https://doi.org/10.1001/archsurg.2010.178.

43. Wroński M, Cebulski W, Karkocha D, et al. Ultrasound-guided percutaneous drainage of infected pancreatic necrosis. Surg Endosc. 2013;27(8):2841–8. https://doi.org/10.1007/s00464-013-2831-9.

44. Park D, Lee S, Moon S-H, et al. Endoscopic ultrasound-guided versus conventional transmural drainage for pancreatic pseudocysts: a prospective randomized trial. Endoscopy. 2009;41(10):842–8. https://doi.org/10.1055/s-0029-1215133.

45. Varadarajulu S, Phadnis MA, Christein JD, Wilcox CM. Multiple transluminal gateway technique for EUS-guided drainage of symptomatic walled-off pancreatic necrosis. Gastrointest Endosc. 2011;74(1):74–80. https://doi.org/10.1016/j.gie.2011.03.1122.

46. Varadarajulu S, Bang JY, Phadnis MA, Christein JD, Wilcox CM. Endoscopic transmural drainage of peripancreatic fluid collections: outcomes and predictors of treatment success in 211 consecutive patients. J Gastrointest Surg. 2011;15(11):2080–8. https://doi.org/10.1007/s11605-011-1621-8.

47. Siddiqui AA, Adler DG, Nieto J, et al. EUS-guided drainage of peripancreatic fluid collections and necrosis by using a novel lumen-apposing stent: a large retrospective, multicenter U.S. experience (with videos). Gastrointest Endosc. 2016;83(4):699–707. https://doi.org/10.1016/j.gie.2015.10.020.

48. Jürgensen C, Neser F, Boese-Landgraf J, Schuppan D, Stölzel U, Fritscher-Ravens A. Endoscopic ultrasound-guided endoscopic necrosectomy of the pancreas: is irrigation necessary? Surg Endosc. 2012;26(5):1359–63. https://doi.org/10.1007/s00464-011-2039-9.

49. Thompson CC, Kumar N, Slattery J, et al. A standardized method for endoscopic necrosectomy improves complication and mortality rates. Pancreatology. 2016;16(1):66–72. https://doi.org/10.1016/j.pan.2015.12.001.

50. Bang JY, Hasan M, Navaneethan U, Hawes R, Varadarajulu S. Lumen-apposing metal stents (LAMS) for pancreatic fluid collection (PFC) drainage: may not be business as usual. Gut. 2017;66(12):2054–6. https://doi.org/10.1136/gutjnl-2016-312812.

51. Basha J, Lakhtakia S, Nabi Z, et al. Impact of disconnected pancreatic duct on recurrence of fluid collections and new-onset diabetes: do we finally have an answer? Gut. 2021;70(3):447–9. https://doi.org/10.1136/gutjnl-2020-321773.

52. Werner J. Management of acute pancreatitis: from surgery to interventional intensive care. Gut. 2005;54(3):426–36. https://doi.org/10.1136/gut.2003.035907.

53. van Brunschot S, Hollemans RA, Bakker OJ, et al. Minimally invasive and endoscopic versus open necrosectomy for necrotising pancreatitis: a pooled analysis of individual data for 1980 patients. Gut.

2018;67(4):697–706. https://doi.org/10.1136/gutjnl-2016-313341.

54. van der Wiel SE, May A, Poley JW, et al. Preliminary report on the safety and utility of a novel automated mechanical endoscopic tissue resection tool for endoscopic necrosectomy: a case series. Endosc Int Open. 2020;08(03):E274–80. https://doi.org/10.1055/a-1079-5015.

55. Worhunsky DJ, Qadan M, Dua MM, et al. Laparoscopic transgastric necrosectomy for the management of pancreatic necrosis. J Am Coll Surg. 2014;219(4):735–43. https://doi.org/10.1016/j.jamcollsurg.2014.04.012.

56. Horvath KD, Kao LS, Wherry KL, Pellegrini CA, Sinanan MN. A technique for laparoscopic-assisted percutaneous drainage of infected pancreatic necrosis and pancreatic abscess. Surg Endosc. 2001;15(10):1221–5. https://doi.org/10.1007/s004640080166.

57. Gibson SC, Robertson BF, Dickson EJ, McKay CJ, Carter CR. 'Step-port' laparoscopic cystgastrostomy for the management of organized solid predominant post-acute fluid collections after severe acute pancreatitis. HPB. 2014;16(2):170–6. https://doi.org/10.1111/hpb.12099.

58. Carter CR, McKay CJ, Imrie CW. Percutaneous necrosectomy and sinus tract endoscopy in the management of infected pancreatic necrosis: an initial experience. Ann Surg. 2000;232(2):175–80. https://doi.org/10.1097/00000658-200008000-00004.

59. Driedger M, Zyromski NJ, Visser BC, et al. Surgical transgastric necrosectomy for necrotizing pancreatitis. Ann Surg. 2020;271(1):163–8. https://doi.org/10.1097/SLA.0000000000003048.

60. Mentula P. Surgical decompression for abdominal compartment syndrome in severe acute pancreatitis. Arch Surg. 2010;145(8):764. https://doi.org/10.1001/archsurg.2010.132.

61. Bugiantella W, Rondelli F, Boni M, et al. Necrotizing pancreatitis: a review of the interventions. Int J Surg. 2016;28:S163–71. https://doi.org/10.1016/j.ijsu.2015.12.038.

62. Flati G, Andrén-Sandberg Å, La Pinta M, Porowska B, Carboni M. Potentially fatal bleeding in acute pancreatitis: pathophysiology, prevention, and treatment. Pancreas. 2003;26(1):8–14. https://doi.org/10.1097/00006676-200301000-00002.

63. Fitzpatrick J, Bhat R, Young JA. Angiographic embolization is an effective treatment of severe hemorrhage in pancreatitis. Pancreas. 2014;43(3):436–9. https://doi.org/10.1097/MPA.0000000000000051.

64. Vanek P, Urban O, Trikudanathan G, Freeman ML. Disconnected pancreatic duct syndrome in patients with necrotizing pancreatitis. Surg Open Sci. 2023;11:19–25. https://doi.org/10.1016/j.sopen.2022.10.009.

65. van Dijk SM, Timmerhuis HC, Verdonk RC, et al. Treatment of disrupted and disconnected pancreatic duct in necrotizing pancreatitis: a systematic review and meta-analysis. Pancreatology. 2019;19(7):905–15. https://doi.org/10.1016/j.pan.2019.08.006.

66. Varadarajulu S, Noone TC, Tutuian R, Hawes RH, Cotton PB. Predictors of outcome in pancreatic duct disruption managed by endoscopic transpapillary stent placement. Gastrointest Endosc. 2005;61(4):568–75. https://doi.org/10.1016/s0016-5107(04)02832-9.

67. Verma S, Rana SS. Disconnected pancreatic duct syndrome: updated review on clinical implications and management. Pancreatology. 2020;20(6):1035–44. https://doi.org/10.1016/j.pan.2020.07.402.

68. Irani S, Gluck M, Ross A, et al. Resolving external pancreatic fistulas in patients with disconnected pancreatic duct syndrome: using rendezvous techniques to avoid surgery (with video). Gastrointest Endosc. 2012;76(3):583–6. https://doi.org/10.1016/j.gie.2012.05.006.

69. Kochhar R, Jain K, Gupta V, et al. Fistulization in the GI tract in acute pancreatitis. Gastrointest Endosc. 2012;75(2):436–40. https://doi.org/10.1016/j.gie.2011.09.032.

70. Ho HS. Gastrointestinal and pancreatic complications associated with severe pancreatitis. Arch Surg. 1995;130(8):817. https://doi.org/10.1001/archsurg.1995.01430080019002.

71. Jiang W, Tong Z, Yang D, et al. Gastrointestinal fistulas in acute pancreatitis with infected pancreatic or peripancreatic necrosis. Medicine (Baltimore). 2016;95(14):e3318. https://doi.org/10.1097/MD.0000000000003318.

72. Timmerhuis HC, Van Dijk SM, Hollemans RA, et al. Perforation and fistula of the gastrointestinal tract in patients with necrotizing pancreatitis: a nationwide prospective cohort. Ann Surg. 2023;278(2):e284–92. https://doi.org/10.1097/SLA.0000000000005624.

73. Sikora SS, Khare R, Srikanth G, Kumar A, Saxena R, Kapoor VK. External pancreatic fistula as a sequel to management of acute severe necrotizing pancreatitis. Dig Surg. 2005;22(6):446–52. https://doi.org/10.1159/000091448.

74. Al-Diery H, Phillips A, Evennett N, Pandanaboyana S, Gilham M, Windsor JA. The pathogenesis of nonocclusive mesenteric ischemia: implications for research and clinical practice. J Intensive Care Med. 2019;34(10):771–81. https://doi.org/10.1177/0885066618788827.

75. Sissingh NJ, Groen JV, Koole D, et al. Therapeutic anticoagulation for splanchnic vein thrombosis in acute pancreatitis: a systematic review and meta-analysis. Pancreatology. 2022;22(2):235–43. https://doi.org/10.1016/j.pan.2021.12.008.

76. Szatmary P, Grammatikopoulos T, Cai W, et al. Acute pancreatitis: diagnosis and treatment. Drugs. 2022;82(12):1251–76. https://doi.org/10.1007/s40265-022-01766-4.

77. van Brunschot S, van Grinsven J, Voermans RP, et al. Transluminal endoscopic step-up approach versus minimally invasive surgical step-up approach in patients with infected necrotising pancreatitis (TENSION trial): design and rationale of a randomised controlled multicenter trial [ISRCTN09186711]. BMC Gastroenterol. 2013;13(1):161. https://doi.org/10.1186/1471-230X-13-161.

Managing Organ Failure in Acute Pancreatitis

Lu Ke, Wenjian Mao, and Weiqin Li

Key Points

1. The presence and duration of organ failure determine the severity and classification of acute pancreatitis.
2. Organ failure is preceded by organ dysfunction, and this can occur in a single organ system or as multiple organ dysfunction syndrome (MODS).
3. Important systemic contributors to organ failure include inflammation, microcirculatory dysfunction, and coagulopathy.
4. Additional factors contribute to different organ failure, for instance, respiratory (increased intra-abdominal pressure and restricted diaphragmatic excursion), renal (hypovolemia), cardiovascular (hypovolemia and distributive shock), and intestinal (ischemia and iatrogenic factors).
5. Each organ system requires specific management, including ventilation, dialysis, inotropes, and enteral nutrition, respectively.

L. Ke · W. Li (✉)
Department of Critical Care Medicine, Jinling Hospital, Medical School of Nanjing University, Nanjing, Jiangsu, China

National Institute of Healthcare Data Science, Nanjing University, Nanjing, Jiangsu, China
e-mail: ctgkelu@nju.edu.cn

W. Mao
Department of Critical Care Medicine, Jinling Hospital, Medical School of Nanjing University, Nanjing, Jiangsu, China

1 Introduction

Organ failure (OF) is the key determinant of mortality in patients with acute pancreatitis (AP) and is the key criterion for grading the severity of AP [1, 2]. Previously, it was considered that OF and infected pancreatic necrosis (IPN) were equivalent determinants of mortality [3], but there has been considerable progress in the management of IPN, including drainage-first strategy and a step-up approach to laparoscopic and endoscopic necrosectomy [4, 5]. This has resulted in a decreased incidence of new-onset OF and mortality compared with open surgical necrosectomy, which means that OF is the most important determinant of severity and mortality, while IPN is still associated with increased morbidity but it has less impact on mortality [6].

Organ failure is preceded by organ dysfunction and can involve single or multiple organ systems. Most patients with OF require intensive care unit (ICU) admission, leading to considerable utilization of healthcare resources. Failure of different organ systems are not equivalent in terms of prognosis. The outcome is worse with multiple (rather than single) OF [6], longer duration OF [7], and certain combinations of individual OFs [8].

The genesis of OF during AP was previously attributed to acinar cell-initiated cytokine-mediated systemic inflammation and the release of activated digestive enzymes [9]. Over the last two decades, there have been important discoveries that have provided new insights into the

© The Author(s), under exclusive license to Springer Nature Singapore Pte Ltd. 2024
J. A. Windsor et al. (eds.), *Acute Pancreatitis*, https://doi.org/10.1007/978-981-97-3132-9_17

pathophysiology and evolution of OF. These include increased capillary permeability (with tissue and organ edema) [10], reflex splanchnic vasoconstriction with impaired organ perfusion (including kidneys, pancreas, and intestine) [11], and extensive coagulopathy [12] and lipotoxicity (Chap. 6). These factors all contribute to the development of OF and have implications for management strategies. Newer concepts, including the gut-lymph model of organ failure, will likely result in new specific treatment strategies [13].

The management of AP requires accurate prediction of severe AP (i.e., persistent OF, lasting >48 h), monitoring of the clinical course, and definition of severity, which vary among studies [14–16]. The Revised Atlanta Classification (RAC) [1] recommends the modified Marshall scoring system to be used to define the severity of AP, but this is not entirely suitable for patients in ICU because it does not take into account the need for mechanical ventilation and the importance of different doses of inotropes or include the intestine as an organ that not only fails but also contributes to the severity of OF. The preference is to use the Sequential Organ Failure Assessment (SOFA) score, especially for critically ill AP patients [17].

The aim of this chapter is to provide a practical guide to the intensive care management of the most common types of OF in severe AP.

2 Prediction of Persistent Organ Failure

When treating a patient with initial/mild organ dysfunction in the ward/emergency room, it is crucial to identify those at high risk of developing persistent OF to ensure timely ICU admission. There are several diagnostic tools available in clinical practice. Mounzer et al. compared a series of clinical scoring systems for predicting persistent OF and found that all the conventional scores for AP prognosis assessment, including the Ranson score, APACHE II score, and BISAP score, had only modest sensitivity and overall predictive performance [18].

Apart from these commonly used scoring systems in AP, the quick Sequential Organ Failure Assessment (qSOFA) score, developed for rapid identification of patients with suspected infection outside ICU, consists of only three items: respiratory rate, altered mentation, and systolic blood pressure [19]. Rasch et al. tested the qSOFA score in a cohort of 203 AP patients in the emergency room and found it has moderate accuracy in predicting ICU admission with an area under the curve (AUC) of 0.73 [20]. The authors also developed a new scoring system called the emergency room assessment of acute pancreatitis (ERAP) score by adding two rapidly available laboratory parameters: blood urea nitrogen and C-reactive protein (CRP). The ERAP score, compared with the original qSOFA, increases the AUC in predicting ICU admission to approximately 0.79. In a large cohort of more than 2000 patients, Shi et al. developed a nomogram to predict persistent OF, consisting of 6 items: age, respiratory rate, albumin, lactate dehydrogenase, oxygen support, and pleural effusion [21]. The nomogram demonstrates an AUC of 0.814 in external validation, although it is more complex to use, requiring laboratory data and additional examination. The advent of artificial intelligence has resulted in the application of machine learning algorithms to the prediction of AP severity, including organ failure. This approach results in improved predictive validity and accuracy and is covered in Chap. 8.

Taken together, repeated clinical assessment should be carried out when treating early AP patients in the ward/emergency room since all the available scoring systems have only modest accuracy. Special attention should be paid when the patients show increased respiratory rate or significantly altered laboratory measures like CRP.

3 Management of Acute Respiratory Failure

Respiratory failure is the most common type of OF in AP patients [14]. A recent cohort study found that respiratory failure occurred in 92% of acute necrotizing pancreatitis patients with OF, and the incidence peaked during the first week. Of the three most frequently affected organ systems (respiratory, renal, and cardiovascular), the respiratory system was the first to fail and persisted for the longest time [14]. In a large cohort study involving more than 800,000 hospitalized AP patients, Gajendran et al. found that 5.4% of AP patients developed respiratory failure, with a mortality rate of 26.5%. Important predictors of respiratory failure were pleural effusion and pneumonia, and the presence of respiratory failure significantly increased hospital stay and risk of mortality [22]. For the occurrence of persistent respiratory failure, Li et al. developed a simplified Lung Injury Prediction Score (sLIPS) incorporating oxygen requirement, hypoalbuminemia, and obesity. They demonstrated that sLIPS could accurately predict persistent respiratory failure with an AUC of 0.81 in an external validation cohort [23].

3.1 Oxygen Therapy

Hypoxemia is common in AP mainly because of ventilation/perfusion (V/Q) mismatch. In this regard, the UK guidelines recommended that oxygen supplementation be provided to patients with a diagnosis of AP regardless of severity in 2005 [24]. Since there is no additional evidence either for or against this recommendation in recent years, it has been practiced variably worldwide. Oxygen therapy can be implemented through nasal prongs or a face mask. In recent years, non-invasive high-flow oxygen therapy has attracted significant attention as a bridge between simple oxygen supplementation and mechanical ventilation (i.e., to delay or avoid the need for this) [25]. In a small cohort study involving 69 patients with AP-associated respiratory failure, the use of high-flow oxygen therapy, compared to conventional oxygen therapy, was associated with a lower intubation rate and shortened intensive care unit stay [26]. The clinical value of high-flow oxygen therapy should be assessed in future prospective trials.

3.2 Anti-Inflammatory Therapy

Since AP is an inflammatory disease by its nature, the use of anti-inflammatory therapy makes sense. In severe cases of AP, local injury and inflammation in the pancreas proceeds to systemic inflammation (see Chap. 5). Platelet-activating factor (PAF) is an important inflammatory mediator, recruiting white cells into inflammatory sites. Animal studies showed that PAF participated in the progression of AP by activating the interleukin system in endothelial cells and promoting tissue damage in multiple organs, including the lung [27]. Lexipafant, which is a PAF inhibitor, was tested in AP patients in the hope of reducing the incidence of organ failure. However, the multicenter, double-blind, phase III trial conducted in patients with predicted severe acute pancreatitis failed to show benefit from lexipafant therapy in preventing any type of new organ failure [28]. However, the evidence did show clinical benefit if PAF was administered within 48 h of admission [29], but this has not been confirmed in a subsequent adequately powered randomized controlled trial. Despite multiple trials evaluating a range of anti-inflammatory therapies, there are no evidence-based recommendations in management guidelines for anti-inflammatory or other specific treatments for AP [30]. There is now evidence of the equivalence of non-steroidal anti-inflammatory medication and opioids in treating pain, at least in patients with non-severe AP (see Chap. 9), but an impact on organ failure incidence and severity has not been demonstrated.

3.3 Mechanical Ventilation

Mechanical ventilation is a lifesaving treatment for patients with severe respiratory failure. In patients with AP-related respiratory failure, it is noteworthy that intra-abdominal hypertension (IAH), which is relatively common in severe AP [31], is a vital contributor to the underlying pathophysiology, which must be considered when implementing mechanical ventilation in this cohort. Pelosi et al. described the effect of IAH on respiratory mechanics using obese patients as the study group [32] and found that increased intra-abdominal pressure (IAP) led to increased chest wall elastance (impaired compliance), consequently reducing lung volume and promoting atelectasis formation. In a physiological animal model incorporating AP and IAH, the addition of 20 or 30 mmHg resulted in significantly dropped arterial PO_2 and decreased venous oxygen saturation, suggesting impaired tissue oxygen delivery [33]. Given the unique pathophysiology of respiratory failure in AP, the management strategy of acute respiratory failure in AP is technically different from that used in patients with acute respiratory distress syndrome (ARDS), although the underlying philosophy is the same: maintain adequate oxygenation and ventilation while protecting the lung from unnecessary mechanical injury.

For patients requiring mechanical ventilation for ARDS, the lung-protective strategy was proposed by ARDSnetwork and widely adopted worldwide [34]. Back in 2000, a well-designed and well-conducted large trial conclusively demonstrated the benefits of mechanical ventilation with low tidal volumes in patients with ARDS

[35]. The clinical benefits include reduced mortality and shorter duration of mechanical ventilation. In recently published guidelines, the recommendation is strong for the lung-protective strategy, which advocates low tidal volumes (4–8 mL/kg predicted body weight) and lower inspiratory pressures (airway plateau pressure $\leq$ 30 cmH$_2$O). However, increased IAP can lead to cranial shift of the diaphragm, which is the key and unique extrapancreatic factor contributing to the development of respiratory failure in AP (Fig. 1). Therefore, the mechanical ventilation strategy needs to be modified to address this issue.

First of all, when considering implementation of mechanical ventilation in AP patients, IAP should be routinely measured and at least daily. Moreover, if available, esophageal pressure, as a surrogate for intrathoracic pressure, should be measured to calculate trans-pulmonary pressure, which is one of the main determinants in ventilator-induced lung injury [36]. For the lung-protective strategy, it is of note

Fig. 1 The key mechanisms for acute respiratory failure associated with acute pancreatitis. Increased abdominal pressure leads to a headlong shift of the diaphragm, thereby increasing intrathoracic pressure. Esophageal pressure can be seen as a surrogate of intrathoracic pressure and used to calculate trans-pulmonary pressure

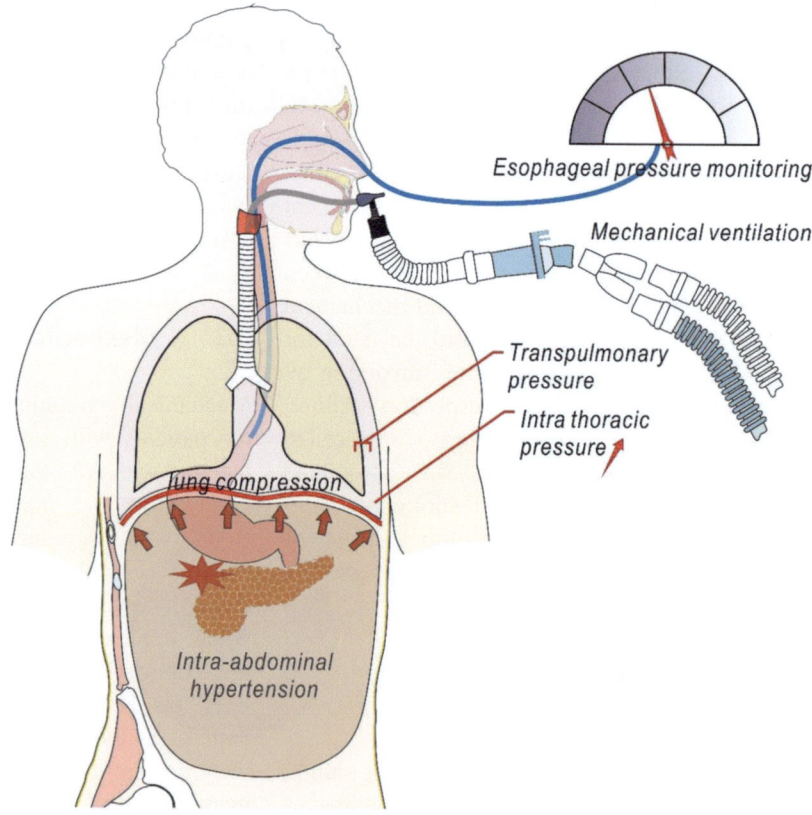

that the recommendation of using an upper limit for plateau pressures does not take IAP into account. The fundamental rationale for this recommendation is to avoid excess trans-pulmonary pressure, which needs to be reassessed in patients with increased IAP. When targeting trans-pulmonary plateau pressure at 30 cmH$_2$O, the measured plateau pressure should be 30 cmH$_2$O plus the intrathoracic pressure, which could be either measured by esophageal pressure or calculated [37].

3.4 Other Treatments

Because of the role that IAH plays in the pathophysiology of AP-related respiratory failure, efforts should be made to lower the IAP. Initial treatment may include reduction in hollow-viscera volume like nasogastric drainage, reduction in intra−/extravascular fluid content like restrictive fluid therapy (de-escalation, see Chap. 10), ultrafiltration or diuretics, and improvement of abdominal wall compliance, e.g., adequate analgesia and sedation [38]. Invasive interventions such as percutaneous catheter drainage (PCD) or even open surgery should be considered when medical management fails [39]. Moreover, extracorporeal membrane oxygenation (ECMO), a lifesaving therapy for patients with severe respiratory failure, may be of potential value in the management of AP, though quality studies assessing the efficacy and safety of ECMO in AP patients are absent in the literature [40]. More studies are needed before any formal recommendation can be made.

---

4 Management of Acute Renal Failure

Acute renal failure or acute kidney injury (AKI) is common in AP, with varied prevalence in previous reports. In a large, national observational study, the overall AKI prevalence was 7.9% in hospitalized AP patients, and it was associated with poor outcomes. Apart from direct disease-induced kidney injury, inappropriate patient management also plays an important role in AKI associated with AP.

4.1 Fluid Management

During the acute phase of AP, fluid therapy is one of the mainstay treatments (Chap. 10). However, there are major uncertainties about fluid type, volume, rate, and duration of intravenous fluid [41].

For fluid type, there has been an overall consensus that isotonic crystalloid should be the primary choice in the initial treatment of AP, and Ringer's lactate is recommended in some guidelines [42]. However, the evidence for this is modest. A recent meta-analysis showed that compared with saline, Ringer's lactate did not reduce the incidence of SIRS, which is supposed to be the major clinical benefit it confers. Still, the studies were largely small or observational [43]. The main difference between Ringer's lactate, other balanced solutions, and saline lies in their chloride levels. An ongoing large stepped-wedge trial may provide evidence as to whether the different chloride levels in different solutions impact plasma chloride levels sufficiently to have a clinically meaningful impact [44]. Current evidence regarding the effect of different types of crystalloids on clinical outcomes in AP patients is summarized in Table 1.

For fluid rate, the association between large-volume fluid resuscitation and renal complications in AP is not clear due to the lack of high-quality evidence. An observational study of 179 patients with moderately severe or severe AP showed that aggressive fluid resuscitation (4 L or over in the first 24 h) was associated with increased incidence and duration of AKI [45]. In a recent meta-analysis comparing aggressive (from 3 mL/kg/h to 5 mL/kg/h in first 24 h) and nonaggressive fluid strategy in AP, patients receiving aggressive fluid therapy had a higher rate of AKI [46]. Thus, although early fluid resuscitation is indicated for AP patients, excessive fluid administration may be harmful in terms of causing kidney injury. However, high-quality evidence is required to draw a firm conclusion.

Table 1 RCTs assessing the effect of balanced solution compared to saline on clinical outcomes in acute pancreatitis

First author (year), country	Study design	n	Population	Age	Group 1	Group 2	Group 3	Group 4	Primary outcome	Main findings
Wu et al. (2011) [84], USA	Multicenter factorial RCT	40	AP patients	52.1 ± 19.8 years	Goal-directed fluid resuscitation with LR	Goal-directed fluid resuscitation with NS	Standard resuscitation with LR	Standard resuscitation with NS	Prevalence of SIRS at 24 h post-randomization	There was a significant reduction in SIRS after 24 h among subjects resuscitated with lactated Ringer's solution, compared with normal saline (84% reduction vs. 0%, respectively; $P = 0.035$); administration of lactated Ringer's solution also reduced levels of CRP, compared with normal saline (51.5 vs. 104 mg/dL, respectively; $P = 0.02$)
Choosakul et al. (2018) [85], Thailand	Single-center RCT	47	AP patients	51.6 ± 17.0 years	Received NS	Received LR			SIRS reduction at 24 h and 48 h compared to levels prior to resuscitation	Lactated Ringer's solution was superior to NS in SIRS reduction in acute pancreatitis only in the first 24 h. SIRS at 48 h and mortality were not different between LR and NS
Lee et al. (2021) [86], USA	Single-center RCT	121	MAP patients	42.90 ± 14.05 years	Received NS	Received LR			Change in SIRS prevalence at 24 h after randomization	While this trial did not show a difference in SIRS prevalence at 24 h, LR appears to reduce the need for intensive care and shortens the length of hospitalization for acute pancreatitis

de Madaria et al. (2018) [87], Spain	Single-center RCT	40	First episode of AP	62.54 ± 17.12 years	Received NS and 1000 mL of 10% dextrose solution	Received LR and 1000 mL of 10% dextrose solution	The number of SIRS score levels of CRP at 24 h, 48 h, and 72 h	The median (p25–p75) number of SIRS criteria at 48 h was 1 (1–2) for NS vs. 1 (0–1) for LR, $p = 0.060$. CRP levels (mg/l) were as follows: At 48 h NS 166 (78–281) vs. LR 28 (3–124), $p = 0.037$; at 72 h NS 217 (59–323) vs. LR 25 (3–169), $p = 0.043$. LR inhibited the induction of inflammatory phenotype of macrophages and NF-kB activation
Karki et al. (2022) [88], Nepal	Single-center RCT	51	AP within 48 h from the onset of the symptoms	41.33 ± 14.17 years	Received NS and 1000 mL of 5% dextrose solution per 24 h	Received LR and 1000 mL of 5% dextrose solution per 24 h	The difference in CRP level and SIRS score at admission and subsequently	LR was associated with a reduction in systemic inflammation compared to NS. Incidence of SIRS at 72 h and occurrence of local complications were similar in both groups
Kayhan et al. (2021) [89], Turkey	Single-center RCT	132	AP patients and had abdominal pain less than 24 h	55.4 ± 17.5 years	Received 1000 mL of NS within the first hour and 3 mL/kg/h until oral feeding	Received 1000 mL of LR within the first hour and 3 mL/kg/h until oral feeding	Measure systemic inflammatory response and CRP, pH, and HCO3 levels 48 h after randomization	Resuscitation with LR is associated with decreased severity of AP. It may derive from how it causes lower CRP levels

RCT randomized controlled trials, *AP* acute pancreatitis, *NS* normal saline, *LR* lactated Ringer's, *CRP* C-reactive protein

4.2 Renal Replacement Therapy

When AKI has already developed, the principles of management are largely similar to AKI in other disease settings, namely, supportive and replacement treatment when necessary. For the timing and indication of renal replacement therapy (RRT), since there is no high-quality evidence supporting the use of RRT for nonrenal replacement purposes (including a promising role in removing Inflammatory mediators and maintenance of acid-base status, for instance), the application of RRT should be limited to patients with severe AKI, evidenced by anuria (negligible urine output for 6 h), severe metabolic acidosis (pH <7.2 with normal arterial PCO_2), severe volume overload (pulmonary edema), and pronounced azotemia (blood urea nitrogen >30 mmol/L or creatinine >300 mol/L) [47]. In recent years, with the emergence of new evidence, there has been a trend toward postponing RRT in critically ill patients with AKI since the delay strategy can significantly reduce the requirement of RRT without impacting clinical outcomes [48] . However, since there are no studies addressing this question in AP patients, no recommendations can be given regarding delaying RRT.

5 Management of Acute Cardiovascular Failure

During AP, acute cardiovascular (CVS) failure or shock is often caused by noncardiac factors and usually a combination of hypovolemia and distributive shock (Fig. 2). On the one hand, fluid sequestration due to third spacing is typical in AP, resulting in ascites and pleural effusion, which are well-recognized early events during AP [49]. Moreover, nausea and vomiting may also contribute to volume depletion in AP. Several parameters representing hemoconcentration, like increased hematocrit, blood urea nitrogen, or creatinine levels, have been found to predict a more severe course of AP [50]. Further, local pancreatic inflammation results in the release of cytokines, pro-inflammatory mediators, and

other vasodilators like substance P and nitric oxide [51], which can exacerbate inadequate intravascular volume. Another factor is the marked decrease in response to endogenous vasopressors observed in AP [52], thought to be due to endothelin and renin occupying receptors for endogenous vasoconstrictors. In summary, CVS failure in AP is caused by multiple pathophysiological processes and, therefore, needs to be addressed with a multimodel approach to management.

5.1 Fluid Resuscitation/Therapy

The treatment of acute CVS failure should start with fluid replacement since hypovolemia and shock are common features of the pathogenesis of AP. Current guidelines recommend a moderately aggressive and goal-directed fluid approach, initiating a rate of 5–10 mL/kg of body weight [42]. The goals recommended for this approach include heart rate, mean arterial pressure, urine output, and hematocrit [42]. A major safety concern with fluid resuscitation is overload and the development of pleural effusion, pulmonary edema, and ascites, in addition to edema within end organs themselves. A recently published large trial (the WATERFALL trial) in mainly patients with mild AP confirmed that early aggressive fluid resuscitation (which was a bolus of 20 mL/kg in the first 2 h followed by 3 mL/kg/h), despite it being a previous standard of care, resulted in a higher incidence of fluid overload and did not improve outcomes [53]. There are several previous studies that had previously demonstrated that aggressive fluid resuscitation increased rates of organ failure and mortality in patients with AP [54–56]. The conclusion from these studies is that a moderate fluid rate (5–10 mg/kg) should be used to address hypovolemia in the initial stage of resuscitation. Determining ongoing fluid requirements beyond that, the so-called optimization phase of fluid resuscitation [57], requires more research, especially with the development of capillary leak syndrome [10] and the adverse clinical consequences of excess interstitial fluid.

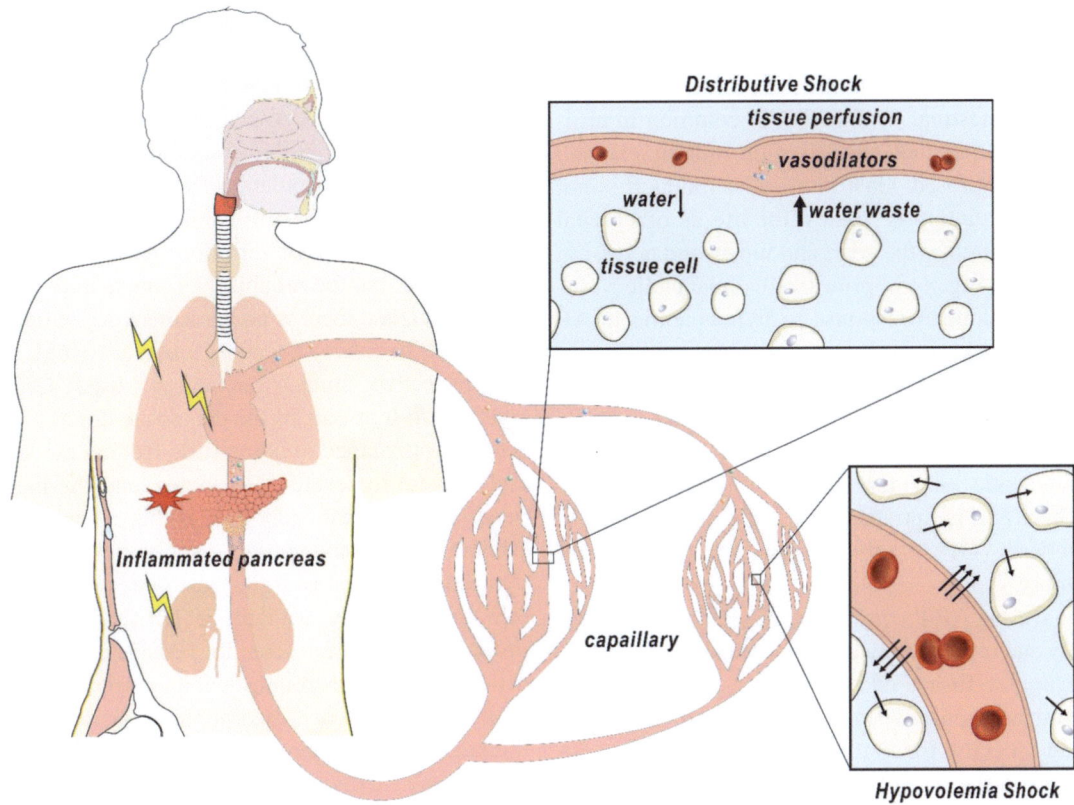

Fig. 2 Combined distributive shock and hypovolemic shock in acute pancreatitis. The circulatory failure during acute pancreatitis results from both mechanisms. Multiple vasodilators like nitric oxide and substance P are released into the circulation from the pancreas in acute pancreatitis, leading to a fall in arterial pressure. In addition, due to the increased vascular permeability, "third spacing" is a common phenomenon in acute pancreatitis, which exacerbates circulatory failure

5.2   The Use of Vasoactive Drugs

As CVS failure in AP has characteristics of both hypovolemia and vasodilation, vasopressors are commonly applied after initial fluid resuscitation. There are some controversies regarding the use of vasoactive drugs in AP patients, especially in regard to the optimal timing of administration. In light of the consequences of aggressive fluid resuscitation [53], the early addition of vasopressors may help reduce the volume of fluid resuscitation required and may result in better outcomes [58]. However, vasopressors can compromise gastrointestinal perfusion [59] in patients who are already at risk of mucosal ischemia secondary to reflex splanchnic vasoconstriction in hypovolemic AP patients. This gut injury contributes to systemic inflammation, bacterial translocation, secondary infection, and end-organ dysfunction/failure and is mediated through the lymphatic system more than the portal venous system [13].

For the specific selection of available vasopressors, based on evidence across multiple shock populations (including septic, hemorrhagic, and cardiogenic shock [59]), norepinephrine should be the first-line choice mainly because it improves coronary blood flow and microcirculation [60]. Overall, due to the lack of evidence specifically in AP patients, the use of vasopressors mostly depends on local practice and the treating clinician (timing and type), and studies are urgently needed in this field.

6 Gastrointestinal Failure and Management

Gastrointestinal dysfunction is common in critically ill patients and is often subclinical and underdiagnosed. Gastrointestinal function is not as immediately necessary for life as other vital organs, such as the heart and lungs, and perfusion of these organs is prioritized. Splanchnic vasoconstriction, in response to hypovolemia in AP patients, causes ischemic gut injury, resulting in gastrointestinal dysfunction, the loss of barrier function, and systemic exposure to toxic inflammatory mediators from the microbiome, activated pancreatic enzymes, and the injured gut wall. There is a reciprocal and damaging relationship between OF in other organ systems and gut injury.

During AP, the gastrointestinal tract is inevitably and immediately affected by the local inflammatory effusion of the pancreas. The released pancreatic enzymes and inflammatory mediators can directly track through the mesentery and involve the bowels. In a magnetic resonance imaging (MRI) study conducted by Ji et al., it was found that thickened bowel walls, mural stratification, and dilation of the gastrointestinal tract are common in AP patients and related to clinical outcomes [61]. When the mesenteric vessels get involved by the inflammatory process initiated from the pancreas, blood supply to the corresponding bowel segment is impaired, compounding ischemia and occasionally leading to life-threatening bowel necrosis. In a single-center prospective clinical study, Rahman et al. demonstrated that gastrointestinal failure, as reflected by the gastrointestinal failure score [62], was a common organ failure in AP, and its severity was associated with mortality [63].

6.1 Diagnosis, Monitoring, and Severity Assessment

Although not included in RAC as a named organ failure, gastrointestinal failure is an important and outcome-related organ failure worth more atten-tion. The difficulty might lie in the lack of assessment tools, and the recently established Gastrointestinal Dysfunction Score (GIDS) may help improve the objectivity for both research and clinical use. The feasibility and accuracy of the GIDS in the AP population should be tested in future studies [64]. Gastric residual volume (GRV) is a traditional marker reflecting gastrointestinal dysfunction, but the reliability of this marker was questioned, and there is no agreement on the optimal cutoff to diagnose feeding intolerance [65]. In a prospective study, Lin et al. used GRV >500 mL/6 h as part of the diagnostic criteria for feeding intolerance in nasogastric feeding moderately severe to severe AP patients, and the incidence was approximately 25% in this cohort [66]. Abdominal ultrasonography may be helpful as a convenient tool for assessing gastrointestinal function and is widely available in ICUs. Gao et al. proposed a quantitive score for bedside evaluation called the acute gastrointestinal injury ultrasonography (AGIUS) score, incorporating the diameter, thickness, and movement of the intestine [67]. Their results showed that the AGIUS score correlated well with the conventional gastrointestinal failure score [62] and may serve as a useful tool for point-of-care evaluation.

6.2 Drugs Associated with Gastrointestinal Dysfunction

Antibiotics are widely used in managing AP for either prophylactic or therapeutic purposes and are essential for treating infected pancreatic necrosis [68]. However, long-course antibiotics are associated with potential adverse events, including increased prevalence of multidrug-resistant bacteria, higher risk of fungal infection, and dysbiosis, which might be associated with short-term and long-term detrimental effects [69]. In this regard, prophylactic antibiotics are not recommended in patients with AP because they were not associated with improved clinical outcomes [70] and because of the potential risks mentioned above (Chap. 12).

On the other hand, analgesic therapy is a cornerstone in the early treatment of AP, and opioids are commonly prescribed, especially for those requiring mechanical ventilation. However, opioids can cause significant and varying gastrointestinal symptoms, including nausea, vomiting, immotility, and diarrhea [71], and a large cohort study showed that increased opioid use was associated with prolonged hospital stay (Chap. 9). Therefore, non-opioids should be considered for analgesic therapy in AP. A recent meta-analysis showed that nonsteroidal anti-inflammatory drugs (NSAIDs) and epidural administration of local anesthetics might be effective adjuncts to opioids in the pain management of AP patients [72], though the evidence level is still low and future large studies are warranted.

6.3 Drainage of Ascites

Ascites is a common occurrence in AP patients during the first week of disease onset, with an incidence varying from 38.5% [73] to 60% [74], depending on the severity of the patients. The presence of ascites was associated with increased mortality and longer duration of mechanical ventilation [73]. A retrospective cohort study of 102 patients showed that drainage of ascites was associated with reduced inflammatory markers, delayed or less organ failure, and reduced need for retroperitoneal intervention. Moreover, another observational study addressed the most significant safety concern of early paracentesis by showing that it did not increase the incidence of infectious complications and infection-related mortality [75]. However, since there is a lack of randomized controlled trials concerning this topic, early paracentesis is not recommended in routine practice. For peritoneal lavage, which used to be a common practice in the early treatment of AP, a meta-analysis found that early lavage may not confer clinical benefits and may be associated with increased complications [76]. Therefore, lavage should not be routinely applied to AP patients before new evidence emerges.

6.4 Early Enteral Nutrition

In the management of AP, early enteral nutrition (EN) is considered essential because it helps maintain the function and structure of the gastrointestinal mucosa, preserving the integrity of intestinal barrier function and preventing bacterial translocation [77] (see Chap. 11). This "EN-first" approach goes against the conventional "pancreatic rest" and "bowel rest" theories, which state that EN increases the secretion of pancreatic enzymes to increase the severity of AP [78]. However, it is shown that pancreatic exocrine function is diminished proportionally to the morphologic destruction of the pancreas during AP episodes, especially severe in patients with pancreatic necrosis [79]. Based on this evidence, EN should not stimulate pancreatic secretion, especially in acute necrotizing pancreatitis. More importantly, numerous studies have shown that compared with early parenteral nutrition or delayed EN, early EN is associated with lower mortality, organ failure, infection of pancreatic necrosis and extrapancreatic sites, and the requirement for invasive interventions (Table 2).

In practice, due to the frequent presence of IAH and impaired gastrointestinal motility, the implementation of EN in AP can be challenging, and caution is advised. The 2020 ESPEN guidelines divided AP patients into predicted "mild to moderate" and "severe" and recommended different approaches. Severe AP is considered at nutrition risk regardless of pre-admission nutrition status due to enhanced catabolism. In patients who cannot be orally fed, the guidelines recommend that EN should be started early, within 24–72 h of admission. During the acute phase of AP, EN intake should gradually increase over the first 3 to 4 days to reach the feeding target [80]. Because EN can cause an increase in IAP, caution is needed when IAP reaches 15 mmHg and over. In this population, the majority of the patients have different degrees of gastrointestinal failure characterized by the absence of bowel movement, abdominal distention, and high gastric residual volumes, and the guidelines recommend that the

Table 2 Randomized trials comparing enteral nutrition vs. parenteral nutrition in acute pancreatitis

First author (year), country	Study design	n	Population	Age	Group 1	Group 2	Primary outcome	Main findings
Kalfarentzos et al. (1997) [90], Greece	Single-center RCT	38	Severe necrotizing pancreatitis	65.2 ± 9.9	EN (18 pts)	PN (20 pts)	Not stated	• Patients who received enteral feeding experienced fewer total complications ($P < 0.05$) and were at a lower risk of developing septic complications ($P < 0.01$) than those receiving parenteral nutrition • The cost of nutritional support was three times higher in patients who received parenteral nutrition
Louie et al. (2005) [91], Vancouver, BC	Multicenter RCT	28	AP with a Ranson score of 3 or greater	61.25 ± 16.4	EN (10 pts)	PN (18 pts)	Days to achieve a 50% reduction in C-reactive protein levels	• C-reactive protein in EN patients was reduced by 50% faster than PN patients ($p = 0.09$) • Both groups received a similar number of kilojoules and achieved near normal prealbumin and 24-h urinary nitrogen values • Overall mortality was 4.9% (3 patients in the PN group) • Nine EN patients dislodged the nasojejunal tube
Petrov et al. (2006) [92], Russia	Single-center RCT	70	Predicted SAP within 72 h of the onset of symptoms	Median (range): 51 (42–67) for TEN patients, 52 (41–70) for TPN patients	TEN (35 pts)	TPN (34 pts)	Incidence of pancreatic infectious complications	• The incidence of pancreatic infectious complications was significantly lower in the enterally fed group (7 vs. 16, $p = 0.02$) • Overall mortality was 20% with 2 deaths in the TEN group and 12 in the TPN group ($p < 0.01$)
Casas et al. (2007) [93], Spain	RCT	22	SAP (Atlanta criteria)	58.4 ± 16	TPN (11 pts)	TEN (11 pts)	Not stated	• No significant differences were found between the two groups in the APACHE II score; in CRP, TNF-α, and IL-6 concentrations; or in prealbumin and albumin levels over the first 10 days • Length of hospital stay was alike in the two groups • Two patients from group 1 died in the course of the hospitalization
Doley et al. (2009) [94], India	A single-center, prospective clinical trial	50	SAP (Atlanta criteria) with a CTSI equal to or greater than 7	39.75 ± 12.6	EN (25 pts)	PN (25 pts)	Not stated	• There was a significant decrease in serum C-reactive protein values in both the enteral nutrition group and the total parenteral nutrition group at 1 week and 2 weeks ($P < 0.001$ for both) • There was no significant difference in surgical intervention (56.0 vs. 60.0%; $P = 1.000$), infective complications (64.0 vs. 60.0%; $P = 1.000$), or mortality (20.0 vs. 16.0%; $P = 1.000$) in enteral nutrition vs. total parenteral nutrition, respectively

Study	Study type	N	Inclusion criteria	Age	Group	Group	Outcome measure	Findings
Gupta et al. (2003) [95], UK	Single-center RCT	21	Predicted SAP with the presence of an APACHE II of 6 or more	Median (range): 65 (56–89) for EN patients, 57 (38–86) for PN patients	TEN (8 pts)	TPN (9 pts)	Not stated	• All patients tolerated the feeding regime well with few nutrition-related complications • In the TPN group, 3 patients developed respiratory failure and 3 developed non-respiratory single organ failure. There were no such complications in the TEN group • The cost of TEN was considerably less than that of TPN
Eckerwall et al. (2006) [96], Sweden	A single-center, prospective randomized study	50	Predicted SAP	Median (IQR): 71 (58–80) for EN patients, 68 (60–80) for PN patients	EN (24 pts)	TPN (26 pts)	Intestinal permeability measured by excretion of polyethylene glycol (PEG) in urine	• PEG, EndoCAb, CRP, IL-6, APACHE II score, severity according to the revised Atlanta classification (22 patients), and gastrointestinal symptoms or abdominal pain did not significantly differ between the groups • Total complications (25 vs. 52; $P = 0.04$) and pulmonary complications (10 vs. 21; $P = 0.04$) were significantly more frequent in EN patients, although complications were diagnosed dominantly within the first 3 days
Olah et al. (2002) [97], Hungary	Single-center RCT	89	AP admitted within 24 to 72 h after the onset of symptoms	47.2 (mean) for EN patients, 43.8 (mean) for PN patients	EN (41 pts)	PN (48 pts)	Not stated	• The rate of septic complications (infected pancreatic necrosis, abscess) was lower in the enteral group ($P = 0.08$)
Windsor et al. (1998) [98], UK	RCT	34	AP within 48 h after admission	Median (IQR): 63 (47–76) for EN patients, 63 (52–73) for PN patients	EN (16 pts)	PN (18 pts)	Incidence of the systemic inflammatory response syndrome	• SIRS, sepsis, organ failure, and ICU stay were globally improved in the enterally fed patients • Enterally fed patients showed no change in the level of EndoCAb antibodies and an increase in TAC
Wu et al. (2010) [99], China	Single-center RCT	107	ANP within 48 h after the onset of the disease	53 ± 11.6	TEN (53 pts)	TPN (54 pts)	None	• Eighty percent of the patients developed organ failure in the group with total parenteral nutrition, which was higher than that in the group with total enteral nutrition (21%) • The incidence of pancreatic septic necroses in the group with total enteral nutrition (23%) was lower than that in the group with total parenteral nutrition (72%, P G 0.05)

RCT randomized controlled trials, *AP* acute pancreatitis, *SAP* severe acute pancreatitis, *EN* enteral nutrition, *PN* parenteral nutrition, *TEN* total enteral nutrition, *TPN* total parenteral nutrition

nasojejunal route is preferred over the nasogastric route despite the RCTs showing no difference between nasojejunal and nasogastric routes in severe AP patients [81]. Taken together, when implementing early EN in AP patients, always keep IAP and gastrointestinal dysfunction in mind and monitor them frequently.

6.5 Assessment and Treatment of Enteral Feeding Intolerance

Feeding intolerance is common when implementing EN [66] or taking oral diet [82] in AP patients and is associated with more severe disease and unfavorable outcomes. There is no universal tool to assess feeding intolerance in AP; thus the definitions of intolerance varyes between different studies. Generally, patients who report worsening symptoms (including abdominal distension, pain, vomiting) had increased IAP, and/or cannot reach the nutrition target, and an alternative approach to nutritional support should be considered.

The use of prokinetics appears to make sense in patients with feeding intolerance. In critically ill patients, a meta-analysis showed that prokinetic agents could reduce feeding intolerance, but its impact on clinical outcomes like mortality and length of ICU stay remains unclear [83]. However, the evidence for prokinetics in AP patients is sparse, and further studies are needed.

7 Hepatic and Other Organ Failures

For other organ systems, liver failure and central nervous system failure are relatively uncommon in AP and are usually due to extrapancreatic causes. The management of these organ failures should follow the relevant guidelines for critically ill patients.

8 Conclusion

In conclusion, the development, number and duration of organ failure are the most important determinants of severity and outcome in AP. Although

the clinical characteristics are similar to organ failure in other critical illnesses, AP-associated organ failure has a unique combination of challenges, including systemic inflammation, intra-abdominal pressure, compromised mesenteric perfusion associated with gastrointestinal failure, hypovolemia, and distributive shock. The management of AP-associated organ failure requires expertise to optimize organ function and avoid iatrogenic injury, especially as there is an urgent need for better quality evidence in a number of areas highlighted in this chapter.

References

1. Banks PA, Bollen TL, Dervenis C, et al. Classification of acute pancreatitis—2012: revision of the Atlanta classification and definitions by international consensus. Gut. 2013;62:102–11.
2. Dellinger EP, Forsmark CE, Layer P, et al. Determinant-based classification of acute pancreatitis severity: an international multidisciplinary consultation. Ann Surg. 2012;256:875–80.
3. Petrov MS, Shanbhag S, Chakraborty M, et al. Organ failure and infection of pancreatic necrosis as determinants of mortality in patients with acute pancreatitis. Gastroenterology. 2010;139:813–20.
4. van Santvoort HC, Besselink MG, Bakker OJ, et al. A step-up approach or open necrosectomy for necrotizing pancreatitis. N Engl J Med. 2010;362:1491–502.
5. van Brunschot S, van Grinsven J, van Santvoort HC, et al. Endoscopic or surgical step-up approach for infected necrotising pancreatitis: a multicentre randomised trial. Lancet. 2018;391:51–8.
6. Sternby H, Bolado F, Canaval-Zuleta HJ, et al. Determinants of severity in acute pancreatitis: a nation-wide multicenter prospective cohort study. Ann Surg. 2019;270:348–55.
7. Shi N, Liu T, de la Iglesia-Garcia D, et al. Duration of organ failure impacts mortality in acute pancreatitis. Gut. 2020;69:604–5.
8. Machicado JD, Gougol A, Tan X, et al. Mortality in acute pancreatitis with persistent organ failure is determined by the number, type, and sequence of organ systems affected. United European Gastroenterol J. 2021;9:139–49.
9. Raraty MG, Connor S, Criddle DN, et al. Acute pancreatitis and organ failure: pathophysiology, natural history, and management strategies. Curr Gastroenterol Rep. 2004;6:99–103.
10. Komara NL, Paragomi P, Greer PJ, et al. Severe acute pancreatitis: capillary permeability model linking systemic inflammation to multiorgan failure. Am J Physiol Gastrointest Liver Physiol. 2020;319:G573–83.
11. Kinnala PJ, Kuttila KT, Gronroos JM, et al. Splanchnic and pancreatic tissue perfusion in experimental acute pancreatitis. Scand J Gastroenterol. 2002;37:845–9.

12. Cuthbertson CM, Christophi C. Disturbances of the microcirculation in acute pancreatitis. Br J Surg. 2006;93:518–30.

13. Windsor JA, Trevaskis NL, Phillips AJ. The gut-lymph model gives new treatment strategies for organ failure. JAMA Surg. 2022;157:540–1.

14. Schepers NJ, Bakker OJ, Besselink MG, et al. Impact of characteristics of organ failure and infected necrosis on mortality in necrotising pancreatitis. Gut. 2019;68:1044–51.

15. Qu C, Zhang H, Chen T, et al. Early on-demand drainage versus standard management among acute necrotizing pancreatitis patients complicated by persistent organ failure: the protocol for an open-label multicenter randomized controlled trial. Pancreatology. 2020;20:1268–74.

16. Bang JY, Arnoletti JP, Holt BA, et al. An endoscopic transluminal approach, compared to minimally invasive surgery, reduces complications and costs for patients with necrotizing pancreatitis. Gastroenterology. 2019;156(4):1027–40.

17. Lambden S, Laterre PF, Levy MM, et al. The SOFA score-development, utility and challenges of accurate assessment in clinical trials. Crit Care. 2019;23:374.

18. Mounzer R, Langmead CJ, Wu BU, et al. Comparison of existing clinical scoring systems to predict persistent organ failure in patients with acute pancreatitis. Gastroenterology. 2012;142:1476–82; quiz e15–6

19. Seymour CW, Liu VX, Iwashyna TJ, et al. Assessment of clinical criteria for sepsis: for the third international consensus definitions for sepsis and septic shock (Sepsis-3). JAMA. 2016;315:762–74.

20. Rasch S, Pichlmeier EM, Phillip V, et al. Prediction of outcome in acute pancreatitis by the qSOFA and the new ERAP score. Dig Dis Sci. 2022;67:1371–8.

21. Shi N, Zhang X, Zhu Y, et al. Predicting persistent organ failure on admission in patients with acute pancreatitis: development and validation of a mobile nomogram. HPB (Oxford). 2022;24:1907–20.

22. Gajendran M, Prakash B, Perisetti A, et al. Predictors and outcomes of acute respiratory failure in hospitalised patients with acute pancreatitis. Frontline Gastroenterol. 2021;12:478–86.

23. Li L, Liu S, Zhang X, et al. Predicting persistent acute respiratory failure in acute pancreatitis: the accuracy of two lung injury indices. Dig Dis Sci. 2023;68:2878–89.

24. Working Party of the British Society of G, Association of Surgeons of Great B, Ireland, et al. UK guidelines for the management of acute pancreatitis. Gut. 2005;54 Suppl 3:iii1–9.

25. Paraskevas T, Oikonomou E, Lagadinou M, et al. The role of high flow nasal oxygen in the management of severe COVID-19: a systematic review. Acta Medica Port. 2022;35:476–83.

26. Ji X, Zhou J, Wu W, et al. Application of high-flow oxygen therapy in acute pancreatitis complicated with acute respiratory dysfunction. Turk J Med Sci. 2022;52:707–14.

27. Chen C, Xia SH, Chen H, et al. Therapy for acute pancreatitis with platelet-activating factor receptor antagonists. World J Gastroenterol. 2008;14:4735–8.

28. Johnson CD, Kingsnorth AN, Imrie CW, et al. Double blind, randomised, placebo controlled study of a platelet activating factor antagonist, lexipafant, in the treatment and prevention of organ failure in predicted severe acute pancreatitis. Gut. 2001;48:62–9.

29. Abu-Zidan FM, Windsor JA. Lexipafant and acute pancreatitis: a critical appraisal of the clinical trials. Eur J Surg. 2002;168:215–9.

30. Szatmary P, Grammatikopoulos T, Cai W, et al. Acute pancreatitis: diagnosis and treatment. Drugs. 2022;82:1251–76.

31. Ke L, Ni HB, Sun JK, et al. Risk factors and outcome of intra-abdominal hypertension in patients with severe acute pancreatitis. World J Surg. 2012;36:171–8.

32. Pelosi P, Quintel M, Malbrain ML. Effect of intra-abdominal pressure on respiratory mechanics. Acta Clin Belg Suppl. 2007;62:78–88.

33. Ke L, Tong ZH, Ni HB, et al. The effect of intra-abdominal hypertension incorporating severe acute pancreatitis in a porcine model. PLoS One. 2012;7:e33125.

34. Fan E, Del Sorbo L, Goligher EC, et al. An Official American Thoracic Society/European Society of Intensive Care Medicine/Society of Critical Care Medicine Clinical Practice Guideline: Mechanical Ventilation in Adult Patients with Acute Respiratory Distress Syndrome. Am J Respir Crit Care Med. 2017;195:1253–63.

35. Acute Respiratory Distress Syndrome N, Brower RG, Matthay MA, et al. Ventilation with lower tidal volumes as compared with traditional tidal volumes for acute lung injury and the acute respiratory distress syndrome. N Engl J Med. 2000;342:1301–8.

36. *Talmor D, Sarge T, Malhotra A, et al. Mechanical ventilation guided by esophageal pressure in acute lung injury. N Engl J Med 2008;359:2095–2104. *This study showed that a ventilator strategy using esophageal pressures to estimate the trans-pulmonary pressure significantly improves oxygenation and compliance.

37. Regli A, Pelosi P, Malbrain M. Ventilation in patients with intra-abdominal hypertension: what every critical care physician needs to know. Ann Intensive Care. 2019;9:52.

38. Kirkpatrick AW, Roberts DJ, De Waele J, et al. Intra-abdominal hypertension and the abdominal compartment syndrome: updated consensus definitions and clinical practice guidelines from the World Society of the Abdominal Compartment Syndrome. Intensive Care Med. 2013;39:1190–206.

39. Jena A, Singh AK, Kochhar R. Intra-abdominal hypertension and abdominal compartment syndrome in acute pancreatitis. Indian J Gastroenterol. 2023;42:455–66.

40. Schmandt M, Glowka TR, Kreyer S, et al. Secondary ARDS following acute pancreatitis: is extracorporeal

membrane oxygenation feasible or futile? J Clin Med. 2021;10:1000.

41. Machicado JD, Papachristou GI. Intravenous fluid resuscitation in the management of acute pancreatitis. Curr Opin Gastroenterol. 2020;36:409.

42. Working Group IAPAPAAPG. IAP/APA evidence-based guidelines for the management of acute pancreatitis. Pancreatology. 2013;13:e1–15.

43. Vedantam S, Tehami N, de Madaria E, et al. Lactated ringers does not reduce SIRS in acute pancreatitis compared to normal saline: an updated meta-analysis. Dig Dis Sci. 2022;67(7):3265–74.

44. Ye B, Huang M, Chen T, et al. The impact of normal saline or balanced crystalloid on plasma chloride concentration and acute kidney injury in patients with predicted severe acute pancreatitis: protocol of a phase II, multicenter, stepped-wedge, cluster-randomized, controlled trial. Front Med (Lausanne). 2021;8:731955.

45. Ye B, Mao W, Chen Y, et al. Aggressive resuscitation is associated with the development of acute kidney injury in acute pancreatitis. Dig Dis Sci. 2019;64:544–52.

46. Gad MM, Simons-Linares CR. Is aggressive intravenous fluid resuscitation beneficial in acute pancreatitis? A meta-analysis of randomized control trials and cohort studies. World J Gastroenterol. 2020;26:1098–106.

47. Bellomo R, Kellum JA, Ronco C. Acute kidney injury. Lancet. 2012;380:756–66.

48. Li X, Liu C, Mao Z, et al. Timing of renal replacement therapy initiation for acute kidney injury in critically ill patients: a systematic review of randomized clinical trials with meta-analysis and trial sequential analysis. Crit Care. 2021;25:15.

49. Maringhini A, Ciambra M, Patti R, et al. Ascites, pleural, and pericardial effusions in acute pancreatitis. A prospective study of incidence, natural history, and prognostic role. Dig Dis Sci. 1996;41:848–52.

50. Haydock MD, Mittal A, Wilms HR, et al. Fluid therapy in acute pancreatitis: anybody's guess. Ann Surg. 2013;257:182–8.

51. Garcia M, Calvo JJ. Cardiocirculatory pathophysiological mechanisms in severe acute pancreatitis. World J Gastrointest Pharmacol Ther. 2010;1:9–14.

52. Garcia M, Hernandez-Barbachano E, Hernandez Lorenzo MP, et al. Cardiovascular homeostasis in hypotension associated with initial stages of severe acute pancreatitis. Pancreas. 2008;37:432–9.

53. de Madaria E, Buxbaum JL, Maisonneuve P, et al. Aggressive or moderate fluid resuscitation in acute pancreatitis. N Engl J Med. 2022;387:989–1000.

54. Jin T, Jiang K, Deng L, et al. Response and outcome from fluid resuscitation in acute pancreatitis: a prospective cohort study. HPB (Oxford). 2018;20:1082–91.

55. Mao EQ, Fei J, Peng YB, et al. Rapid hemodilution is associated with increased sepsis and mortality among patients with severe acute pancreatitis. Chin Med J. 2010;123:1639–44.

56. de Madaria E, Soler-Sala G, Sanchez-Paya J, et al. Influence of fluid therapy on the prognosis of acute pancreatitis: a prospective cohort study. Am J Gastroenterol. 2011;106:1843–50.

57. Hoste EA, Maitland K, Brudney CS, et al. Four phases of intravenous fluid therapy: a conceptual model. Br J Anaesth. 2014;113:740–7.

58. Russell JA. Vasopressor therapy in critically ill patients with shock. Intensive Care Med. 2019;45:1503–17.

59. Jozwiak M, Geri G, Laghlam D, et al. Vasopressors and risk of acute mesenteric ischemia: a worldwide pharmacovigilance analysis and comprehensive literature review. Front Med (Lausanne). 2022;9:826446.

60. Georger JF, Hamzaoui O, Chaari A, et al. Restoring arterial pressure with norepinephrine improves muscle tissue oxygenation assessed by near-infrared spectroscopy in severely hypotensive septic patients. Intensive Care Med. 2010;36:1882–9.

61. Ji YF, Zhang XM, Mitchell DG, et al. Gastrointestinal tract involvement in acute pancreatitis: initial findings and follow-up by magnetic resonance imaging. Quant Imaging Med Surg. 2017;7:641–53.

62. Reintam A, Parm P, Kitus R, et al. Gastrointestinal failure score in critically ill patients: a prospective observational study. Crit Care. 2008;12:R90.

63. Rahman A, Hasan RM, Agarwala R, et al. Identifying critically-ill patients who will benefit most from nutritional therapy: further validation of the "modified NUTRIC" nutritional risk assessment tool. Clin Nutr. 2016;35:158–62.

64. Reintam Blaser A, Padar M, Mandul M, et al. Development of the gastrointestinal dysfunction score (GIDS) for critically ill patients—a prospective multicenter observational study (iSOFA study). Clin Nutr. 2021;40:4932–40.

65. Elke G, Felbinger TW, Heyland DK. Gastric residual volume in critically ill patients: a dead marker or still alive? Nutr Clin Pract. 2015;30:59–71.

66. Lin J, Lv C, Wu C, et al. Incidence and risk factors of nasogastric feeding intolerance in moderately-severe to severe acute pancreatitis. BMC Gastroenterol. 2022;22:327.

67. Gao T, Cheng MH, Xi FC, et al. Predictive value of transabdominal intestinal sonography in critically ill patients: a prospective observational study. Crit Care. 2019;23:378.

68. Severino A, Varca S, Airola C, et al. Antibiotic utilization in acute pancreatitis: a narrative review. Antibiotics (Basel). 2023;12:1120.

69. Patangia DV, Anthony Ryan C, Dempsey E, et al. Impact of antibiotics on the human microbiome and consequences for host health. Microbiol Open. 2022;11:e1260.

70. Leppaniemi A, Tolonen M, Tarasconi A, et al. 2019 WSES guidelines for the management of severe acute pancreatitis. World J Emerg Surg. 2019;14:27.

71. Camilleri M, Lembo A, Katzka DA. Opioids in gastroenterology: treating adverse effects and creating therapeutic benefits. Clin Gastroenterol Hepatol. 2017;15:1338–49.

72. Thavanesan N, White S, Lee S, et al. Analgesia in the initial management of acute pancreatitis: a systematic review and meta-analysis of randomised controlled trials. World J Surg. 2022;24:S241.

73. Samanta J, Rana A, Dhaka N, et al. Ascites in acute pancreatitis: not a silent bystander. Pancreatology. 2019;19:646–52.

74. Dugernier T, Laterre PF, Reynaert MS. Ascites fluid in severe acute pancreatitis: from pathophysiology to therapy. Acta Gastroenterol Belg. 2000;63:264–8.

75. Liu L, Yan H, Liu W, et al. Abdominal paracentesis drainage does not increase infection in severe acute pancreatitis: a prospective study. J Clin Gastroenterol. 2015;49:757–63.

76. Dong Z, Petrov MS, Xu J, et al. Peritoneal lavage for severe acute pancreatitis: a systematic review of randomised trials. World J Surg. 2010;34:2103–8.

77. Jablonska B, Mrowiec S. Nutritional support in patients with severe acute pancreatitis-current standards. Nutrients. 2021;13:1498.

78. Petrov MS. Gastric feeding and "gut rousing" in acute pancreatitis. Nutr Clin Pract. 2014;29:287–90.

79. O'Keefe SJ, Lee RB, Li J, et al. Trypsin secretion and turnover in patients with acute pancreatitis. Am J Physiol Gastrointest Liver Physiol. 2005;289:G181–7.

80. Arvanitakis M, Ockenga J, Bezmarevic M, et al. ESPEN guideline on clinical nutrition in acute and chronic pancreatitis. Clin Nutr. 2020;39:612–31.

81. Nally DM, Kelly EG, Clarke M, et al. Nasogastric nutrition is efficacious in severe acute pancreatitis: a systematic review and meta-analysis. Br J Nutr. 2014;112:1769–78.

82. Pothoulakis I, Nawaz H, Paragomi P, et al. Incidence and risk factors of oral feeding intolerance in acute pancreatitis: results from an international, multicenter, prospective cohort study. United European Gastroenterol J. 2021;9:54–62.

83. Lewis K, Alqahtani Z, McIntyre L, et al. The efficacy and safety of prokinetic agents in critically ill patients receiving enteral nutrition: a systematic review and meta-analysis of randomized trials. Crit Care. 2016;20:259.

84. Wu BU, Hwang JQ, Gardner TH, et al. Lactated Ringer's solution reduces systemic inflammation compared with saline in patients with acute pancreatitis. Clin Gastroenterol Hepatol. 2011;9:710–717 e1.

85. Choosakul S, Harinwan K, Chirapongsathorn S, et al. Comparison of normal saline versus lactated Ringer's solution for fluid resuscitation in patients with mild acute pancreatitis, a randomized controlled trial. Pancreatology. 2018;18:507.

86. Lee A, Ko C, Buitrago C, et al. Lactated ringers vs normal saline resuscitation for mild acute pancreatitis: a randomized trial. Gastroenterology. 2021;160:955–957 e4.

87. de Madaria E, Herrera-Marante I, Gonzalez-Camacho V, et al. Fluid resuscitation with lactated Ringer's solution vs normal saline in acute pancreatitis: a triple-blind, randomized, controlled trial. United European. Gastroenterol J. 2018;6:63–72.

88. Karki B, Thapa S, Khadka D, et al. Intravenous ringers lactate versus normal saline for predominantly mild acute pancreatitis in a Nepalese tertiary hospital. PLoS One. 2022;17:e0263221.

89. Kayhan S, Selcan Akyol B, Ergul M, et al. The effect of type of fluid on disease severity in acute pancreatitis treatment. Eur Rev Med Pharmacol Sci. 2021;25:7460–7.

90. Kalfarentzos F, Kehagias J, Mead N, et al. Enteral nutrition is superior to parenteral nutrition in severe acute pancreatitis: results of a randomized prospective trial. Br J Surg. 1997;84:1665–9.

91. Louie BE, Noseworthy T, Hailey D, et al. 2004 MacLean-Mueller prize enteral or parenteral nutrition for severe pancreatitis: a randomized controlled trial and health technology assessment. Can J Surg. 2005;48:298–306.

92. Petrov MS, Kukosh MV, Emelyanov NV. A randomized controlled trial of enteral versus parenteral feeding in patients with predicted severe acute pancreatitis shows a significant reduction in mortality and in infected pancreatic complications with total enteral nutrition. Dig Surg. 2006;23:336–44; discussion 344–5

93. Casas M, Mora J, Fort E, et al. Total enteral nutrition vs. total parenteral nutrition in patients with severe acute pancreatitis. Rev Esp Enferm Dig. 2007;99:264–9.

94. Doley RP, Yadav TD, Wig JD, et al. Enteral nutrition in severe acute pancreatitis. JOP. 2009;10:157–62.

95. Gupta R, Patel K, Calder PC, et al. A randomised clinical trial to assess the effect of total enteral and total parenteral nutritional support on metabolic, inflammatory and oxidative markers in patients with predicted severe acute pancreatitis (APACHE II > or =6). Pancreatology. 2003;3:406–13.

96. Eckerwall GE, Axelsson JB, Andersson RG. Early nasogastric feeding in predicted severe acute pancreatitis: a clinical, randomized study. Ann Surg. 2006;244:959–65; discussion 965–7

97. Olah A, Pardavi G, Belagyi T, et al. Early nasojejunal feeding in acute pancreatitis is associated with a lower complication rate. Nutrition. 2002;18:259–62.

98. Windsor AC, Kanwar S, Li AG, et al. Compared with parenteral nutrition, enteral feeding attenuates the acute phase response and improves disease severity in acute pancreatitis. Gut. 1998;42:431–5.

99. Wu XM, Ji KQ, Wang HY, et al. Total enteral nutrition in prevention of pancreatic necrotic infection in severe acute pancreatitis. Pancreas. 2010;39:248–51.

Correction to: Acinar Cell Events Initiating Acute Pancreatitis

Anna S. Gukovskaya and Ilya Gukovsky

Correction to:
Chapter 3 in: J. A. Windsor et al. (eds.), *Acute Pancreatitis*,
https://doi.org/10.1007/978-981-97-3132-9_3

Due to an unfortunate oversight on the part of production, the chapter was published with errors.

The following corrections have been made to the original publication:

1. Figure 3: The special characters and symbols are missed out. The figure has been updated as below.

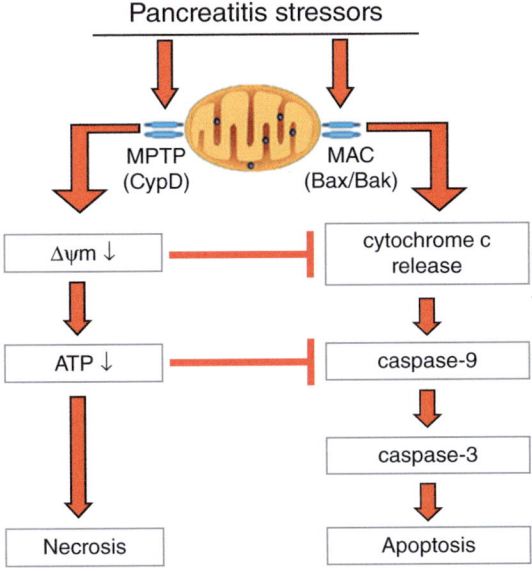

2. Table 1: The reference to the Agent 'TRO40303' has been updated in the last column as Preclinical models (Ref. 146).

The updated version of this chapter can be found at https://doi.org/10.1007/978-981-97-3132-9_3

© The Author(s), under exclusive license to Springer Nature Singapore Pte Ltd. 2024
J. A. Windsor et al. (eds.), *Acute Pancreatitis*, https://doi.org/10.1007/978-981-97-3132-9_18

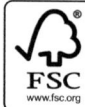

MIX
Papier aus verantwortungsvollen Quellen
Paper from responsible sources
FSC® C105338

If you have any concerns about our products,
you can contact us on
ProductSafety@springernature.com

In case Publisher is established outside the EU,
the EU authorized representative is:
Springer Nature Customer Service Center GmbH
Europaplatz 3, 69115 Heidelberg, Germany

Printed by Libri Plureos GmbH
in Hamburg, Germany